Awake Thoracic Surgery

Edited By

Eugenio Pompeo

Tor Vergata University
Rome, Italy

CONTENTS

Foreword   *i*

Preface   *ii*

List of Contributors   *iii*

Acknowledgement   *v*

CHAPTERS

1. **Awake Thoracic Surgery: A Historical Perspective**   **3**
    Eugenio Pompeo and Tommaso Claudio Mineo

2. **Pathophysiology of Surgical Pneumothorax in the Awake Patient**   **9**
    Eugenio Pompeo

3. **Systemic Host Response in Awake Thoracic Surgery**   **19**
    Federico Tacconi, Gianluca Vanni and Eugenio Pompeo

4. **Adverse Effects of General Anesthesia in Thoracic Surgery**   **34**
    Mario Dauri, Ludovica Celidonio, Sarit Nahmias, Florencia Della Badia, Filadelfo Coniglione and Eleonora Fabbi

5. **Anesthesia Techniques in Awake Thoracic Surgery**   **44**
    Mario Dauri, Sarit Nahmias, Ludovica Celidonio, Elisabetta Sabato, Maria Beatrice Silvi and Eleonora Fabbi

6. **Awake Resection of Solitary Pulmonary Nodules**   **74**
    Eugenio Pompeo, Francesco Sellitri, Benedetto Cristino and Tommaso Claudio Mineo

7. **Awake Non-Resectional Lung Volume Reduction Surgery**   **88**
    Eugenio Pompeo, Ilaria Onorati and Tommaso Claudio Mineo

8. **Awake Lung Biopsy for Interstitial Lung Disease**   **105**
    Luca Frasca, Vincenzo Ambrogi, Paola Rogliani, Cesare Saltini and Eugenio Pompeo

9. **Awake Videothoracoscopic Treatment of Pleural Effusion**   **119**
    Francesco Sellitri, Federico Tacconi, Benedetto Cristino and Eugenio Pompeo

10. **Awake Thoracoscopic Treatment of Spontaneous Pneumothorax**   **130**
    Gianluca Vanni, Federico Tacconi, Tommaso Claudio Mineo and Eugenio Pompeo

11. **Awake Pleural Decortication for Empyema Thoracis**   **141**
    Federico Tacconi and Eugenio Pompeo

12. **Awake Thymectomy**   **155**
    Isao Matsumoto, Makoto Oda and Go Watanabe

13. Awake Thoracoscopic Biopsy of Anterior Mediastinal Masses   **165**

Eugenio Pompeo, Alessandra Picardi, Maria Cantonetti and Tommaso Claudio Mineo

14. Awake Thoracoscopic Sympathectomy   **177**

Maria Elena Cufari, Eugenio Pompeo, Tommaso Claudio Mineo and Vincenzo Ambrogi

15. Video-Assisted Thoracic Surgery Utilizing Local Anesthesia and Sedation   **191**

Mark Katlic

16. Awake Thoracic Surgery: Future Perspectives   **199**

Eugenio Pompeo

Subject index   **202**

FOREWORD

Minimally invasive thoracic surgery has been demonstrated to achieve superior outcomes for patients with basic and complex thoracic conditions. Advantages of thoracoscopic surgery include less postoperative pain, faster return to full activity, preserved pulmonary function, shorter length of hospitalization, reduced inflammatory response, and a lower rate of postoperative complications. With increasing experience, the boundaries of thoracoscopy have dissolved and the strategies of minimally invasive surgery have expanded. In particular, the concept of awake thoracic surgery has emerged as an important novel strategy to optimize the advantages of minimally invasive surgery.

Awake thoracoscopic surgery encompasses the advantages of limiting the invasiveness of both anesthesia and surgery, which may magnify the known benefits of minimally invasive thoracic surgery. Although initially applicable to only the most basic procedures, awake thoracoscopic strategies are currently used to successfully complete advanced procedures as well, including lung volume reduction, decortication, and thymectomy. Whereas the recognition of the advantages of thoracoscopic surgery has been slow in evolution, it is hoped that the strategy of awake thoracoscopic surgery is more promptly understood and embraced. This monograph by Dr. Eugenio Pompeo outlines both the theoretical and proved advantages of the anesthetic and surgical techniques that are employed in awake surgery. In addition, the results of a spectrum of awake thoracoscopic surgery, including both basic and complex procedures, are described in detail by the recognized experts in the field. Awake thoracic surgery will eventually be included in thoracic surgery training programs, but until then the practicing thoracic surgeon should learn this important strategy, and this monograph represents a comprehensive and valuable summary.

Thomas A. D'Amico
Professor of Surgery
Duke University Medical Center
Durham, North Carolina

PREFACE

Health care in our era is dominated by an increasing attention to patients' quality of life and cost to benefit ratio of therapies. For these reasons, interest towards minimally invasive surgery procedures that are typically associated with minor postoperative pain and morbidity, short hospitalization and optimal cosmesis, continues to grow. Awake thoracic surgery is being developed according to the idea that making thoracic surgery procedures less and less aggressive can be a feasible task. Theoretically, the avoidance of well known adverse effects of general anesthesia and one-lung ventilation could translate into some advantages including a smoother postoperative course, a more rapid resumption of daily-life activities, and even an opportunity to offer surgical treatment to patients in whom this would be denied because of a high-risk for standard surgery.

The reader will have the opportunity to acknowledge that, though awake thoracic surgery is a totally explorable novel surgical field, many of the concepts we advocate today had already been hypothesized in the past by pioneer surgeons, whereas some of the fears of yesterday now prove either groundless, thanks to a better knowledge in cardiopulmonary physiology, or easily surmountable by our current technology. However, despite the enthusiasm and encouraging initial results, there is still a long way to go. Many pathophysiologic aspects as well as real advantages and cost-effectiveness of these novel options need to be better elucidated. Alternative non-surgical treatment procedures are being developed to cure a number of thoracic conditions and it is likely that many valid surgical procedures of today will become obsolete within a few years.

Awake thoracic surgery might represent one strong answer to this challenge and the aim of this e-Book is to provide a first overview on current advances matured in this exciting surgical field. Following some historical notes, the main pathophysiologic aspects of epidural anesthesia and the surgical pneumothorax in the awake patient, are focused to provide insights on intraoperative changes in oxygenation, ventilation and the main cardiopulmonary variables. In addition, the low impact of awake thoracic surgery on postoperative immunologic and stress hormone responses is also analyzed in detail. Chapters on surgical techniques include a description of the advantages, indications, technical details and results of several surgical procedures including the promising non-resectional awake lung volume reduction surgery technique for the treatment of end-stage emphysema, pulmonary resections and thymectomy.

This monograph is the result of a multi-mind effort and I want to thank all the authors for their excellent contributions. Some of them are talented young researchers from our own University, whereas others are well-known thoracic surgeons from other countries who are actively involved in awake thoracic surgery programs. I greatly thank my mentor, Prof. Mineo, who has given me the opportunity to be fully involved in advanced videothoracoscopic surgery, to apply my ideas and to develop our awake thoracic surgery clinical program. He constantly guided me in the art of surgery with his advice and constructive comments arising from an unexceptionable 40-year based full-time academic practice in thoracic surgery.

I am particularly grateful to Bentham Science Publishers that believed in this project and allowed its realization. The modern formula of an e-monograph has made it possible to include rich iconographic and multimedia material that will facilitate diffusion and understanding of the various topics.

Enjoy your reading

Eugenio Pompeo
Associate Professor
Department of Thoracic Surgery
Policlinico Tor Vergata University
Rome, Italy

List of Contributors

Vincenzo Ambrogi	Associate Professor, Department of Thoracic Surgery, Tor Vergata University, Rome, Italy
Maria Cantonetti	Associate Professor, Department of Onco-Hematology, Tor Vergata University, Rome, Italy
Ludovica Celidonio	Resident, Department of Anesthesiology and Intensive Care, Tor Vergata University, Rome, Italy
Filadelfo Coniglione	Assistant Professor, Department of Anesthesiology and Intensive Care, Tor Vergata University, Rome, Italy
Benedetto Cristino	Assistant Professor, Department of Thoracic Surgery Tor Vergata University, Rome, Italy
Maria Elena Cufari	Resident, Department of Thoracic Surgery Tor Vergata University, Rome, Italy
Thomas A. D'Amico	Professor, Section of Thoracic Surgery, Duke University Medical Center, Durham, North Carolina, USA
Mario Dauri	Associate Professor, Department of Anesthesiology and Intensive Care, Tor Vergata University, Rome, Italy
Florencia Della Badia	Resident, Department of Anesthesiology and Intensive Care, Tor Vergata University, Rome, Italy
Eleonora Fabbi	Department of Anesthesiology and Intensive Care, Tor Vergata University, Rome, Italy
Luca Frasca	Resident, Department of Thoracic Surgery, Tor Vergata University, Rome, Italy
Marc Katlic	Chairman, Department of Surgery and Surgeon-in-Chief, Sinai Hospital, MD, USA
Isao Matsumoto	Associate Professor, Department of General and Cardiothoracic Surgery, Kanazawa University, Kanazawa, Japan
Tommaso C Mineo	Professor and Head, Department of Thoracic Surgery, Tor Vergata University, Rome, Italy
Sarit Nahmias	Resident, Department of Anesthesiology and Intensive Care, Tor Vergata University, Rome, Italy
Ilaria Onorati	Department of Thoracic Surgery, Tor Vergata University, Rome, Italy

Makoto Oda	Professor, Department of General and Cardiothoracic Surgery, Kanazawa University, Kanazawa, Japan
Alessandra Picardi	Assistant Professor, Department of Onco-Hematology, Tor Vergata University, Rome, Italy
Eugenio Pompeo	Associate Professor, Department of Thoracic Surgery, Tor Vergata University, Rome, Italy
Paola Rogliani	Associate Professor, Department of Pneumology, Tor Vergata University, Rome, Italy
Elisabetta Sabato	Resident, Department of Anesthesiology, and Intensive Care, Tor Vergata University, Rome, Italy
Cesare Saltini	Professor and Head, Department of Pneumology, Tor Vergata University, Rome, Italy
Francesco Sellitri	Assistant Professor, Department of Thoracic Surgery, Tor Vergata University, Rome, Italy
Maria Beatrice Silvi	Assistant Professor, Department of Anesthesiology and Intensive Care, Tor Vergata University, Rome, Italy
Federico Tacconi	Assistant Professor, Department of Thoracic Surgery, Tor Vergata University, Rome, Italy
Gianluca Vanni	Department of Thoracic Surgery, Tor Vergata University, Rome, Italy
Go Watanabe	Professor and Chairman, Department of General and Cardiothoracic Surgery, Kanazawa University, Kanazawa, Japan

Acknowledgement

We thank Mrs. Susan West for linguistic revision, Mr. Carmine Paciolla for precious help in video-editing, and Dr. Giuseppe Rodia, for artistic set-up of Fig. 1 in chapter 3.

CHAPTER 1

Awake Thoracic Surgery: A Historical Perspective

Eugenio Pompeo* and Tommaso Claudio Mineo

Department of Thoracic Surgery, Policlinico Tor Vergata University; Rome, Italy

Abstract: During the early twentieth century, thoracic surgery procedures were frequently attempted through local anesthesia, although the pneumothorax created after opening of the chest wall was deemed invariably fatal. During the ensuing decades, some surgeons started performing awake thoracic surgery procedures taking into account the experience matured during the World War I, which suggested that soldiers with severe open thoracic traumas could eventually survive.

In the 1940s, a multi-step analgesia protocol entailing multiple local blocks with Novocaine was developed in Russia. Using this technique, hundreds of major thoracic surgery procedures including major lung resections and esophagectomies, were carried out. Subsequently, Buckingham first reported on major surgery procedures using sole thoracic epidural anesthesia in awake patients.

The introduction of double-lumen tube ventilation in the 1950s led to the birth of modern thoracic surgery and general anesthesia with one-lung ventilation is still considered mandatory to allow accomplishment of more complex surgical procedures including lung resections.

Awake thoracic surgery fell into disuse until recent years when, thanks to the better knowledge of potential adverse effects of general anesthesia, some surgeons again started to investigate the possibility of performing thoracic surgery operation in awake patients

Awake thoracic surgery could not have been developed without the previous experience of pioneering thoracic surgeons. Moreover, continuing technological advances and the increased knowledge in cardiopulmonary physiology, are leading to a potentially revolutionary strategy capable of minimizing both surgical and anesthesiological trauma to eventually offer patients comprehensive non-invasive surgical management.

Keywords: Awake thoracic surgery, history, VATS, local anesthesia, epidural anesthesia.

AWAKE ANESTHESIA IN OPEN THORACIC SURGERY

During the early twentieth century, thoracic surgery procedures were frequently attempted through local anesthesia, although the pneumothorax created after opening of the chest wall was deemed invariably fatal [1]. However, since the pioneering experiences of Reclus [2], who is credited as one of the most important forefathers of topical anesthesia in surgery, the possibility of operating on the chest without the use of general anesthesia has historically attracted thoracic surgeons.

In 1923, the american surgeon George J. Heuer stated with regard to the surgical treatment of pleural empyema: *we have some evidence that the kind of anesthesia is a contributing factor in mortality .... local anesthesia is the safest and therefore the best whenever it can be used* [3]. At that time, a consistent part of thoracic surgeons' daily practice was represented by management of suppurative processes so that surgical procedures were limited to simple evacuation of fluid collections. In this historical context, the US army surgeon William Gorgas established the first international Empyema Commission, in which eminent surgeons such as Evart Graham and Richard Bell [4, 5] were actively involved. Although these surgeons were able to establish some of the basic principles of modern thoracic surgery, such as the usefulness of

*Address correspondence to Eugenio Pompeo: Department of Thoracic Surgery, Policlinico Tor Vergata University, Rome, Italy; E-mail: pompeo@med.uniroma2.it

postoperative physiotherapy in optimizing patients' recovery, the development of more aggressive awake procedures was limited by concerns about the supposed disastrous physiologic effects of iatrogenic pneumothorax in spontaneously ventilating patients.

In particular, Graham reported that this event could lead to a mortality rate of up to 30% in patients with active pneumonia, and could be lethal even in individuals with normal vital capacity after creation of a pleural opening larger than 51.5 cm^2 [5].

Since 1920, prominent surgeons, including Berkley Moyinah and Pierre Duval, established that, provided optimized pharmacological support was given, an iatrogenic pneumothorax could be tolerated without remarkable risks. This assumption was based on the observation that, during World War I, soldiers with large chest openings but with no concomitant injuries could survive, even in the case of bilateral trauma. These innovative theories, alongside the increased knowledge on anesthesiology practice, led to the birth of a more aggressive way of thinking about awake thoracic surgery, which contributed to extend the indication for local anesthesia to more complex operations [6].

Local anesthesia with multiple intercostal nerve blocks was electively used by Eloesser [7, 8] and Sauerbruch [9] as well as by Schede who developed his own method of thoracoplasty [10]. In particular, in a review over the merits of topical anesthesia, Eloesser centered on one of the main advantages of this approach, namely the preservation of cough reflexes which could prevent retained bronchial secretion in the perioperative period [9].

Birbeck [11] reported a case of bullet extraction from the right ventricle performed by thoracotomy with local anesthesia. It is worth noting that immediately after the creation of the surgical pneumothorax and subsequent lung collapse, his patient developed acute respiratory distress, which promptly resolved after closing the thoracotomy with a gauze allowing the operation to be safely completed. This behavior anticipated what we commonly do today when patients undergoing awake operations complain of some dyspnea along with anxiety symptoms, which usually resolve after light sedation and transient restoration of intrapleural negative pressure.

A further contribution to the development of awake thoracic surgery came from the refinements of regional analgesia techniques, through which a more efficient control of pain and disturbing reflexes could be achieved.

In 1946, Overholt first developed a method of paravertebral anesthesia with local infiltration of novocaine [12]. In the meantime, Vischnevski [12] developed a multi-step analgesia protocol, which consisted in the block of both phrenic and vague nerves at the neck, followed by extensive intercostals and lung hilum blocks with up to 900 mL of Novocaine. The rationale of phrenic nerve block was to avoid diaphragmatic motion during the operation, while the parasympathetic block was aimed at limiting the possibility of dangerous vagal reflexes, which could be triggered by surgical manipulation, iatrogenic pneumothorax, or both. Using this technique, Vischnevski was able to perform more than 600 major thoracic surgery procedures, including major lung resections and even esophagectomies [13]. The same procedures were subsequently refined by his colleague Boris Ossipov, who in 1960 published a comprehensive experience including more than 3000 operations performed during a 20-year period [14].

The use of thoracic epidural anesthesia to perform awake thoracic procedures was first proposed by the American surgeon Buckingham [15], who reported on a series of 607 patients who underwent major surgery using this method. Interestingly, inhalation anesthesia was used in a limited number of patients in that study, and mainly for experimental purposes [16].

Subsequently, the development of double-lumen tube ventilation by Bjork and Carlens in the 1950s [17] led to the birth of modern thoracic surgery. Due to the possibility of operating on a immobile and collapsed lung, the use of general anesthesia and single-lung ventilation rapidly became the gold-standard. Subsequent refinements of the basic device, alongside the introduction of bronchial blockers, made it possible to reduce the risk of tracheal-bronchial ruptures [18, 19] and to extend the use of one-lung ventilation even in patients with unfavorable central airway anatomy.

In 1976, Djohar [20] was still reporting on his experience with 215 patients receiving open thoracic surgery under just local anesthesia including major lung resections. Nonetheless, the use of local or regional anesthesia progressively fell into disuse, though it maintained a certain role in minimally-invasive procedures.

In recent years, the potential adverse effects of general anesthesia have been increasingly investigated leading to a renewed interest for awake thoracic surgery and allowing lung resection [21, 22], thymectomy [23] and even tracheal resection [24] to be successfully carried out by this approach.

AWAKE ANESTHESIA IN MINI-INVASIVE THORACIC SURGERY

The remote origins of thoracoscopy can be dated back to a long-lasting process that took more than 6 centuries to evolve and started with the invention of corrective lenses in the 14th century. The subsequent three main steps ahead could be attributed to the development of the telescope by Galileo in the 17th century; the proposal of a light conduction system (a candle) added to a speculum to allow exploration of body cavities, by Bozzini in 1804; and, finally, to the evolution of the first medical instrument called 'endoscope', the Désormeaux cystoscope proposed in 1853 [25].

The first thoracoscopy probably dates back to 1865 when the Irish physician Francis Richard Cruise employed a modified Désormeaux cystoscope to perform a binocular thoracoscopy in an 11-year old girl with empyema [26].

Nonetheless, the Swedish internist Hans Jacobaeus is rightfully credited as the forefather of modern thoracoscopy, which he initially employed to sever pleural adhesions and help lung collapse during the Forlanini artificial pneumothorax [26, 27].

It is worth noting that thoracoscopy was initially performed by local anesthesia in awake patients. However, for several decades it remained underused, being relegated to a minor role in the management of undetermined pleural diseases and effusions.

Buchanan and coworkers [28] first reported on thoracoscopic biopsy in patients with pleural effusion of unknown origin. Similarly, Bergqvist and Nordenstein [29] reported a diagnostic yield of over 90% in patients undergoing thoracoscopy for pleural effusions of either tubercular or malignant etiology.

LeRoux [30] used thoracoscopy as a preoperative staging tool in 139 patients with lung cancer, reporting metastatic pleural spread in 82 of them. Brandt and Mai [31] used thoracoscopy to rule-out cancer recurrence in a patient with post-resectional bronchial fistula. Thoracoscopy was also employed in the 1940s by Branco for management of traumatic hemithorax. Babischev and coworkers first employed it for diagnostic purposes in spontaneous pneumothorax whereas pleurodesis by talc insufflation was advocated by Swieringa and coworkers [30]. In 1976, Brun and coworkers [32] reported on 93 patients undergoing thoracoscopic lung biopsy. At that time, local anesthesia and spontaneous ventilation with or without sedation were universally accepted as the elective type of anesthesia to perform thoracoscopy.

Use of one-lung ventilation in thoracoscopy was reported in the early 1970s by Friedel and coworkers [30], Maasen and coworkers [33], and Bloomberg [34]. Hence, the indication for local anesthesia remained confined to minor thoracoscopic procedures, namely the so-called medical thoracoscopy, which entered the diagnostic armamentarium of interventional pneumologists [35]. Amongst a few anecdotal reports on local anesthesia in mini-invasive thoracic surgery at that time, Ward [36] and Selby [37] employed local anesthesia to perform cervical mediastinoscopy in the 1970s whereas some years later, Rusch and Mountain [38] advocated insertion of the mediastinoscope in the pleural cavity to manage patients with complex pleural effusions and empyemas.

Despite the abovementioned anecdotal reports, thoracoscopy remained underused until the early 1990's when the introduction of video-technology and magnified imaging led to the explosive birth of Video-Assisted Thoracic Surgery (VATS). This novel surgical approach was thought to mandate general anesthesia and one-lung ventilation to allow adequate surgical manipulation of the lung and an easy accomplishment of more complex surgical procedures, including lung resections.

Wedge resection by VATS under local anesthesia and sedation was first reported in 1997 by Nezu and coworkers [39] to resect blebs in patients with spontaneous pneumothorax. More recently, we reported on a series of VATS operations including videothoracoscopic resection of pulmonary nodules [21], surgery for emphysema [40-42], and pleural decortication for empyema thoracis [43] performed in awake, spontaneously ventilating patients through thoracic epidural anesthesia.

Rendina and coworkers [44] inserted an optical mediastinoscope parasternally under local anesthesia for diagnosis of anterior mediastinal masses. Other recently suggested indications for awake videothoracoscopic surgery include cardiac bypass [45], sympathectomy [46, 47], management of complex pneumothorax [48, 49], and thymectomy [50].

Awake VATS is now credited as a valuable tool in the management of pleural effusions such that the British Thoracic Society recently inserted VATS under local anesthesia in its current guidelines for surgical management of pleural diseases [49].

CONCLUSION

Our surgical heritage presents us with the opportunity to both moderate the improper feeling of being promoters of something really innovative and at the same time re-interpret more properly what has been done by pioneer surgeons, taking advantage of their well done *piece of work*.

Nonetheless, awake thoracic surgery could be erroneously considered as a return to the past. Instead, we believe that the increased knowledge in cardiopulmonary physiology as well as the relentlessly growing demand of non-traumatizing therapeutic options is leading to a renewed interpretation of awake anesthesia techniques in thoracic surgery.

As a result, a potentially revolutionary strategy can evolve, making it possible to minimize both surgical and anesthesiological trauma in order to offer patients a highly reliable but comprehensive non-invasive surgical management.

REFERENCES

[1]   Sauerbruch F, O'Shaughnessy L. Thoracic Surgery. London: Edward Arnold & Co, 1937; pp. 324-86.
[2]   No author listed. Report on the scientific titles and works of Prof. Paul Reclus. Can Anesthesiol 1984;6:439-42.
[3]   Heuer GJ. Empyema of the pleural cavity. Ann Surg 1923;78:711-24.
[4]   Graham EA, Bell R.D. Open pneumothorax: its relation to the treatment of empyema. Am J Med Sc 1918;46:839.
[5]   Graham EA, Berck M. Principles versus details in the treatment of acute empyema. Ann Surg 1933;98:520-7.
[6]   Kergin FG. The treatment of chronic pleural empyema. Ann R Coll Surg Engl 1995;17:271-90.
[7]   Eloesser L. Local anesthesia in major surgery: its uses and limitations. Cal State Med J 1923;21:412-5.
[8]   Eloesser L. Recent advances in regional (local) anesthesia. Can State Med J 1912;10:90-7.
[9]   Sauerbruch F. The nature and history of the treatment of tuberculosis. Zentralbl Chir 1951;76:421-30.
[10]   Lambert A. Axillary approach to Schede thoracoplasty. Surg Gynecol Obstet 1947;84:56-61.
[11]   Birbeck LH, Lorimer GM, Gray HM. Removal of a bullet from the right ventricle of the heart under local anesthesia. Br Med J 1915;2:561-2.
[12]   Petrovsky BV. Role of local anesthesia according to Vischnevsky in thoracic surgery. Anesth Analg 1952;9:75-9.
[13]   Vischnevski AA. Local anesthesia in thoracic surgery: lungs, heart, and esophagus. Minerva Anestesiol 1954;20:432-5.

[14]   Ossipov BK. Local anesthesia in thoracic surgery: 20 years experience with 3265 cases. Anesth Analg 1960;39:327-32.

[15]   Buckingham WW, Beatty AJ, Brasher CA, Ottosen P. The technique of administering epidural anesthesia in thoracic surgery. Dis Chest 1950;17:561-8.

[16]   Buckingham WW, Beatty AJ, Brasher CA, Ottosen P. An analysis of 607 surgical procedures done under epidural anesthesia. Mo Med 1950;47:485-7.

[17]   Bjork VO, Carlens E. The prevention of spread during pulmonary resections by the use of a double-lumen catheter. J Thorac Surg 1950;20:151-7.

[18]   Borm D. Tracheo-bronchial ruptures during intubation anesthesias using the Carlens tube. Chirurg 1977;48:793-5.

[19]   Bricard H, Sillard B, Leroy G, *et al*. Rupture of the trachea following endotracheal intubation by Carlens tube. Ann Chir 1979;33:238-41.

[20]   Djohar A. Thoracotomy under local anesthesia: personal experiences in 215 cases. Arch Chir Neerl 1976;28:233-41.

[21]   Pompeo E, Mineo TC. Awake operative videothoracoscopic resections. Thorac Surg Clin 2008;18:311-20.

[22]   Al-Abdullatief M, Wahood A, Al-Shirawi N, *et al*. Awake anesthesia for major thoracic surgical procedures: an observational study. Eur J Cardiothorac Surg 2007;32:346-50.

[23]   Matsumoto I, Oda M, Watanabe G. Awake endoscopic thymectomy via an infrasternal approach using sternal lifting. Thorac Cardiovasc Surg 2008;56:311-3.

[24]   Macchiarini P, Rovira I, Ferrarello S. Awake upper airway surgery. Ann Thorac Surg 2010;89:387-90.

[25]   Moisiuc FV, Colt HG. Thoracoscopy: origins revisited. Respiration 2007;74:344-55.

[26]   Hocksh B, Birken-Bertsch H, Muller JM. Thoracoscopy before Jacobaeus. Ann Thorac Surg 2002;74:1288-90.

[27]   Hatzinger M, Kwon ST, Langblein S, *et al*. Hans Christian Jacobaeus: inventor of human laparoscopy and thoracoscopy. J Endourol 2006;20:848-50.

[28]   Buchanan G, Fleishman SJ, Lichter AI, Sichel RJ. Investigation on idiopathic pleural effusion by thoracoscopy. Thorax 1956;11:324-7.

[29]   Bergqvist S, Nordenstein H. Thoracoscopy and pleural biopsy in the diagnosis of pleurisy. Scand J Respir Dis 1966;47:64.

[30]   Bloomberg AE. Thoracoscopy in perspective. Surg Gynecol Obstet 1978;147:433-43.

[31]   Brandt HJ, Mai J. Differential diagnosis of pleural effusion using thoracoscopy. Pneumonologie 1971;145:192-203.

[32]   Brun J, Magnin F, Perrin-Fayolle M, Pozzeto H. Surgical pulmonary biopsy under local anesthesia and its results (based on 93 cases). Poumon Coeur 1975;31:343-6.

[33]   Maasen W. Thoracoscopy and lung biopsy without initial pneumothorax. Poumon Coeur 1981;37:317-20.

[34]   Bloomberg AE. Thoracoscopy in diagnosis of pleural effusions. NY State J Med 1970;70:1974-7.

[35]   Boutin C, Astoul P. Diagnostic thoracoscopy. Clin Chest Med 1998;19:295-309.

[36]   Ward PH. Mediastinoscopy under local anesthesia. A valuable diagnostic technique. Calif Med 1970;112:15-22.

[37]   Selby JH, Leach CL, Heath BJ, Neely WA. Local anesthesia for mediastinoscopy: experience with 450 consecutive cases. Am Surg 1978;44:679-82.

[38]   Rusch VW, Mountain C. Thoracoscopy under regional anesthesia for diagnosis and management of pleural disease. Am J Surg 1987;154:274-8.

[39]   Nezu K, Kushibe K, Tojo T, Takahama M, Kitamura S. Thoracoscopic wedge resections of blebs under local anesthesia with sedation for treatment of a spontaneous pneumothorax. Chest 1997;111:230-35.

[40]   Pompeo E, Tacconi F, Frasca L, Mineo TC. Awake thoracoscopic bulloplasty. Eur J Cardiothorac Surg 2011;39:1012-17.

[41]   Mineo TC, Pompeo E, Mineo D, *et al*. Awake nonresectional lung volume reduction surgery. Ann Surg 2006;243:131-6.

[42]   Tacconi F, Pompeo E, Forcella D, *et al*. Lung volume reduction reoperations. Ann Thorac Surg 2008;85:1171-7.

[43]   Tacconi F, Pompeo E, Fabbi E, Mineo TC. Awake video-assisted pleural decortication for empyema thoracis. Eur J Cardiothorac Surg 2010;37:594-601.

[44]   Rendina EA, Venuta F, De Giacomo T, *et al*. Biopsy of anterior mediastinal masses under local anesthesia. Ann Thorac Surg 2002;74:1720-2.

[45]   Byhahn C, Meininger D, Kessler P. Coronary artery bypass grafting in conscious patients: a procedure with a perspective? Anaesthesist 2008;57:1144-54.

[46]   Elia S, Guggino G, Mineo D, *et al*. Awake one-stage bilateral thoracoscopic sympathectomy for palmar hyperhydrosis: a safe outpatient procedure. Eur J Cardiothorac Surg 2005;28:312-7.

[47]   Jeong JY, Park HJ. Sympathectomy under local anesthesia: a simple way to treat palmar hyperhydrosis. Ann Thorac Surg 2010;90:1730-1.

[48]   Tacconi F, Pompeo E, Mineo TC. Late-onset occult pneumothorax after lung-volume reduction surgery. Ann Thorac Surg 2005;80:2008-12.

[49]   Mukaida T, Andou A, Date H, Aoe M, Shimizu N. Thoracoscopic operations for secondary pneumothorax under local anesthesia in high-risk patients. Ann Thorac Surg 1998;65:924-6.

[50]   Rahman NM, Ali NJ, Brown G, *et al.* Local anaesthetic thoracoscopy: British Thoracic Society Pleural Disease Guideline 2010. Thorax 2010;65:S54-S60.

CHAPTER 2

Pathophysiology of Surgical Pneumothorax in the Awake Patient

Eugenio Pompeo[*]

Department of Thoracic Surgery, Policlinico Tor Vergata University, Rome, Italy

Abstract: Surgical pneumothorax makes awake thoracic surgery procedures feasible. This iatrogenic event is followed by a complex cascade of physiologic changes in both lung ventilation and perfusion, as well as in mechanical interaction between lungs, pleural cavity, diaphragm and mediastinum.

In most instances, the newly developed intrapleural atmospheric pressure environment leads to a drop in lung volume, thus assuring an adequate space for easy surgical maneuvering. The extent of this effect, however, varies considerably and is related to the conditions of lung tissue, airways and pleural cavity.

During surgical pneumothorax, ventilation-to-perfusion mismatch increases shunt fraction. Mechanical changes may include mediastinal shifting towards the dependent ventilated lung, and paradoxical respiration with collapse of non-dependent lung during inspiration and expansion during exhalation, leading to alveolar hypoventilation and hypoxemia. Mediastinal shift and paradoxical respiration decrease the efficiency of spontaneous ventilation with re-breathing of exhaled gases. Hemodynamic changes include an increase in vascular resistance due to mechanical limitation to flow and hypoxemia, which accompanies collapse of the lung and may enhance this effect by inducing pulmonary vasoconstriction. Administration of oxygen can usually prevent hypoxemia but permissive hypercapnia can develop, particularly in patients with severe emphysema.

Hence, though well tolerated by the majority of patients, hypoxemia, hypercapnia and hypoventilation are all common findings during awake thoracic surgery and need to be carefully taken into account by physicians who decide to be involved in this novel surgical field.

Keywords: Open pneumothorax, awake thoracic surgery, VATS, ventilation, paradoxical respiration.

At the end of the XIX century it was believed [1] that only general anesthesia could permit thoracic surgery procedures to be performed and avoid a fatal outcome, which was deemed to be inevitably triggered by a surgically created open pneumothorax in awake subjects.

At that time, ingenious and yet unreliable methods aimed at avoiding lung collapse during thoracotomy were proposed [2, 3] and rapidly abandoned thereafter until general anesthesia with endotracheal intubation became the accepted method of artificial respiration [4].

The birth of modern thoracic surgery eventually coincided with the clinical application of one-lung ventilation by double-lumen endobronchial intubation [5, 6]. This proved a revolutionary advance and is still considered mandatory for most thoracic surgery procedures.

Thereafter, attention was mainly focused on elucidating the pathophysiology of one-lung ventilation and on refining general anesthesia techniques, whereas little effort was devoted to investigate the effects of surgical pneumothorax. In recent years, the greatly expanded use of epidural- and local anesthesia techniques in various surgical fields, the improved knowledge in pathophysiology of one-lung ventilation and the development of minimally invasive, thoracoscopic approaches, represented the bases that have made it possible to start performing various awake thoracic surgery procedures in a safe manner [7-9]. Nonetheless, during this type of surgery, creation of an open pneumothorax can lead to alveolar

*Address correspondence to Eugenio Pompeo:** Department of Thoracic Surgery, Policlinico Tor Vergata University, Rome, Italy; E-mail: pompeo@med.uniroma2.it

hypoventilation and hypoxemia resulting from a complex cascade of physiologic changes whose underlying mechanisms still need to be fully elucidated.

In this chapter we have sought to revise the current knowledge regarding the physiologic effects of surgical pneumothorax, taking into account data arising from both clinical and experimental work in the literature as well as from our own clinical research in this field.

EFFECTS ON VENTILATION

In physiologic conditions, during quiet breathing, the elastic recoil of the lung is balanced by the tendency of the thoracic wall to spring out. This equilibrium maintains a negative intrapleural pressure with respect to atmospheric and alveolar pressure [10]. However, pleural pressures are not uniform in erect subjects and an apex-to-base gradient of approximately 0.25 cm H_2O per cm exists with a more negative pressure being present at the apex of the pleural cavity due to the effects of gravity on the lung. In a similar manner, gradients of regional lung volumes compatible with those of pleural surface pressure and esophageal (intrapleural) pressure also exist [11].

Pneumothorax, either caused by a communication between the lung and pleural cavity (closed pneumothorax) or between the opened chest wall and the pleural cavity (open or surgical pneumothorax), consists in the passage of atmospheric air into the pleural cavity. This allows the thoracic wall to bow out and the lung to collapse, significantly altering distribution of ventilation.

Closed pneumothorax. Anthonisen [12] investigated regional lung function in 3 awake men with spontaneous pneumothorax. He found that, as expected, Total Lung Capacity (TLC) was decreased in collapsed lungs. Further, he observed a different behavior of regional volume distribution amongst collapsed lungs and contralateral expanded lungs. In particular, he found a distinct apex-to-base gradient of regional volume in the lungs without pneumothorax, which contrasted with a uniform decrease of lung expansion with no volume gradients in lungs with pneumothorax. This finding resembled what was observed in isolated animal lungs and led to the interpretation that, by abolishing pleural pressure gradients, pneumothorax also abolished regional volume gradients [12]. Pneumothorax also modified airway closure in the lungs so that regional residual volumes were relatively uniform with virtually the whole lung being closed at a low lung volume. Conversely, other studies have suggested the persistence of apex-to-base gradients of regional volume even in supine recumbency [13, 14] when pleural pressure gradient is assumed to be absent. This finding led to hypothesize the existence of differences in elastic properties between upper and lower lobes [14].

Gilmartin *et al.* [15] compared the effects of pneumothorax and pleural effusion on pulmonary function. They showed that both these conditions behaved in a similar manner producing a restrictive ventilatory defect with reductions in Vital Capacity (VC), Functional Residual Capacity (FRC), Residual Volume (RV) and TLC. In particular, when looking to the flow-volume curves, they suggested that the lungs emptied slightly faster during forced expiration in the presence of pleural air or fluid. One theoretical explanation was that if pleural air or fluid reduces the number of functioning compliant lung units, airway size will remain appropriate for the lung recoil pressure but will be inappropriately large for the lung volume, so that the slope of the flow-volume curve appears supranormal.

What is clinically evident is that with a closed pneumothorax, the degree of derangement from physiologic ventilation is related to the degree of the lung collapse, which can vary considerably and is, in turn, dependent on the quantity of air that moves into the pleural space, the size of the communication with atmospheric air, its patency, and the possibility of development of a valve mechanism allowing unidirectional passage of air into the pleural cavity with eventual creation of a tension pneumothorax. Experimental data have led to assume that significant ventilatory changes do occur when pneumothorax becomes greater than 25% in volume [16].

Open pneumothorax. Surgically-induced pneumothorax represents the first physiologic change that allows awake thoracic surgery procedures to be feasible. In fact, following opening of the thorax, atmospheric air enters into the pleural cavity and induces an immediate collapse of the non-dependent lung.

In most instances, the newly developed intrapleural, atmospheric pressure environment leads to a drop of lung volume thus assuring an adequately large space for easy surgical maneuvering. The extent of this effect, however, varies considerably and is correlated to the size of the chest opening, the conditions of the lung tissue and airways as well as to those of the pleural cavity. In patients with normal or nearly normal lung elastic recoil, an open pneumothorax is followed by a nearly complete collapse of the lung whereas this can be hampered by some pathologic conditions.

Diffuse pleural adhesions anchoring the lung to the chest wall can greatly limit lung collapse; moreover, in patients with chronic obstructive pulmonary disease and emphysema, the reduced lung elastic recoil with increased expiratory airway resistance, lead to increased end-expiratory pressures and trapped lung gases that tend to counterbalance atmospheric pressure and thus oppose the lung collapse.

Lateral position. With the assumption of a lateral position in an awake subject, the non-dependent lung behaves like the superior portion of the upright lung whereas the dependent one behaves like the inferior portion of the upright lung. The dependent lung is thus on a steep portion of the pulmonary compliance curve and the non-dependent lung is on a less compliant portion on the curve. The shape of the dependent hemidiaphragm is altered and is subjected to increased loading from the abdominal contents that improve its efficiency with increased ventilation [17].

As regards the effect of body posture on spirometric variables, Masumi *et al.* [18] found a significant decrease in the forced inspiratory flow measured between 25% and 75% of VC upon recumbency.

Meysman and Vincken [19] found that in normal subjects in lateral recumbency, forced expiratory volume in one second (FEV_1), Forced Vital Capacity (FVC) and peak expiratory flow decreased by 5%-10% compared with measurements in the sitting posture.

These authors attributed the recumbency-induced changes in flow rates to a decrease in lung volume. Recumbency also produced a significant reduction in VC, RV and TLC that were deemed to be related mainly to an increase in intrathoracic blood volume [20, 21].

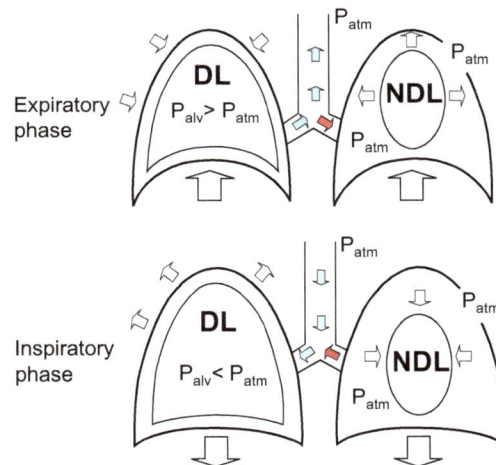

Fig. 1. Distribution of ventilated gases in a subject lying in lateral decubitus with a surgical pneumothorax created in the non-dependent pleural cavity. During expiration, air moves out (sky-blue arrows) from the Dependent Lung (DL) since alveolar pressure (P_{alv}) becomes higher than atmospheric pressure (P_{atm}). Part of the exhaled gases inflate (red arrow) the Non-Dependent Lung (NDL), in which alveolar pressure equalizes atmospheric pressure. Instead, during inspiration, atmospheric air inflate the DL in which P_{alv} becomes sub-atmospheric whereas the NDL deflates, contributing (red arrow) to ventilate the DL.

Opening the non-dependent hemithorax of an awake, laterally positioned subject, leads to redirection of ventilation to the dependent lung. However, the dependent lung is exposed to the full weight of the mediastinum because this is no longer held in place by the negative intrapleural pressure of the non-dependent hemithorax [22]. Thus, theoretically, an open pneumothorax could lead to mediastinal shifting with compression of the dependent lung eventually resulting in functional compromise. Further, spontaneous ventilation leads to paradoxical respiration, the extent of which is related to the degree of collapse of the non-dependent lung induced by the surgical pneumothorax. In fact, with an open chest, descent of the diaphragm leads to decreased intrathoracic pressure only in the closed, dependent hemithorax. The continuous atmospheric pressure environment in the open hemithorax leads to mediastinal movement toward the dependent hemithorax during inspiration and the contrary during expiration. Tidal volume to the dependent lung is reduced. Paradoxical respiration is due to non-dependent lung collapse during inspiration and expansion during exhalation. As the pressure decreases in the dependent hemithorax during inspiration, volume to the dependent lung is partially entrained from the non-dependent lung. The process is reversed during expiration, and part of the dependent lung tidal volume is exhaled into the non-dependent lung, causing paradoxical expansion (*i.e.* pendular ventilation) (Fig. **1**) [17]. Mediastinal shift and paradoxical respiration decrease the efficiency of spontaneous ventilation with re-breathing of exhaled gases [22].

However, in most patients, the modified pattern of ventilation induced by the open pneumothorax is relatively well tolerated. This is mainly attributable to the maintained diaphragmatic motion, which contrasts compressive effects of abdominal pressure against the dependent lung and assures an effective ventilation [23].

To better investigate changes in spirometric variables induced by surgical pneumothorax, we performed intra-operative spirometry in patients undergoing various awake thoracic surgery procedures. Spirometric measurements were obtained in lateral recumbency, with closed versus opened chest immediately after creation of the surgical pneumothorax in patients with relatively normal lung, interstitial lung disease, or emphysema. We found that the rate of change in FEV_1 was -52%, -49% and -30%, respectively whereas changes in FVC were -45%, -46% and -34%, respectively (Fig. **2**). Such findings suggest that in patients with severe ventilatory obstruction and hyperinflation, the ventilatory impairment associated with surgical pneumothorax can be of lesser extent than that observed in patients with either relatively normal function or restrictive ventilatory defect.

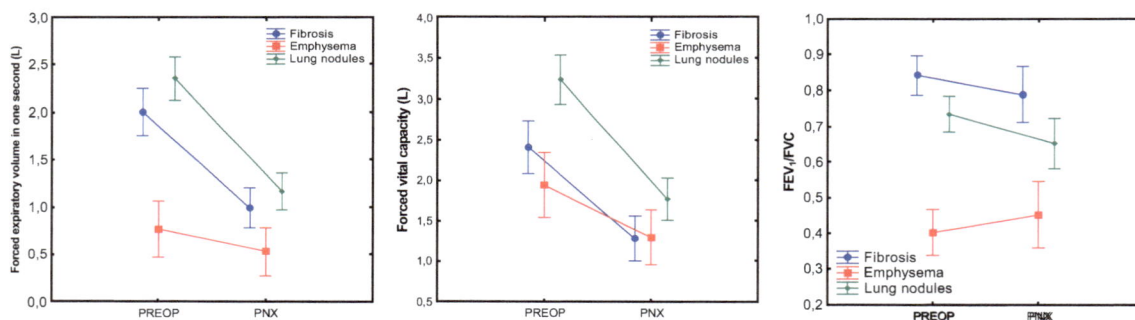

Fig. 2. Spirometric changes induced by surgical pneumothorax (PNX) in awake subjects lying in lateral decubitus. Preoperative measurements (PREOP) are performed in lateral decubitus with closed chest.

EFFECTS ON PULMONARY HEMODYNAMICS AND OXYGENATION

Closed pneumothorax. During closed pneumothorax, a decrease in lung volume leads to an increase in pulmonary vascular resistance [24]. In addition, unilateral pneumothorax causes mild hypoxemia in subjects with normal lung function [25]. Hypoxemia may be secondary to a regional imbalance between alveolar ventilation and pulmonary capillary perfusion. Atelectasis leads immediately to an increased pulmonary shunt fraction and hypoxemia that are secondary to relative overperfusion of the atelectatic areas. Normally, the pulmonary vasculature responds to regional atelectasis by selectively increasing vascular tone, decreasing blood flow to the atelectatic areas and restoring the balance between ventilation and perfusion. This local phenomenon occurs within 1 minute, is maximal at 15 minutes and is reversible, its magnitude being proportional to the amount of hypoxic lung [17, 26, 27].

Norris *et al.* [16] showed that in patients with spontaneous pneumothorax, the more extensive the pneumothorax, the larger the anatomical veno-arterial shunt and the higher the level of hypoxemia. In particular, they observed that when the lung to intrapleural space ratio was greater than 75%, the anatomical shunt did not exceed the normal value of 2% of the cardiac output, whereas for a ratio of about 65% or more the shunt started to increase meaningfully.

Moran *et al.* [28] investigated changes in respiratory and cardiovascular function, including regional ventilation and perfusion, during unilateral pneumothorax in awake dogs. They found that following induction of pneumothorax, respiratory rate increased by 124%, while alveolar ventilation remained unchanged. Pulmonary shunt fraction rose by 93% during pneumothorax, causing a fall in arterial oxygen tension (PaO_2) from 86 to 51 mmHg. Arterial carbon dioxide tension ($PaCO_2$), pH and cardiac output were not affected by the pneumothorax. In addition, pneumothorax induced a relative underventilation of the collapsed lung and an overventilation of the expanded lung.

Central nervous mechanisms for maintaining a constant $PaCO_2$ increase the respiratory rate to compensate for the decreased volume per breath during collapse of one lung.

However, Dale and Rahn [29] had previously shown that the loss in tidal volume was not linearly correlated to the amount of the pneumothorax, probably due to mechanical factors that increased the volume of the contralateral lung slightly.

In the aforementioned study, cardiac output and systemic vascular resistance did not change during unilateral pneumothorax, a finding that had been previously reported also by other authors [30]. The increase of up to 80% in pulmonary vascular resistance (PVR) also confirmed findings of other investigators [24, 31] although regional distribution of pulmonary perfusion was unchanged in the study by Moran *et al.* [28]. This suggested that a diffuse increase in PVR occurred in both lungs, possibly due to systemic hypoxemia acting on chemoreceptors in the aortic body and increased sympathetic stimulation during stress as shown by the rise in heart rate and local hypoxia in the partially collapsed underventilated lung [27, 32-34].

This behavior contrasts with that of regional atelectasis from bronchial occlusion that results in decreased perfusion of the atelectatic area [27, 35].

Rapid re-expansion of a unilateral pneumothorax occasionally leads to unilateral pulmonary edema [36] that has been attributed to an adverse re-perfusion effect [37, 38], which also results in radical-oxygen-species-related injury [39, 40]. Nonetheless, in the study by Moran *et al.* [28] no animal developed unilateral pulmonary edema for up to 2 hours after acute re-expansion of the collapsed lung.

Bennett and coworkers [41] investigated cardiopulmonary changes occurring in conscious dogs with induced progressive pneumothorax. They found that cardiac function remained relatively unchanged whereas a linear increase occurred in central venous pressure accompanying a progressive increase of afterload in the right heart resulting from pulmonary hypertension [31, 42]. In this study, pulmonary hypertension was thought to reflect the combined effect of mechanical collapse of pulmonary vessels caused by increased intrapleural pressure and hypoxic vasoconstriction [42, 43].

Alveolar ventilation was maintained during progressive pneumothorax as shown by normal $PaCO_2$ values, although a linear decrease in PaO_2 developed. Diffusion impairment, ventilation to perfusion mismatch, and intrapulmonary shunting of blood are all potential causes of lowered PaO_2 in the face of maintained ventilation. In the study by Bennett and coworkers [41], the accompanying linear increase in the alveolar to arterial oxygen tension and shunt fraction during progressive pneumothorax suggested that collapsed alveoli continued to be perfused, creating areas of low ventilation to perfusion ratio and pulmonary shunt. Hypoxemia during pneumothorax was therefore deemed more dependent on ventilation to perfusion imbalance and intrapulmonary shunting rather than on alveolar hypoventilation.

In response to low alveolar oxygen tension, resistance vessels of lungs undergo vasoconstriction. The net effect is to divert blood away from hypoxic regions of lungs in order to reduce ventilation to perfusion inequality and maintain PaO$_2$. The stimulus-response curve to the vasoconstriction is not linear since marked vasoconstriction develops only when PaO$_2$ falls below 70 mmHg. Generalized pulmonary hypoxic vasoconstriction can induce an increase in pulmonary arterial pressure and an increase in right ventricle work [33, 41].

Open pneumothorax. Similarly to what has been reported in closed pneumothorax, following creation of surgical pneumothorax, lung collapse induced by intrathoracic atmospheric pressure results in an increase in PVR due to mechanical limitation to flow. Furthermore, hypoxemia which accompanies collapse of the lungs may enhance this effect by causing pulmonary vasoconstriction [44].

Cary *et al.* [44], in an experimental study conducted on mongrel dogs and monkeys, failed to find an increased filling gradient between great veins and the right heart, findings that contrasted with the hypothesis of an interference with cardiac output due to caval kinking or obstruction. Furthermore, the authors of this study found a different behavior between dogs and monkeys, with the latter tolerating thoracotomy for up to 40 minutes during spontaneous ventilation without any marked hemodynamic disturbance except for an increase in PVR and the development of a moderate hypoxemia.

These effects seem to resemble those currently observed in humans, whereas they were less pronounced than in dogs in which severe hypoxemia and respiratory arrest occurred after only 5 minutes.

The effect of open pneumothorax on oxygenation in the clinical setting is based on anecdotal clinical studies. Simple physiologic data of awake thoracoscopy had been reported by Oldenburg and Newhouse [45]. In their 41 patients operated on through sole local anesthesia, they found that during simple thoracoscopic procedures, no significant electrocardiographic changes were noted and the decrease in oxygen saturation was small.

They attributed the relatively good conservation of arterial oxygen saturation to the vasoconstrictive response of the pulmonary vasculature to the alveolar hypoxia produced at the time of the induced atelectasis. Positioning of the patient in the lateral decubitus, with the affected lung in a non-dependent position, helped minimize changes in the ventilation-perfusion ratio.

In a further study, Faursschou *et al.* [46] found a significant increase in respiratory rate and a reduction in PaCO$_2$ with no significant changes in PaO$_2$, pH, cardiac rhythm and rate. Also these results, however, were observed during short diagnostic thoracoscopic procedures lasting not more than 15 minutes.

We found that the decrease in arterial oxygenation that occurs following the surgical pneumothorax is usually limited and can be easily corrected by simple oxygen administration through a Venturi mask. It is likely that, in most instances, a sufficient degree of compensatory ventilation and oxygenation is assured by the dependent lung whose respiratory efficiency is increased by the maintained diaphragmatic function.

Katz *et al.* [47] found that in patients undergoing one-lung ventilation there was an inverse relationship between preoperative FEV$_1$ and development of hypoxemia. Explanations for this apparently paradoxical effect may include slow non-dependent lung collapse following one-lung ventilation; preexisting reduced perfusion in the non-dependent lung secondary to intrinsic pathology or chronic hypoxic pulmonary vasoconstriction; kinked pulmonary vessels in the deflated, non-dependent lung that inhibit perfusion; and development of intrinsic positive end-expiratory pressure in dependent lung, increasing FRC and decreasing atelectasis. Moreover, Sling *et al.* [48] identified three factors that predicted oxygen desaturation during one lung ventilation. Namely: the side of surgery, since the right lung receives 10% more blood flow and can thus be more subject to hypoxemia during one lung ventilation; PaO$_2$ during total lung ventilation; and the percentage of FEV$_1$ that was inversely correlated with hypoxemia.

This latter feature introduces the attractive hypothesis that patients with severe obstructive ventilatory defect may develop lower degrees of hypoxemia during surgical pneumothorax.

Our clinical data seem to support these findings, since we found that the drop in the arterial oxygen tension to fraction of inspired oxygen ratio that followed creation of surgical pneumothorax was 38 mmHg in emphysema patients undergoing awake lung volume reduction surgery, 74 mmHg in patients with interstitial lung disease, and 91 mmHg in those with lung nodules and relatively normal lung function (Fig. **3**).

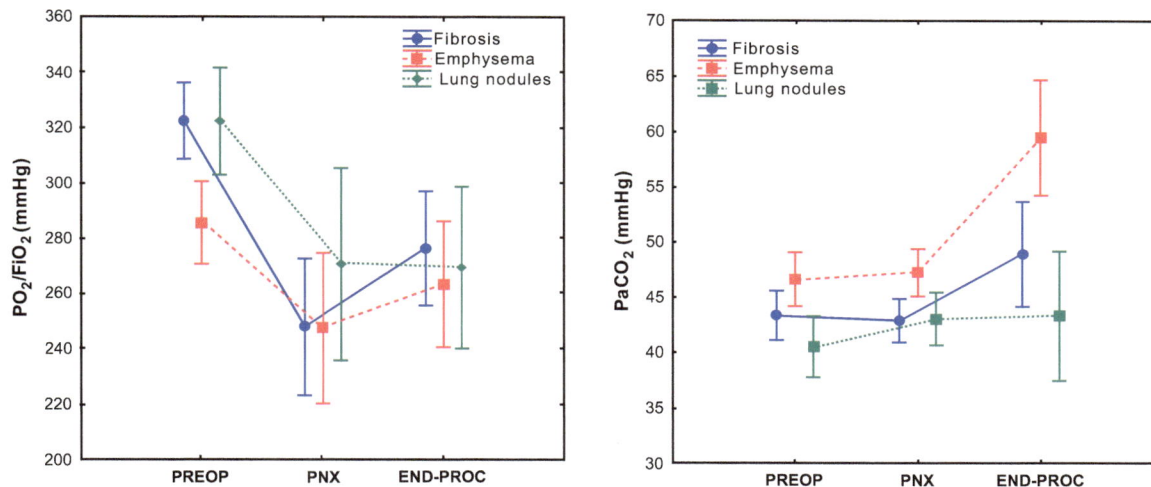

Fig. 3. Behavior of arterial oxygen tension to fraction of inspired oxygen ratio (PO_2/FiO_2) and arterial carbon dioxide tension ($PaCO_2$) measured preoperatively (PREOP), after creation of a surgical pneumothorax (PNX) and at end-procedure (END-PROC) in patients with interstitial lung disease (fibrosis), emphysema and normal lung function (lung nodules).

We hypothesize that in patients with emphysema and severe gas trapping, the effect of atmospheric pressure on ventilation is limited due to the existence of positive end-expiratory pressures in peripheral alveolar regions. This might lead to uneven pressure gradients between different regions of the same lung resulting in a certain maintained ventilation in both lungs. Furthermore, prolonged exhalation times that are typical of patients with emphysema might counteract the between-lung pendular ventilation.

On the other hand, collapse of the non-dependent lung due to the presence of an intra-pleural atmospheric pressure environment increases the inspiratory load and might thus negatively affect respiration. However, we found that in patients with baseline PaO_2 as low as 55 mmHg, simple administration of oxygen through a Venturi mask made it possible to maintain oxygenation to satisfactory levels throughout the procedure. To support this hypothesis, some recently reported data suggest that suprapontine compensatory mechanisms are active in defending ventilation in awake subjects challenged with an inspiratory load [49].

PERMISSIVE HYPERCAPNIA

During awake thoracic surgery, administration of oxygen can prevent hypoxemia in the majority of patients although permissive hypercapnia sometimes develops, particularly in patients with severe emphysema.

The pathophysiology of this event is not fully understood although hypoventilation due to partial collapse of the operated lung and a rebreathing effect due to between-lung pendular ventilation seem reasonable hypotheses.

Permissive hypercapnia rarely becomes clinically dangerous and may even exert some potentially beneficial effects including increased parenchymal compliance and improved ventilation/perfusion matching [50-52]. In fact, the hypercapnic-mediated sympathicoadrenal effects of increased preload, decreased afterload, and increased heart rate lead to a net increase in cardiac output. However, for these reasons, the development of hypercapnia must be carefully monitored in patients on β-adrenergic antagonists or those with heart failure or coronary artery disease. Furthermore, the increase in cerebral blood flow that is associated with hypercapnic acidosis must be taken into account as a potential risk for raised intracranial pressure [53]. Finally, the marked sympathetic activation of hypercapnic acidosis, particularly when combined with arterial hypoxemia, can reduce glomerular filtration and increase fluid retention [54].

CONCLUSION

There is increased evidence that several thoracic surgical procedures can be reliably performed in awake patients through thoracic epidural or other non-general anesthesia techniques. Surgical creation of an open pneumothorax is necessary to collapse the lung and obtain adequate space for surgical maneuvering. However, this iatrogenic event is followed by a complex cascade of physiologic changes on lung ventilation, perfusion and mechanical interaction between lungs, pleural cavity, diaphragm and mediastinum.

Useful data is continuing to be accumulated to better elucidate mechanisms underlying these effects although it has already become evident that even patients with severe respiratory impairment can safely undergo an awake surgical operation.

Nonetheless, though well tolerated by the majority of patients, hypoxemia, hypercapnia and hypoventilation are all common findings with this type of surgery and need to be clearly taken into account by physicians who decide to be actively involved in this novel field of thoracic surgery.

REFERENCES

[1]   Sauerbruch F, O'Shaughnessy L, Eds. Thoracic Surgery. London: Edward Arnold & Co 1937; pp. 324-86.
[2]   Brauer L. Die ausschaltung der pneumothoraxfolgen mit hilfe des ueberdruckverfahrens. Mitteilungen aus den Grenzgebieten der Medizin und Chirurgie 1904;13:483-500.
[3]   Sauerbruch F. Zur pathologie des offenen pneumothorax und die grundlagen meinees verfahrens zu seiner ausschaltung. Mitteilungen aus den Grenzgebieten der Medizin und Chirurgie 1904;13:399-482.
[4]   Hagopian EJ, Mann C, Galibert L, *et al.* The history of thoracic surgical instruments and instrumentation. Chest Surg Clin North Am 2000;10:9-43.
[5]   Zavod WA. Bronchospirography 1. Description of the catheter and the technique of intubation. J Thorac Surg 1940;10:27-31.
[6]   Björk VO, Carlens E. The prevention of spread during pulmonary resection by use of a double-lumen catheter. J Thorac Surg 1950;20:151-7.
[7]   Pompeo E, Mineo D, Rogliani P, *et al.* Feasibility and results of awake thoracoscopic resection of solitary pulmonary nodules. Ann Thorac Surg 2004;78:1761-8.
[8]   Pompeo E, Mineo TC. Awake pulmonary metastasectomy. J Thorac Cardiovasc Surg 2007;133:960-6.
[9]   Pompeo E, Mineo TC. Two-year improvement in multidimensional body-mass index, airflow obstruction, dyspnea and exercise capacity index after nonresectional lung volume reduction surgery in awake patients. Ann Thorac Surg 2007;84:1862-9.
[10]   Benumof JL. Respiratory physiology and respiratory function during anesthesia. In: Miller Ed. Miller's Anesthesia. New York, Churchill-Livingstone, 1986; pp. 1115-62.
[11]   Milic-Emili J, Henderson JA, Dolovich MB, Trop D, Kaneko K. Regional distribution of inspired gas in the lung. J Appl Physiol 1966;21:749-59.
[12]   Anthonisen NR. Regional lung function in spontaneous pneumothorax. Am Rev Respir Dis 1977;11:873-6.
[13]   Grassino AE, Bake B, Martin RR, Anthonisen NR. Voluntary change of thoracoabdominal shape and regional lung volumes in humans. J Appl Physiol 1975;39:997-1003.
[14]   Bake B, Bjure J, Grimby G, Milic-Emili J, Nilsson NJ. Regional distribution of inspired gas in supine man. Scand J Respir Dis 1967;48:189-96.
[15]   Gilmartin JJ, Wright AJ, Gibson GJ. Effects of pneumothorax or pleural effusion on pulmonary function. Thorax 1985;40:60-5.
[16]   Norris RM, Jones JG, Bishop JM. Respiratory gas exchange in patients with spontaneous pneumothorax. Thorax 1968;21:427-33.
[17]   Benumof JL. Chapter 2:distribution of ventilation and perfusion. In: Benumof JL, Ed. Anesthesia for thoracic surgery. 2nd edition. Philadelphia, WB Saunders, 1995; pp. 35-52.
[18]   Masumi S, Nishigawa K, Willimas AJ, *et al.* Effect of jaw position and posture on forced inspiratory airflow in normal subjects and patients with sleep apnea. Chest 1996;109:1484-9.
[19]   Meysman M, Vincken W. Effect of body posture on spirometric values and upper airway obstruction indices derived from the flow-volume loop in young nonobese subjects. Chest 1998;114:1042-7.

[20]   Agostoni E, D'Angelo E. Statics of the chest wall. In: Russos C, Macklem PT, Eds. The Thorax. New York, Marcel Dekker, 1985; pp. 259-95.

[21]   Agostoni E, Hyatt RE. Static behaviour of the respiratory system. In: Fishman AP, Macklem PT, Mead J, Eds. Hand-book of physiology. Section 3: The respiratory system. Volume III. Mechanics of breathing, part 1. Bethesda, American Physiological Society, 1986; pp. 118-22.

[22]   Grichnik KP, Clark JA. Pathophysiology and management of one-lung ventilation. Thorac Surg Clin 2005;15:85-103.

[23]   Mineo TC, Pompeo E, Mineo D, *et al.* Awake nonresectional lung volume reduction surgery. Ann Surg 2006;243:131-6.

[24]   Simmons DH, Hemingway A. The pulmonary circulation following pneumothorax and vagotomy in dogs. Circ Res 1959;7:93-100.

[25]   Guz A, Noble MIM, Eisele JH, Trenchard D. The effect of lung deflation on breathing in man. Clin Sci 1971;40:451-61.

[26]   Leach RM, Treacher DF.Clinical aspects of hypoxic pulmonary vasoconstriction. Exp Physiol 1995;80:865-75.

[27]   Fishman AP. Respiratory gases in the regulation of the pulmonary circulation. Physiol Rev 1961;41:214-80.

[28]   Moran JF, Jones RH, Wolfe WG. Regional pulmonary function during experimental unilateral pneumothorax in the awake state. J Thorac Cardiovasc Surg 1977;74:396-402.

[29]   Dale WA, Rahn H. Experimental pulmonary atelectasis. Changes in chest mechanics following block of one lung. J Appl Physiol 1956;9:359-66.

[30]   Kilburn H. Cardiorespiratory effects in conscious and anesthetized dogs. J Appl Physiol 1963;18:279-83.

[31]   Rutheford RB, Hurt HH Jr, Brickman RD, Tubb JM. The pathophysiology of progressive tension pneumothorax. J Trauma 1968;8:212-27.

[32]   Comroe JH Jr. Ed. Physiology of respiration, 2nd Edition. Chicago: Year Book Medical Publisher Inc 1974; p. 155.

[33]   West JB, Ed. Respiratory Physiology. Baltimore: The Williams & Wilkins Company 1974; pp. 40-6.

[34]   Velez-Roa S, Ciarka A, Najem B, *et al.* Increased Sympathetic Nerve Activity in Pulmonary Artery Hypertension. Circulation. 2004;110:1308-12.

[35]   Kersten TE, Humphrey EW. Pulmonary Shunt mechanism in atelectasis. Surg Forum 1975;26:211-13.

[36]   Carlson RI, Classen KL, Gollan F, Gobbel WG Jr, Sherman DE, Christensen RO. Pulmonary edema following the rapid re-expansion of a totally collapsed lung due to a pneumothorax. A clinical and experimental study. Surg Forum 1958;9:367-71.

[37]   Poulias GE, Prombonas E. Massive unilateral pulmonary edema as arapid re-expansion sequel (the post-expansion syndrome). Scand J Thorac Cardiovasc Surg 1974;8:67-9.

[38]   Saini GS. Unilateral pulmonary oedema after drainage of spontaneous pneumothoax. Br Med J 1974;1:615.

[39]   Misthos P, Katsaragakis S, Theodorou D, Milingos N, Skottis I. The degree of oxidative stress is associated with major adverse effects after lung resection. 2006;29:591-5.

[40]   Yin K, Gribbin E, Emanuel S, *et al.* Histochemical alterations in one-lung ventilation. J Surg Res 2007;137:16-20.

[41]   Bennett RA, Orton EC, Tucker A, Heiller CL. Cardiopulmonary changes in conscious dogs with induced progressive pneumothorax. Am J Vet Res 1989;50:280-4.

[42]   Bjorling DE, Whitfield JB. High-frequency jet ventilation during pneumothorax in dogs. Am J Vet Res 1986;47:1984-7.

[43]   Hemingway A, Simmons DH. Respiratory response to acute progressive pneumothorax. J Appl Physiol 1958;13:165-70.

[44]   Carey JS, Huges RK. Hemodynamic studies in open pneumothorax. J Thorac Cardiovasc Surg 1968;55:538-45.

[45]   Oldemburg FA, Newhouse MT. A safe, accurate diagnostic procedure using the rigid thoracoscope and local anesthesia. Chest 1979; 75:45-50.

[46]   Faurschou P, Madsen F, Viskum K. Thoracoscopy: influence of the procedure on some respiratory and cardiac values. Thorax 1983; 38:341-3.

[47]   Katz JA, Laverne RG, Fairley HB, *et al.* Pulmonary oxygen exchange during endobronchial anesthesia: effect of tidal volume and PEEP. Anesthesiology 1982;56:164-72.

[48]   Singer P, Suissa S, Triolet W. Predicting arterial oxygenation during one-lung anesthesia. Can J Anaesth 1992;39:1030-5.

[49]   Raux M, Straus C, Redolfi S, *et al.* Electroencephalographic evidence for pre-motor cortex activation during inspiratory loading in humans. J Physiol 2007;578:569-78.

[50]   Kregenow DA, Swenson ER. The lung and carbon dioxide: implications for permissive and therapeutic hypercapnia. Eur Respir J 2002;20:6-11.

[51]   Wildeboer- Venema F. The influences of temperature and humidity upon the isolated surfactant film of the dog. Respir Physiol 1980;39:63-71.

[52]   Brogan TV, Robertson HT, Souders JE, Swenson ER. Carbon dioxide added to the latter half of inspiration improves Va/Q matching without causing respiratory acidosis. FASEB J 2002;16:A876.

[53]   Feihl F, Perret C. Permissive hypercapnia: How permissive should we be? Am J Respir Crit Care Med 1994;150:1722-37.

[54]   DiBona GF, Kopp UC. Neural control of renal function. Physiol Rev 1997;77:175-97.

CHAPTER 3

Systemic Host Response in Awake Thoracic Surgery

Federico Tacconi[*], Gianluca Vanni and Eugenio Pompeo

Department of Thoracic Surgery, Policlinico Tor Vergata University Rome, Italy

Abstract: Systemic response to surgery entails the activation of hormonal, metabolic and inflammatory pathways, and may affect postoperative outcome due to interaction with host's immunity, metabolism, organ function, coagulation, and wound healing.

In recent years, we have being actively involved with video-assisted thoracoscopic surgery performed on spontaneously ventilating patients (awake VATS), with the use of just local- or locoregional anesthesia techniques. Amongst the expected advantages of this approach, an attenuation of postoperative response has been hypothesized, potentially contributing to a more physiological recovery. In particular, our recent observation has showed that avoidance of one-lung ventilation may result into attenuated release of stress hormones and systemic inflammation biomarkers including C-reactive protein and interleukin-6 in patients undergoing awake videothoracoscopic procedure. In this chapter, we review the basic knowledge on systemic host response after surgery, whit particular reference to our most recent evidences in this setting.

Keywords: Local anesthesia, thoracic epidural anesthesia, SIRS, stress response, VATS.

INTRODUCTION

Systemic response to surgery entails the activation of hormonal, metabolic and inflammatory pathways, which interact in a complex network1 [1-4]. Its goal is to combat this non-physiologic event, which calls for prompt availability of energetic substrates and recruitment of antimicrobial defenses. In some instances, this ancestral biologic answer may become uncontrolled and can translate into a further deterioration of the host's steady-state. A clinical manifestation of this paradigm comes from the so-called *Systemic Inflammation Response Syndrome* (SIRS), which entails dysregulation of proinflammatory mediators ultimately leading to organ injury [5, 6]. In a similar manner, the derangement in cytokine and hormone production may lead to transient inhibition of cell-mediated immunity [4, 7], thus facilitating postoperative infections and even cancer progression.

In recent years, Video-Assisted Thoracicc Surgery (VATS) has become widely accepted for surgical management of a number of thoracic conditions and has been shown to reduce the postoperative systemic response when compared to open approaches [9-11]. A further contribution to the development of minimally-invasive thoracic surgery has derived from the introduction of the so-called *lung protective* ventilation strategies, alongside the renewed interest for locoregional anesthesia techniques in spontaneously ventilating awake patients. All these methods are thought to allow a more physiologic perioperative response that could eventually lessen postoperative complications.

This chapter has a twofold profile. In the first part, we review the basic knowledge on systemic host response to both surgery- and anesthesia-related trauma. In the second part, we focus on the pattern of systemic host response following awake VATS procedures, taking into account our recent experience with this novel surgical approach.

BASIC MECHANISMS OF RESPONSE TO SURGERY AND ANESTHESIA

The *primum movens* of the host's response to surgery is the local production of soluble mediators, which is

*****Address correspondence to Federico Tacconi:** Department of Thoracic Surgery, Policlinico Tor Vergata University, Rome, Italy; Email: tacconifederico@libero.it

stimulated by tissue wounding, vasodilatation and subsequent migration of circulating leukocytes. Soluble mediators mostly entail cytokines, which regulate a series of biological activities by interacting with target cells expressing specific receptors. At the surgical site, they are promoters of antimicrobial response and wound healing [12].

A local increase of soluble mediators is followed by their spillover towards the systemic circulation, so that they can act at distant sites. For example, interleukins-1 and -6 can enhance the release of Adrenal-Corticotropic Hormone (ACTH) from the pituitary gland, eventually increasing plasma cortisol level [13]. They also modulate the hepatic production of a series of *acute response factors,* which include C-Reactive Protein (CRP), fibrinogen, α2-microglobulin and leptin.

An uncontrolled production of pro-inflammatory cytokines can lead to both acute and chronic complications including hemodynamic instability, increased catabolism with muscle wasting, and even multiple organ failure (MOF). The concurrent increase of anti-inflammatory cytokines may partly counterbalance these adverse effects. However, excessive production of anti-inflammatory factors, can be responsible for transient immunodeficiency, with increased likelihood of perioperative infections [1, 4, 13].

The other pathway of systemic response to surgical trauma entails the neuraxial signaling of noxious stimuli, which reach the thalamus *via* the dorsal nerve roots and the spinal-thalamic chord. This signal is primarily activated by specific receptors of mechanical injury, which are sited at the level of sensory neural terminations. Local soluble mediators may enhance or inhibit the activity of these *nociceptors*, thus affecting systemic response. For example, the substance-P, an olygopeptide which is mostly produced by neuroendocrine cells in response to trauma, has been indicated as one of the most important modulators of pain perception and may inhibit the postsurgical increase in cortisol and interleukin-6.

Since a detailed description of the biochemical properties of perioperative systemic response factors and their interaction is beyond the scope of this chapter, herein we briefly review the basic knowledge on this topic.

*Tumor necrosis factor-*α *(TNF-*α*).* This is one of the earliest and most potent mediators of postsurgical host response. The primary source of TNF-α include monocytes/macrophages and T-lymphocytes. Since the latter are abundant in the peritoneum and abdominal organs, a postoperative increase in TNF-α is mostly observed after abdominal surgery. Although the half-life of TNF-α in peripheral circulation is less than 20 minutes, a transient increase is capable of eliciting metabolic and hemodynamic changes, as well as the production of other proinflammatory cytokines. TNF-α also regulates the expression and release of factors involved with coagulation, such as adhesions molecules, prostaglandin E2, platelet-activating factor, glucocorticoids, and eicosanoids [14].

The basic counterbalancing mechanism to TNF-α is represented by the concurrent increase in soluble TNF-receptors (sTNFRs), which are thought to electively bind and thus antagonize TNF-α, although these may also work as a storage mechanism of TNF-α in the circulation.

Interleukin 1 (IL-1). IL-1 is produced by both macrophages and endothelial cells. Two variants exist (IL-1 α and IL-1 β), the latter being the more promptly detectable in the circulation. IL-1 has a synergistic role with TNF-α, and is involved in the febrile response to trauma by stimulating prostaglandin production at the level of anterior hypothalamus. Interestingly, inhibition of pain perception is partly mediated by IL-1 by enhancing the release of β-endorphins from the pituitary gland.

Interleukin 2 (IL-2). IL-2 stimulates a series of immunity functions including T-cell replication and release of immunoglobulin. Inhibition of IL-2 expression as a consequence of major surgery and blood transfusion, can therefore contribute to perioperative immunosuppression [15, 16].

Interleukin 4 (IL-4). IL-4 is produced by activated Th2 lymphocytes and exerts a series of effects on the hematopoietic process and in the antibody-mediated immunity. Indeed, IL-4 stimulates production of IgG and IgE from activated B-lymphocytes, which are important in immunologic memory, as well as allergic response and anti-helminthic defense [17]. IL-4 also has important anti-inflammatory properties due to the antagonizing effect toward IL-1, TNF-α and interleukin-6 cytokines.

Interleukin 6 (IL-6). IL-6 is considered one of the most important indicators of acute response in clinical practice. Its production is induced by IL-1 [18, 19] and TNF-α, and starts 1 hour after skin incision. Its plasmatic peak occurs 2 to 6 hours later and usually returns to preoperative levels 2 to 4 days after the operation, although it can occasionally remain elevated for up to 10 days. One of the hypothesized mechanisms of IL-6-mediated tissue trauma is that IL-6 can inhibit the elimination of senescent neutrophils, thereby prolonging their injurious effects [18]. In the clinical setting, IL-6 has been shown to act as a biomarker of tumor growth and a predictor of postoperative complications after colorectal surgery [20]. Accordingly, Szczesny and coworkers [21] indicated the level of IL-6 in the pleural fluid as an early indicator of postoperative complications after lung cancer resection.

Local and circulating IL-6 levels appear to be strictly related to the global extent of tissue traumatism. In particular, VATS has repeatedly been shown to reduce the perioperative release of IL-6 when compared to open approaches, thus suggesting a role of minimally-invasive surgery in preventing cytokine network derangement [10, 11, 22]. Interestingly, in patients undergoing one-stage bilateral lung-volume reduction surgery for end-stage emphysema, VATS was associated with lesser perioperative IL-6 increase, faster recovery, and reduced morbidity rate when compared to median sternotomy [10].

IL-6 has also been considered a potential pharmacologic target to improve postoperative recovery. In particular, Brivio and coworkers [23] proposed contrasting IL-6 elevation by preoperative administration of IL-2 to prevent both proinflammatory and immunodepressive effects.

Interleukin 8 (IL-8). IL-8 serves as a chemoattractant and activator of neutrophils. Postoperative change of IL-8 resembles that of IL-6, and s cytokine has been considered an adjunctive indicator of postoperative morbidity [24].

Interleukin 10 (IL-10). The main effect of IL-10 is a modulation of TNF-α activity. It has been demonstrated that inactivation of IL-10 during experimental endotoxemia increases monocyte TNF-α production, while restitution of IL-10 reduces TNF-α levels and its associated detrimental effects [25]. In the clinical setting, a reduction of the IL-10 to TNF-α ratio has been shown to be related to increased morbidity rate after abdominal surgery [26].

Interleukin 12 (IL-12). IL-12 has a primary role in cell-mediated immunity and promotes the differentiation of Th1 cells. IL-12 also promotes neutrophil activation and production of coagulation proteins as well as the expression of both proinflammatory and anti-inflammatory mediators. Furthermore, IL-12 toxicity seems to be synergistic with IL-2. Although IL-12 detection after injury or severe infections is variable, there is a mounting evidence that this cytokine contributes to enhance the systemic inflammatory response.

Interleukin 13 (IL-13). IL-13 exerts anti-inflammatory effects similarly to IL-4 and IL-10, as it can inhibit the expression of other proinflammatory cytokines in an early phase of cytokine network activation.

Interleukin 15 (IL 15). IL-15 is mainly produced by macrophages. It enhances IL-8 release of neutrophils and their antifungal function.

Interferon-γ (IFN-γ). An increase of circulating IFN-γ occurs 6 hours after major surgery and may persist for up to 8 days. It has important roles in activating both circulating and resident macrophages. It is thought to have a predominant role in acute lung injury after major surgery or trauma, *via* the activation of alveolar-macrophages.

Nuclear factor k-light-chain-enhancer of activated B-cells (NF-kB). NF-kB is a protein complex that controls the transcription of DNA in a wide series of cell types in response to noxious stimuli. It is involved in resistance to apoptosis, cancer cell growth and inflammatory cell activation. Its expression is triggered by the interaction between the Toll-like receptors with a series of molecules deriving from cell damage and infections, including lipopolysaccharides. Growing evidence exists that NF-kB may mediate activation of alveolar neutrophils in response to mechanical-ventilation-related stimuli, such as airway overstretching and hyperoxia [27], thus playing a potential role in ventilatory-induced lung injury.

The Th1/Th2 paradigm. Surgical injury is associated with transient depression of the immune function that can potentially lead to infective complications as well as cancer spread [4]. This phenomenon is mostly related to impaired cell-mediated immunity and macrophage function.

T-helper lymphocytes are functionally divided into two subtypes, referred to as Th1 and Th2. Each subtype has different secretive properties, and is responsible for a specific subset of immune responses. In particular, the Th1 cell response is characterized by the production of IFN-γ, IL-2, IL-12 and TNF-β as well as activation of cell-mediated immunity. Instead, the Th2 response is primarily characterized by the production of anti-inflammatory cytokines including IL-4, IL-10 and IL-13 along with prevalent activation of antibody-mediated immunity (Fig. **1**).

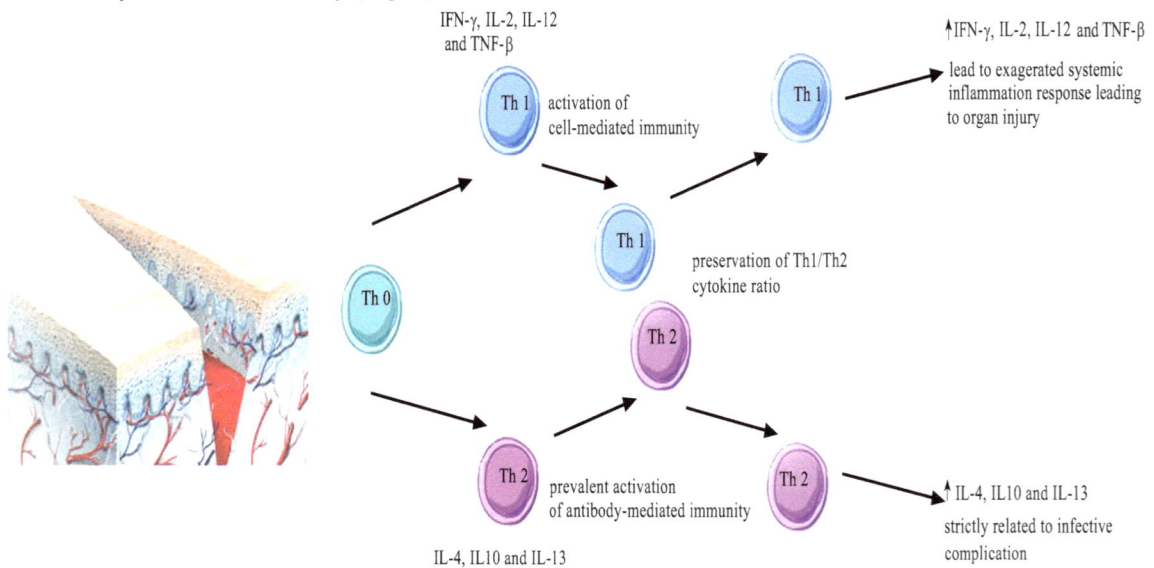

IFN-γ, IL-2, IL-12 and TNF-β

Th 1 activation of cell-mediated immunity

↑IFN-γ, IL-2, IL-12 and TNF-β
lead to exaggerated systemic inflammation response leading to organ injury

Th 0

Th 1

preservation of Th1/Th2 cytokine ratio

Th 2

Th 2 prevalent activation of antibody-mediated immunity

Th 2

↑ IL-4, IL10 and IL-13
strictly related to infective complication

IL-4, IL10 and IL-13

Fig. 1. Main pathways of differentiation of T-helper lymphocyte subsets induced by surgical traumatism. Part of the figure is kindly provided by Hansaplast-Beiersdorf, Hamburg, Germany.

After major surgery, a transient inhibition of Th1 cytokine production does occur, while the shift towards Th2 response suggests inhibition of cell-mediated defense [4]. This phenomenon seems directly related to the degree of surgical stress response and could have important implications in clinical practice. For example, a shift to Th2 cytokine response has been related to infective complication in burn patients [28]. Hence, prevalence of Th2 versus Th1 response could provide a reliable explanation to the finding that some surgical patients are more prone to infections and worse outcome. On the other hand, an excessive Th1 activation might hypothetically trigger an exaggerated systemic inflammation response leading to organ injury, although this phenomenon has not been well documented in surgical or trauma patients. These results suggest that future treatment strategies based on the preservation of the Th1/Th2 cytokine ratio could represent the key to improving postoperative outcomes in different surgical settings [29, 30]. In this regard, use of locoregional anesthesia protocols, either alone or in combination with general anesthesia, might prove useful in this setting since it has been shown that local anesthetics may prevent cancer metastatization to the liver by preserving the Th1/Th2 balance [31] likely due to attenuated activation of the pro-inflammatory cascade.

Endocrine response to surgical stress. The endocrine response to surgery encompasses the activation of both the hypothalamus-pituitary axis and the sympathetic nervous system [1]. The aims of endocrine response are to provide prompt energy substrates *via* the mobilization of stored sources, and to maintain an unaltered fluid balance and cardiac performance.

Cortisol secretion from the adrenal cortex starts early after the beginning of surgical maneuvers as a result of adrenal gland stimulation by ACTH and usually peaks, 4-6 hours later, with a two- to fourfold increase from the baseline values.

In normal conditions, a feedback mechanism exists so that increased plasma concentration of cortisol inhibits further secretion of ACTH. This feedback can become ineffective after surgery, so that concentrations of both hormones can remain high. The main clinically relevant effect of cortisol increase is transient hyperglycemia, which is usually observed after surgery and is considered one of the main indicators of systemic response in daily clinical practice. Although the transient increase in glycemia level is trivial in most patients, it may prove important in diabetic subjects, due to concomitant dysregulation of adaptive mechanisms to hyperglycemia. In particular, a reduction of insulin release may also occur after surgery, partly due to perioperative adrenergic activation which inhibits pancreatic β-cells, alongside an alteration of the normal cell response to insulin.

In addition to its metabolic effects, cortisol has well-known anti-inflammatory and immunodepressive properties. The anti-inflammatory effects of cortisol include decreased expression of some inflammation mediators, such as TNF-α, IL-1, inducible cyclooxygenase (COX-2) and adhesion molecules. In addition, it induces apoptosis in T-lymphocytes, thymocytes and CD8+ cells being more sensitive than CD4+ [32, 33].

Hypothalamic activation of the sympathetic nervous system results in increased secretion of catecholamines from the adrenal medulla, together with a release of norepinephrine from presynaptic nerve terminals. Circulating catecholamines have an inhibitory effect against cell-mediated immunity [34, 35]. The main explanation for this finding is that β-adrenoceptors are expressed on CD4+ helper and CD8+ cytotoxic cell surfaces. Furthermore, it has been shown that patients on long-term therapy with β-blockers have a reduced Th1/Th2 ratio and decreased cytokine production [36].

Effects of general anesthesia on systemic host response. Although the perioperative systemic host response is mostly affected by the extent of surgical trauma, anesthesia may contribute to modulate the degree of response by interacting with cytokine production, lympocyte activity and hormonal release [7, 37, 38]. The mechanisms through which general anesthesia affects systemic host response can differ remarkably depending on the kind of anesthetic drugs used, their plasma concentrations, the type of mechanical ventilation that is employed and the use of adjunctive methods such as locoregional analgesia.

Propofol is a 2, 6-diisopropil-phenolic anesthetic drug which is characterized by rapid hepatic clearance and limited fat-tissue deposit, so that its residual effect is extremely short. Furthermore, since its individual clearance can be estimated by dedicated algorithms based on a patient's body-mass index, the intravenous infusion regimen can be optimized to maintain a constant concentration over time (*target-control infusion*). For these reasons, propofol is widely used in surgical practice either alone or in combination with opioids. Evidence exists that propofol may affect inflammatory response due to it inhibitory effects on neutrophil and monocyte/macrophage functions. However, natural-killer and lymphocyte functions do not seem to be affected by propofol, the use of which may thus be potentially beneficial in immunocompromised patients. In addition, propofol appears to have anti-inflammatory and anti-oxidative properties through its inhibitory effects on neutrophil function.

Morphine has well-known immunosuppressive effects, although the basic mechanisms remain partly misunderstood [39, 40]. The activation of opioid receptors at the level of hypothalamus elicits the production of ACTH, thus enhancing the perioperative glucocorticoid release. Cathecolamines, the release of which is also stimulated by opioids, may contribute to perioperative immunodepression, possibly due to their suppressing activity on lymphocytes, natural-killer cells and macrophages [41]. Most of the inhibitory effects of morphine could be explained by the presence of specific receptors on the surface of different leukocytes [42, 43]. Since synthetic opioids exhibit less affinity for these receptors, they are considered more effective to preserve the postsurgical immunity function although animal studies indicated a suppression of natural-killer activity with high doses of fentanyl [44].

Inhalational anesthesia. A certain amount of evidence exists that inhalational anesthesia attenuates the systemic inflammation response to a greater extent than totally intravenous anesthesia [45, 46]. Therefore, general anesthesia using propofol and fentanyl combined with epidural/spinal analgesia is thought to be advisable in immunocompromised individuals whereas volatile anesthetics should be preferred in patients at risk for SIRS, especially in the cardiac surgery setting.

In thoracic surgery, inhaled anesthetics have been shown to attenuate host response to one-lung ventilation [47]. Nonetheless, data from the literature are controversial. Comparative studies have reported a lower cortisol increase in patients receiving totally-intravenous anesthesia than in those receiving isoflurane, a finding that suggests a more pronounced systemic response in the latter group. In addition, the Th1/Th2 ratio has been reported to decrease significantly with isoflurane anesthesia.

Mechanical ventilation. An interesting field of investigation is whether, and to what extent, mechanical ventilation contributes *per se* to overall surgical traumatism. Mechanical ventilation induces lung damage through different mechanisms (namely, ventilator-related lung injury) which include the stress exerted on the alveolar walls by ventilatory pressures (barotrauma), the overstretching of inflated alveoli (volutrauma), and cyclic closing-reopening of the distal airways (atelectrauma). These different mechanisms of injury can induce, in turn, a compartmental activation of proinflammatory mediators (biotrauma) and their subsequent spillover into the circulation, thus potentially contributing to systemic cytokine unbalance.

Locoregional anesthesia. In recent years, locoregional anesthesia techniques have gained popularity in thoracic surgery and have been shown to reduce postoperative morbidity and length of hospitalization [48, 49]. Potential benefits of locoregional anesthesia include optimal pain control, along with non-analgesic properties including better cardiac performance, protection of gastrointestinal function, lesser perioperative hypercoagulability and a reduction of systemic inflammatory response [48, 49] Furthermore, in a number of clinical studies, the use of epidural anesthetics, alone or in combination with general anesthesia, has proven effective in protecting against perioperative depression of natural-killer cytotoxicity, a finding that has been attributed to the suppression of the cortisol response *via* the blockade of neural signaling. It has also recently been shown in an animal model that the addition of spinal block to inhaled anesthesia can attenuate the surgery-related suppression of anticancer defense function by preserving the Th1/Th2 cytokine response, possibly resulting in a reduced metastatization [31].

CLINICAL EFFECTS OF RESPONSE TO SURGICAL STRESS

Anticancer defense. As previously mentioned, systemic host response is strictly linked to a transient depression of cell-mediated immunity and natural-killer cytotoxicity, which represent the first-line defense against tumor cells [8]. The perioperative period is therefore considered the most vulnerable phase for cancer growth and metastatic spread. The degree of immunosuppression seems related to the extent of surgical trauma. Indeed, in both animal models [50] and clinical settings [10], VATS resections resulted in a lesser impairment in cellular immunity when compared to open approaches, reasonably reflecting a reduced systemic host response.

The loss of defensive properties occurs within hours after surgery and can last for several days [51]. Although the increased cortisol level and the cytokine derangement have a key role in determining perioperative immunosuppression [52], other factors may contribute to the enhanced cancer progression. For example, catecholamines [53] have been shown to increase the invasive properties of ovarian cancer cells *via* an interaction with β1- and β2-adrenergic receptors, which are expressed by tumor cells. Catecholamines also increase the production of vascular endothelial growth factor and fascilitate cell migration by inducing overexpression of matrix-metalloproteinases [54, 55]. Finally, circulating inflammations markers such as cytokines, prostaglandins, and cyclo-oxygenases are also believed to directly promote cancer progression by increasing resistance to apoptosis and enhancement of neo-angiogenesis [56].

Coagulation disorders. The postoperative period is associated with a hypercoagulability state, which can be responsible for thromboembolic events. Although the underlying mechanism is still a matter of investigation, hypercoagulability is thought to be strictly linked to systemic stress response, and it has been related to the extent of surgical trauma [57]. Postoperative changes involve virtually all the steps of the coagulation cascade and include an increased production of pro-coagulative factors, a more rapid clearance of coagulation inhibitors, an enhanced platelet reactivity, and an impaired fibrinolysis.

Different studies have focused on the usefulness of locoregional anesthesia protocols in reducing postoperative hypercoagulability. For example, Bredbacka and coworkers [58] reported a lesser release of factors-VIII and von Willebrand in patients undergoing hysterectomy under epidural anesthesia. Other authors found that epidural anesthesia stimulates fibrinolysis by reducing the postoperative production of plasminogen-activator inhibitor-1 and by increasing the endothelial release of plasminogen activators. In addition, antithrombin-III, the principal inhibitor of thrombin, returns to baseline concentration more promptly in surgical patients receiving just local anesthesia. Although most of these effects can be explained by the attenuation of host response due to blockade of neural signaling, a systemic action of anesthetic drugs can also be ruled in. For example, the inhibition of platelet activity is probably related to the block of Ca^{++} channels by local anesthetic. All these features suggest a protective role of local anesthesia against perioperative thromboembolic accident while so far there is no evidence indicating an increased risk of operative bleeding.

Systemic Inflammation Response Syndrome (SIRS). SIRS was proposed in 1992 by the American College of Chest Physicians-Society of the Critical Care Medicine Consensus Conference Committee as a clinical entity that encompasses the physiological response against stress [5, 6].

It is defined by the presence of abnormal changes in more than 2 out of 4 criteria including body temperature, heart rate, respiratory rate and white blood cell count. It has been suggested that SIRS represents an initiatory step towards the development of more critical pathological stages such as sepsis, multiple organ dysfunction syndrome, and true MOF [59-61]. These conditions seem strictly related to hypercytokinemia in response to surgical stress and are particularly frequent after cardiac surgery under extracorporeal circulation. Some authors [61, 62] have suggested a simple scoring system of SIRS events, which proved a reliable predictor of outcomes in major surgery and ICU settings. In thoracic surgery, the SIRS score has been related to the postoperative increase in IL-6 and has been indicated as a predictive factor for longer hospitalization [6].

SYSTEMIC RESPONSE AFTER AWAKE VATS

The adverse effects of One-Lung Ventilation (OLV) in thoracic surgery have been widely investigated. In particular, there is increasing evidence that OLV may induce a series of anatomic changes in both dependent and non-dependent lungs, which are consistent with a compartmental inflammatory injury [63]. Yin and coworkers [64] showed that vascular congestion and thickening of the alveolar wall occur after 60 minutes of OLV in piglets. Similar observations come from Funakoshi [65] and Kozian [66], who also showed OLV-induced alveolar infiltrates leading to clinically relevant ventilation-to-perfusion mismatch. Most of these changes have been theoretically related to oxidative stress induced by atelectasis and subsequent reoxygenation, which are peculiar features of OLV and may produce adjunctive cellular damage other than traumatism induced by mechanical ventilation itself [66-68]. In addition, recent investigations [69, 70] have highlighted that inflammatory changes can be partly attenuated by the so-called *lung-protective* ventilation strategies, which entails a low tidal volume and preservation of airway patency through the application of a positive end-expiratory pressure. This finding indicates the overstretching, alongside cyclic closure and reopening of the distal airways, as the main factors involved in compartmental lung trauma subsequent to mechanical ventilation and OLV.

We reasoned that OLV-related inflammation could contribute to a variable extent to the overall systemic host response after thoracic surgery, with mechanisms similar to those acting after surgical trauma. We also hypothesized that avoidance of general anesthesia and OLV-related injury together with use of VATS might approximate the ideal goal of *stress-free* thoracic surgery [71-76].

Changes in cytokine release after awake VATS. We analyzed cytokine changes in a series of 24 patients undergoing awake VATS wedge resections under sole thoracic epidural anesthesia (unpublished data). Perioperative changes in IL-6 peaked 3 hours after skin incision with a median increase of 30 pg/dL, while returning toward preoperative levels on postoperative morning 1. This figure differs from what is usually seen in patients undergoing equivalent procedures under general anesthesia in whom the net increase in IL-6 is significantly higher (Fig. **2**) and remains elevated until postoperative day 3. When analyzing the consecutive series of patients undergoing VATS resection regardless of the type of anesthesia received, we found that anesthetic regimen and a diffusion-capacity for carbon monoxide <65% but not age, malignancy, operative time, and use of epidural ropivacaine were related to an absolute increase of IL-6 from baseline over the 75th percentile (>71 pg/dl). This finding is in agreement with the so-called *two-hits* paradigm of the compartmental lung damage. Accordingly, it is reasonable that, in a lung tissue already primed by pre-existing inflammatory changes, any additional injury may trigger an uncontrolled activation of proinflammatory cytokines, ultimately leading to loss of compartmentalization and systemic involvement. However, spillover of proinflammatory factors to systemic circulation could be facilitated in patients with underlying lung disease, due to the increased vascular permeability. Conversely, a remarkable systemic release of cytokines related to mechanical ventilation in patients with normal lungs is less likely to occur [77]. On postoperative day 1, C-reactive protein levels increased less in patients receiving awake analgesia (Fig. **3**), probably reflecting the global attenuation of IL-6 response. On the other hand, no significant changes in TNF-α and other aspecific acute response factor such as white-blood cell count and fibrinogen level occurred at any time point.

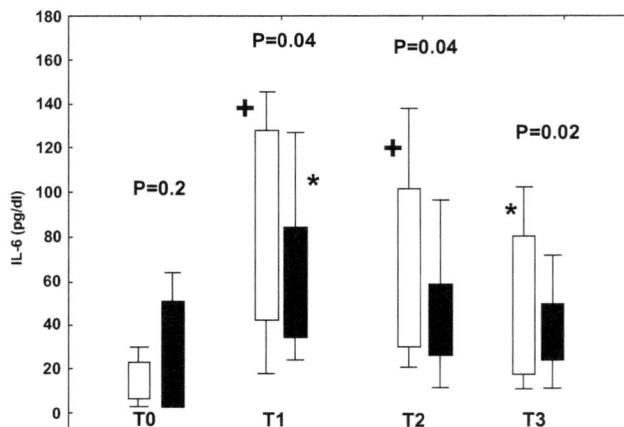

Fig. 2. Postoperative changes in IL-6 after VATS performed under general anesthesia (white) or epidural anesthesia in awake patients (black). +: $p<0.01$ versus preoperative value. *: $p<0.05$ versus preoperative value. T0:preoperative; T1:3h after surgery; T2:postoperative day 1;T3:postoperative day 3.

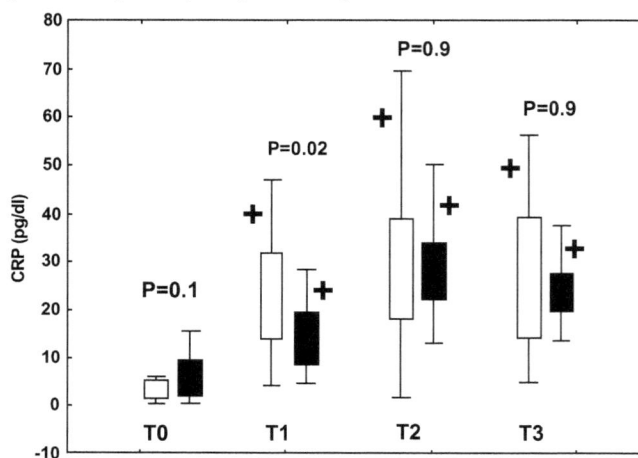

Fig. 3. Postoperative changes in CRP after VATS performed under general anesthesia (white) or epidural anesthesia in awake patients (black). +: $p<0.01$ versus preoperative value. (Time points as in Fig. 2).

SIRS score. We found a different distribution of SIRS scores between patients receiving awake VATS and patients receiving OLV. In particular, awake VATS resulted in a significantly higher number of patients with no SIRS events (Fig. **4**). In addition, although the proportion of patients with a SIRS score ≥ 2 were not affected by the anesthesia type, median SIRS scores on postoperative days 1 and 3 were significantly lower after awake VATS.

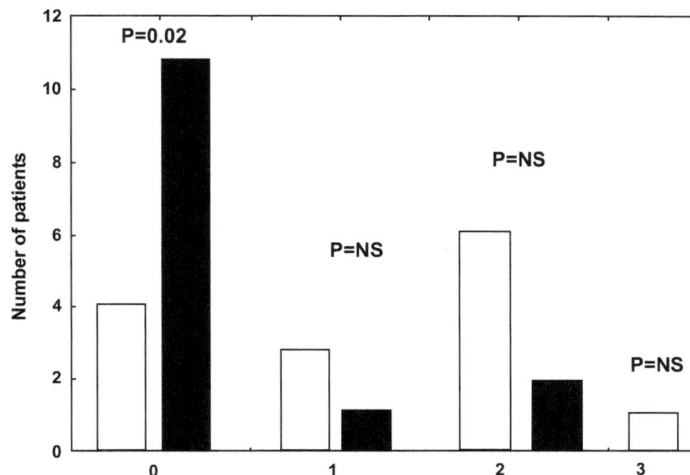

Fig. 4. Number of patients with SIRS-related events (score at x-axis) after VATS performed under general anesthesia (white) or epidural anesthesia in awake patients (black). (Time points as in Fig. **2**).

Changes in hormonal release. Postoperative changes in hormonal release were evaluated in a pilot series of 11 patients undergoing awake VATS for non-malignant disease and were compared with those of a general-anesthesia-group [78]. In patients undergoing awake VATS we failed to observe any significant increase in cortisol, three-hours postoperatively (Fig. **5**) or on postoperative mornings 1 and 3. In addition, perioperative changes in ACTH level were not affected by surgery and its concentrations remained physiologically correlated with cortisol levels, a finding that is not commonly observed after general anesthesia. Changes of catecholamines showed a figure similar to that of cortisol, and appeared clinically negligible.

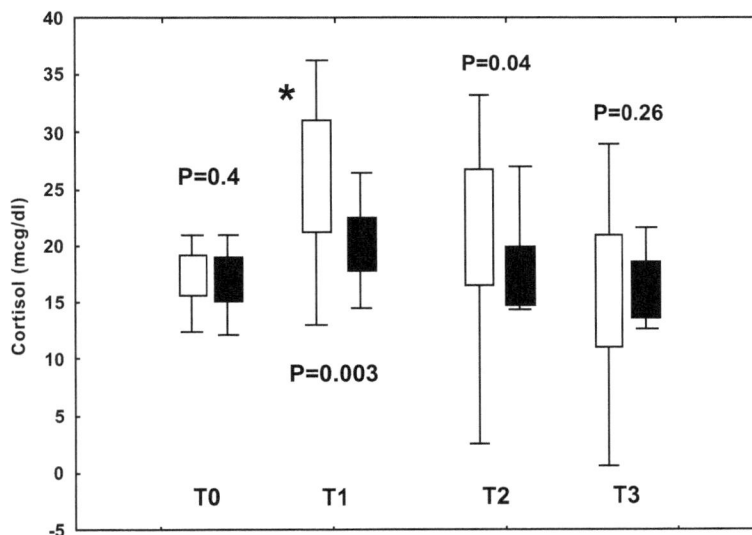

Fig. 5. Postoperative changes in serum cortisol concentration after VATS performed under general anesthesia (white) or epidural anesthesia in awake patients (black). *: p<0.05 versus preoperative value. (Time points as in Fig. **2**).

The type of endocrine response observed in patients undergoing awake VATS might be explained by the avoidance of OLV. Indeed, Tonnesen and coworkers [79] showed that OLV elicits an early increase in epinephrine and cortisol levels, along with a concomitant reduction of natural killer activity.

Since cortisol release is enhanced by pro-inflammatory cytokines including IL-6 and TNF-α, it is conceivable that after awake VATS procedures, reduced cortisol increase may reflect an attenuated inflammatory response. Furthermore, avoidance of OLV could preserve against catecholamine increase by maintaining the endocrine properties of the lung unaltered, which include a reuptake of circulation regulators including endothelin-1, atrial natriuretic peptide, angiotensin II other than catecholamines themselves [80]. To this regard, it was also previously shown that norepinephrine levels remain higher than basal levels until 72 hours postoperatively following general anesthesia and OLV [79], a finding that may indicate a long-lasting detrimental effect of OLV on lung endocrine function.

Inhibition of catecholamine release after awake VATS can be explained by the use of TEA itself, which can inhibit the sympathetic system *via* the blockade of both the afferent and efferent neural pathways [1]. Nonetheless, it has to be reminded that neural signaling blockade with TEA is not complete, since noxious stimuli can be conveyed *via* the phrenic nerves [45]. Another intriguing question is whether stress response could be somewhat increased in awake patients due to psycho-emotive factors since an increased hormone response has been reported using just local anesthesia in other surgical fields [81]. Our findings seem to contradict this hypothesis suggesting that, provided careful patient selection is performed, the psycho-emotional impact of awake VATS is limited, as indirectly shown by the unremarkable intraoperative changes in heart-rate and mean arterial pressure which have been constantly reported in our experience [72-77].

Changes in lymphocyte pattern. The postoperative behavior of lymphocytes distribution was studied prospectively in 59 patients who were randomized to undergo VATS procedures for non-malignant tumors by either awake anesthesia or general anesthesia and OLV [82]. Median operative time was similar in both groups and neither intraoperative complications nor technical difficulties occurred in any patient. Awake surgery resulted in a preservation of the natural-killer cell proportion in the perioperative period (Fig. **6**), while a significant decline was found in patients receiving general anesthesia with the nadir occurring on postoperative day 1. A trend to higher CD4+/CD8+ ratio was also found (Fig. **7**). However, there was a trend to higher total lymphocyte count on postoperative day 3. Conversely, no significant difference was observed between study groups in total lymphocyte count on day 1 and 2, or in the remaining lymphocyte subsets.

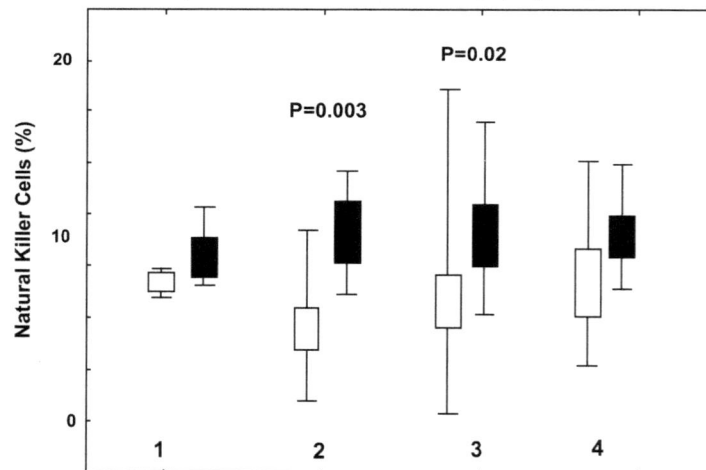

Fig. 6. Postoperative changes in NK count after VATS performed under general anesthesia (white) or epidural anesthesia in awake patients (black). Time points indicate preoperative value (1) and postoperative day 1 (2), 2 (3) and 3 (4).

As previously mentioned, natural-killer cells represent a possible first line of defense against intravascular tumor spread since in the absence of major-histocompatibility-complex restriction, different types of malignant cells can be killed by these cells in a nonspecific way [83-87]. Furthermore, an impairment in immune function and lymphocyte activity has been shown to be associated with several adverse effects including an increased incidence of postoperative infections.

Indeed, data regarding the effect of epidural anesthesia on the lymphocyte activity and immune function remain rather controversial. Papadima and coworkers [88] found that epidural anesthesia did not suppress postoperative lymphocyte apoptosis in patients receiving major abdominal surgery. Beilin *et al.* [89] showed that epidural analgesia may protect against late postoperative lymphocyte suppression but this effect was not found when restricting the analysis to the early postoperative period. Furthermore, Yokoyama *et al.* [90] found that epidural anesthesia is associated with a transient reduction in natural-killer cell activity, a finding that has been found with oral administration of β-adrenoceptor antagonists [91]. These results might be explained by the presence of adrenergic-specific receptors expressed by lymphocytes [92, 93]. Thus, avoidance of general anesthesia and OLV could have been the key factor determining the more physiological lymphocyte response observed in awake patients. In accordance with this hypothesis, Koltun and coworkers [83] found a reduced stress response and an increased natural-killer activity in patients receiving open colectomy under spontaneous ventilation and epidural analgesia.

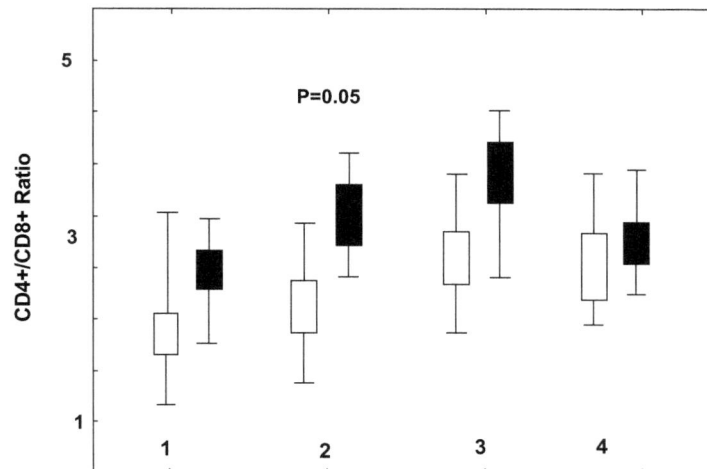

Fig. 7. Postoperative changes in CD4+/CD8+ ratio within days (x-axis) after VATS performed under general anesthesia (white) or epidural anesthesia in awake patients (black). (Time points as in Fig. **6**).

CONCLUSION

Since its introduction, (OLV) has established as gold standard in anesthetic management of thoracic surgery, due to the possibility of operating on an immobile and collapsed lung. Nonetheless, the development of more physiological and less traumatizing surgical and anesthesiology methods is welcome, with the aim to reduce at most the invasiveness of the current procedures. In our recent experience, we have shown that the use of just neuraxial analgesia to perform simple VATS procedures in spontaneously ventilating patients can result into a remarkable reduction of perioperative stress response, as suggested by a lesser increase in several biomarkers of surgical stress including cortisol, IL-6 and CRP. Also, maintainance of perioperative lymphocytes pool has been shown, thus suggesting a potential role for regional anesthesia protocol in preventing from perioperative immunodepression.

On the basis of these observations, we believe that advances in the setting of loco-regional analgesia techniques could represent the first step to approximate, in the future, the ideal goal of a virtually *stress-free* surgery. Future studies aimed to assess the extent of systemic response in large-setting trials are warranted to draw definitive conclusions on this topic.

REFERENCES

[1]   Desborough JP. The stress response to trauma and surgery. Br J Anaesth 2000;85:109-17.

[2]   Baigrie RJ, Lamont PM, Kwiatkowski D, Dallman MJ, Morris PJ. Systemic cytokine response after major surgery. Br J Surg 1992;79:757-60.

[3]   Kashiwabara M, Miyashita M, Nomura T, *et al.* Surgical trauma-induced adrenal insufficiency is associated with postoperative inflammatory responses. J Nippon Med Sch 2007;74:274-83.

[4]   Lin E, Calvano SE, Lowry SF. Inflammatory cytokines and cell response in surgery. Surgery 2000;127:117-26.

[5]   Weigand MA, Horner C, Bardenheuer HJ, Bouchon A. The systemic inflammatory response syndrome. Best Pract Res Clin Anaesth 2004;18:455-75.

[6]   Takenaka K, Ogawa E, Wada H, Hirata T. Systemic inflammatory response syndrome and surgical stress in thoracic surgery. J Crit Care 2006;21:48-55.

[7]   Von Dossow V, Sander M, MacGill M, Spies C. Perioperative cell-mediated immune response. Fronti Biosci 2008;13:3676-84.

[8]   Gottschalk, Sharma S, Ford J, Durieux ME, Tiourirne M. The role of the perioperative period in recurrence after cancer surgery. Anesth Analg 2010;110:1636-42.

[9]   Whitson BA, D'Cunha J, Andrade RS, *et al.* Thoracoscopic versus thoracotomy approaches to lobectomy: differential impairment of cellular immunity. Ann Thorac Surg 2008;12:1735-44.

[10]   Walker WS, Leaver HA. Immunologic and stress responses following video-asisted thoracic surgery and open pulmonary lobectomy in early stage lung cancer. Thorac Surg Clin 2007;17:241-9.

[11]   Friscia ME, Zhu J, Kolff JW, *et al.* Cytokine response is lower after lung volume reduction through bilateral thoracoscopy versus sternotomy. Ann Thorac Surg 2007;83:252-6.

[12]   Christian LM, Graham JE, Padgett DA, Glaser R, Kiecolt-Glaser JK. Stress and wound healing. Neuroimmunomodulation 2006;13:337-46.

[13]   Kurosawa S, Kato M. Anesthetics, immune cells, and immune responses. J Anesth 2008;22:263-77.

[14]   Van der Poll T, Lowry SF. Tumor necrosis factor in sepsis: mediator of multiple organ failure or essential part of host defense? Shock 1995;3:1-12.

[15]   Abraham E; Regan RF. The effect of hemorrhage and trauma on interleukin-2 production. Arch Surg 1983;120:1341-6.

[16]   Oka M, Hirazawa W, Yamamoto K. Induction of Fas-mediated apoptosis on circulating lymphocytes by surgical stress. Ann Surg 1996;223:434-40.17.

[17]   Keegan AD, Ryan JJ, Paul WE. IL-4 regulates growth and differentiation by distinct mechanisms. The Immunologist 1996;4:194-8.

[18]   Biffl WL, Moore EE, Moore FA. Interleukin-6 delays neutrophil apoptosis. Arch Surg 1996;131:24-30.

[19]   Baigrie RJ, Lamont PM, Dallman M, Morris PJ. The release of interleukin-1 beta (IL-1) precedes that of interleukin 6 (IL-6) in patients undergoing major surgery. Lymphokine Cytokine Res 1991;10:253-6.

[20]   Baker EA, El-Gaddal S, Williams L, Leaper DJ. Profiles of inflammatory cytokines following colorectal surgery: relationship with wound healing and outcome. Wound Repair Regen 2006;14:566-72.

[21]   Szczensy TJ, Slotwinski R, Stankiewcz A, *et al.* Interleukin 6 and interleukin 1 receptor antagonist as early markers of complications after lung cancer surgery. Eur J Cardiothorac Surg 2007;31:719-24.

[22]   Sugi K, Kaneda Y, Esato K. Video-assisted thoracoscopic lobectomy reduces cytokine production more than conventional open lobectomy. Jpn J Thorac Cardiovasc Surg 2000;48:161-5.

[23]   Brivio F, Lissoni P, Perego MS, Lissoni A, Fumagalli L. Abrogation of surgery-induced IL-6 hypersecretion by presurgical immunotherapy with IL-2 and its importance in the prevention of postoperative complications. J Biol Regul Homeost Agents 2001;15:370-4.

[24]   Patrick DA, Moore EE, Moore FA, *et al.* The inflammatory profile of interleukin-6, interleukin-8, and soluble intercellular adhesions molecule-1 in postinjury multiple organ failure. Am J Surg 1996;172:425-31.

[25]   Gerard C, Bruyns C, Marchant A, *et al.* Interleukin 10 reduces the release of tumor necrosis factor and prevents lethality in experimental endotoxemia. J Exp Med 1993;177:547-50.

[26]   Dimopoulou I, Armaganidis A, Douka E, *et al.* Tumor necrosis factor –alpha (TNFalpha) and interleukin-10 are crucial mediators in postoperative systemic inflammatory response and determine the occurrence of complications after major abdominal surgery. Cytokine 2007;37:55-61.

[27]   Liu YI, Liao SK, Huang CC, *et al.* Role of nuclear factor-kappa B in augmented lung injury because of interaction between hyperoxia and high stretch ventilation. Transl Res 2009;154:228-40.

[28]   Zedler S, Bone RC, Baue AE, Donnersmarck GH, Faist E. T-cell reactivity and its predictive role in immunosuppression after burns. Crit Care Med 1999;27:66-72.

[29]   Matsuda A, Furukawa K, Suzuki H, *et al.* Does impaired Th1/Th2 balance cause postoperative infectious complications in colorectal cancer surgery? J Surg Res 2007;139:15-21.

[30]   Matsuda A, Furukawa K, Takasaki H, *et al.* Preoperative oral immune-enhancing nutritional supplementation corrects TH1/TH2 imbalance in patients undergoing elective surgery for colorectal cancer. Dis Colon Rectum 2006;49:507-16.

[31]   Wada H, Seki S, Takahashi T, *et al.* Combined spinal and general anesthesia attenuates liver metastasis by preserving TH1/TH2 cytokine balance. Anesthesiology 2007;106:499-506.

[32]　Barber EA, Coyle SM, Marano MA, *et al.* Glucocorticoid therapy alters hormonal and cytokine response to endotoxin in man. J Immunol 1993;150:1999-2006.

[33]　Van der Poll T, Barber EA, Coyle SM, Lowry SF. Hypercortisolemia increases plasma Inteleukin-10 concentration during human endotoxemia-a clinical research center study. J Clin Endocrinol Metab 1996;3604-6.

[34]　Khan MM, Sansoni P, Silverman ED, Engleman EG, Melmon KL. B-adrenergic receptors on human suppressor, helper and cytolytic lymphocytes. Biochem Pharmacol 1986;35:1137-42.

[35]　Swanson MA, Lee WT, Sanders VM. IFN-gamma production by Th1 cells generated from naïve CD4 (+) T cells exposed to norepinehrine. J Immunol 2001;166:232-40.

[36]　Gage JR, Fonarow G, Hamilton M, *et al.* Beta blocker and angiotensin-converting enzyme inhibitor therapy is associated with decreased Th1/Th2 ratios and inflammatory production in patients with chronic heart failure. Neuroimmunomodulation 2004;11:173-80.

[37]　Schneemilch CE, Schilling T, Bank U. Effects of general anaesthesia on inflammation. Best Pract Res Clin Anaesth 2004;18:493-507.

[38]　Kurosawa S, Kato M. Anesthetic immune cells, and immune responses. J Anesth 2008;22:263-77.

[39]　Flores LR, Dretchen KL, Bayer BM. Potential role of the autonomic nervous system in the immunosuppressive effects of the acute morphine administration. Eur J Pharmacol 1996;318:437-46.

[40]　Freier DO, Fucks BA. A mechanism of action for morphine induced immunosuppression: corticosterone mediates morphine induced suppression of NK cell activity. J Pharmacol Exp Ther 1993;270:1127:33.

[41]　Mellon RD, Bayer BM. Evidence for central opioid receptors in the immunomodulatory effects of morphine: review of potential mechanisms of action. J Neuroimmunol 1998;83:19-28.

[42]　Jaeger K, Scheinichen D, Heine J, *et al.* Remifentanil, fentanyl, and alfentanil have no effect on the respiratory burst of neutrophils *in vitro*. Acta Anaesthesiol Scand 1998;42:1110-3.

[43]　Krumholz W, Endrass J, Hempelmann G. Inhibition of phagocytosis and killing of bacteria by anaesthetic agents *in vitro*. Br J Anaesth 1995;75:66-70.

[44]　Shavit Y, Ben-Eliyahu S, Zeidel A, Beilin B. Effects of fentanyl on natural killer cell activity and on resistance to tumor metastasis in rats. Dose and timing study. Neuroimmunomodulation 2004;11:255-60.

[45]　Ihn CH, Joo JD, Choi JW, *et al.* Comparison of stress hormone response, interleukin-6, and anaesthetic characteristics of two anesthetic techniques: volatile induction and maintenance of anaesthesia using sevoflurane versus total intravenous anaesthesia using propofol and remifentanil. J Int Med Res 2009;37:1760-71.

[46]　Kawemura T, Kadosaki M, Nara N, *et al.* Effects of sevoflurane on cytokine balnce in patients undergoing coronary artery bypass graft surgery. J Cardiothorac Vasc Anesth 2009;20:503-8.

[47]　De Conno E, Steurer MP, Wittlinger M, *et al.* Anesthetic-induced improvement of the inflammatory response to one-lung ventilation. Anesthesiology 2009;110:1316-26.

[48]　Hahnekamp K, Herroeder S, Holmann MW. Regional anaesthesia, local anaesthetics and the surgical stress response. Best Pract Res Clin Anaesth 2004;18:509-27.

[49]　Mineo TC. Epidural anesthesia in awake thoracic surgery. Eur J Cardiothorac Surg 2007;32:13-9.

[50]　Ito Y, Oda M, Tsunezuka Y, *et al.* Reduced perioperative immune response in video-assisted versus open surgery in a rat model. Surg Today 2009;39:682-8.

[51]　Page GG. Surgery-induced immunosuppression and postoperative pain management. AACN Clin Issues 2005;16:302-9.

[52]　Goldfarb Y, Ben-Eliyahu S. Surgery as a risk factor for breast cancer recurrence and metastasis: mediating mechanisms and clinical prophylactic approaches. Breast Dis 2006;26:99-114.

[53]　Thaker PH, Sood AK. Neuroendocrine influences on cancer biology. Semin Cancer Biol 2008;18:164-70.

[54]　Masur K, Niggemann B, Zanker KS, Entschladen F. Norepinephrine-induced migration of SW 480 colon carcinoma cells is inhibited by beta-blockers. Cancer Res 2001;61:2866-9.

[55]　Yang EV, Sood AK, Chen M, *et al.* Norepinephrine up-regulates the expression of vascular endothelial growth factor, matrix metalloproteinases (MMP)-2, and MMP-9 in nasopharyngeal carcinoma tumor cells. Cancer Res 2006;66:10357-64.

[56]　Kundu JK, Surh YJ. Inflammation: gearing the journey to cancer. Mutat Res 2008;659:15-30.

[57]　Nguyen NY, Luketich JD, Shurin MR, *et al.* Coagulation modifications after laparoscopic and open cholecystectomy in a swine model. Surg Endosc 1998;12:973-8.

[58]　Bredbacka S, Blomback M, Hagnevik K, Irestedt L, Raabe N. Pre- and postoperative changes in coagulation and fibrinolytic variables during abdominal hysterectomy under epidural or general anaesthesia. Acta Anaesthesiol Scand 1986;30:204-10.

[59]   Pittet D, Rangel-Frausto S, Li N, *et al.* Systemic inflammatory response syndrome, sepsis, severe sepsis and ouctcomes in surgical ICU patients. Intensive Care Med 1995;21:302-9.

[60]   Smail N, Messiah N, Edouard A, *et al.* Role of systemic inflammatory response syndrome and infection in the occurrence of early multiple organ dysfunction syndrome following severe trauma. Intensive Care Med 1995;21:813-6.

[61]   Haga Y, Beppu T, Doi K, *et al.* Systemic inflammatory response syndrome and organ dysfunction following gastrointestinal surgery. Crit Care Med 1997;25:1994-2000.

[62]   Malone D, Kuhls D, Napolitano LM, McCarter R, Scalea T. Back to basic: validation of the admission systemic inflammatory response syndrome score in predicting outcome in trauma. J Trauma 2001;51:458-63.

[63]   Gothart J. Lung injury after thoracic surgery and one-lung ventilation. Curr Opin Anaesthesiol 2006;19:5-10.

[64]   Yin K, Gribbin E, Emanuel S, *et al.* Histochemical alterations in one lung ventilation. J Surg Res 2007;137:16-20.

[65]   Funakoshi T, Ishibe Y, Okazaki N, *et al.* Effect of re-expansion after short-period lung collapse on pulmonary capillary permeability and pro-inflammatory cytokines gene expression in isolated rabbit lung. Br J Anaesth 2004;92:558-63.

[66]   Kozian A, Schilling T, Fredén F, *et al.* One-lung ventilation induces hyperperfusion and alveolar damage in the ventilated lung: an experimental study. Br J Anaesth 2008;100:549-59.

[67]   Misthos P, Katsaragakis S, Theodoru D, Milingos N, Skottis I. The degree of oxidative stress is associated with major adverse effects after lung resection: a prospective study. Eur J Cardiothorac Surg 2006;29:591-5.

[68]   Schilling T, Kozian A, Huth C, *et al.* The pulmonary immune effects of mechanical ventilation in patients undergoing thoracic surgery. Anesth Analg 2005;101:957-65.

[69]   Theroux MC, Fisher AO, Horner LM, *et al.* Protective ventilation to reduce inflammatory injury from one lung ventilation in a piglet model. Paediatr Anaesth 2010;20:356-64.

[70]   Lin WQ, Lu XY, Wen LL, Bai XH, Zhong ZJ. Effects of the lung protective ventilatory strategy on proinflammatory cytokine release during one-lung ventilation. Ai Zheng 2008;27:870-3.

[71]   Pompeo E, Mineo TC. Awake operative videothoracoscopic pulmonary resections. Thorac Surg Clin 2008;18:311-20.

[72]   Mineo TC, Pompeo E, Mineo D, *et al.* Awake nonresectional lung volume reduction surgery. Ann Surg 2006;243:131-6.

[73]   Pompeo E, Tacconi F, Mineo D, Mineo TC. The role of awake video-assisted thoracoscopic surgery in spontaneous pneumothorax. J Thorac Cardiovasc Surg 2007;133:786-90.

[74]   Pompeo E, Tacconi F, Mineo TC. Awake video-assisted thoracoscopic biopsy in complex anterior mediastinal masses. Thorac Surg Clin 2010;20:225-33.

[75]   Tacconi F, Pompeo E, Fabbi E, Mineo TC. Awake videoassisted pleural decortication for empyema thoracis. Eur J Cardiothorac Surg 2010;37:594-601.

[76]   Pompeo E, Mineo TC. Awake pulmonary metastasectomy. J Thorac Cardiovasc Surg 2007;133:960-6.

[77]   Wrigge H, Zinserling J, Stuber F, *et al.* Effects of mechanical ventilation on release of cytokines into systemic circulation in patients with normal pulmonary function. Anesthesiology 2000;93:1413-7.

[78]   Tacconi F, Pompeo E, Sellitri F, Mineo TC. Surgical stress hormones response is reduced after awake videothoracoscopy. Interact Cardiovasc Thorac Surg 2010;10:666-71.

[79]   Tonnesen E, Hohndorf K, Lerbjerg G, *et al.* Immunological and hormonal response to lung surgery during one-lung ventilation. Eur J Anaesth 1993;10:189-95.

[80]   Boldt J, Paspdorf M, Uphus D, Muller M, Hempelmann G. Changes in regulators of the circulation in patients undergoing lung surgery. Br J Anaesth 1997;79:733-9.

[81]   Bachmann MB, Adams HA, Biscoping J, Sokolovski A, Hempelmann G. The sympatho-adrenergic stress reaction in ear surgery using various anesthesia technics. Laryngorhinootologie 1989;68:493.

[82]   Vanni G, Tacconi F, Sellitri F, *et al.* Impact of awake videothoracoscopic surgery on postoperative lymphocyte response. Ann Thorac Surg 2010;90:973-8.

[83]   Koltun WA, Bloomer MM, Tilberg AF, *et al.* Awake epidural anesthesia is associated with improved natural killer cell cytotoxicity and a reduced stress response. Am J Surg 1996;171:68-72.

[84]   Talmadge JE, Meyers KM, Prieur DJ, Starkey JR. Role of NK cells in tumour growth and metastasis in beige mice. Nature 1980;284:622-5.

[85]   Imai K, Matsuyama S, Miyake S, Suga K, Nakachi K. Natural cytotoxic activity of peripheral-blood lymphocytes and cancer incidence: an 11-year follow-up study of a general population. Lancet 2000;356:1795-9.

[86]   Colacchio TA, Yeager MP, Hildebrandt LW. Perioperative immunomodulation in cancer surgery. Am J Surg 1994;167:174-9.

[87]   Trinchieri G, Perussia B. Human natural killer cells: biologic and pathologic aspects. Lab Invest 1984;50:489-513.

[88]   Papadima A, Boutsikou M, Lagoudianakis EE, *et al.* Lymphocyte apoptosis after major abdominal surgery is not influenced by anesthetic technique: a comparative study of general anesthesia versus combined general and epidural analgesia. J Clin Anesth 2009;21:414-21.

[89]   Beilin B, Shavit Y, Trabekin E, *et al.* The effects of postoperative pain management on immune response to surgery. Anesth Analg 2003;97:822-7.

[90]   Yokoyama M, Itano Y, Katayama H, *et al.* The effects of continuous epidural anesthesia and analgesia on stress response and immune function in patients undergoing radical esophagectomy. Anesth Analg 2005;101:1521-7.

[91]   Bachen EA, Manuck SB, Cohen S, *et al.* Adrenergic blockade ameliorates cellular immune responses to mental stress in humans. Psychosom Med 1995;57:266-72.

[92]   Livnat S, Felten SY, Carlson SL, Bellinger DL, Felten DL. Involvement of peripheral and central catecholamine systems in neural-immune interactions. J Neuroimmunol 1985;10:5-30.

[93]   Pirttikangas CO, Perttilä J, Salo M, Vainio O, Liukko-Sipi S. Propofol infusion anaesthesia and immune response in minor surgery. Anaesthesia 1994;49:13-6.

CHAPTER 4

Adverse Effects of General Anesthesia in Thoracic Surgery

Mario Dauri[*], Ludovica Celidonio, Sarit Nahmias, Florencia Della Badia, Filadelfo Coniglione, Eleonora Fabbi

Department of Anesthesiology and Intensive Care, Policlinico Tor Vergata University, Rome, Italy

Abstract: The management of patients for thoracic surgical procedures remains challenging. Not only do patients present with a variety of comorbidites, but they are also subjected to surgical trauma with the requirement for one-lung ventilation and lateral decubitus position, while common intraoperative problems include proper isolation of the lungs utilizing a dual lumen endotracheal tube or bronchial blocker, the potential for dynamic pulmonary hyperinflation and hypoxia. The purpose of this review is to describe the main problems reported in the literature on managing general anesthesia in thoracic surgery, with the aim of choosing the best risk/benefit balance technique.

Mechanical ventilation can produce barotrauma, volotrauma, atelectrauma, and release of a variety of proinflammatory mediators (biotrauma), leading to the development of acute lung injury. Moreover, general anesthesia can lead to an increased risk of pneumonia, impaired cardiac performance, and neuromuscular problems in patients with myasthenia gravis.

Awake anesthesia with thoracic epidural technique, avoids endotracheal intubation, complications such as hypoxia due to double lumen endotracheal tube malposition, hyperinflation of the dependent lung, re-expansion pulmonary edema, and unilateral ventilator-induced lung injury.

Keywords: Local anesthesia, thoracic epidural anesthesia, adverse effect, thoracic surgery.

INTRODUCTION

Nowdays thoracic surgeons routinely perform complex operations on even the most complicated patients. However, just 75 years ago the ability to operate within the chest was strictly limited to only the simplest and quickest procedures. Moreover, it is possible to avoid general anesthesia and One-Lung Ventilation (OLV) for a great number of surgical procedures, managing them with thoracic epidural technique (awake anesthesia) [1, 2]. The choice of an anesthetic technique has always to be the result of a careful risk/benefit balance.

The management of patients for thoracic surgical procedures remains challenging. Not only do patients present with a variety of comorbidites, but they are also subjected to surgical insult with the requirement for one-lung ventilation (OLV) [3]. In addition to the physical considerations of the lateral decubitus position, common intraoperative problems include proper isolation of the lungs utilizing a dual lumen endotracheal tube or bronchial blocker, the potential for dynamic pulmonary hyperinflation and hypoxia [3]. in order to prevent and treat these problems, one must be aware of the potential for causing Acute Lung Injury (ALI) through a variety of mechanisms including barotraumas and volutrauma [4]; OLV can also lead to hypoxia [3].

COMPLICATIONS OF MECHANICAL VENTILATION

One-lung ventilation and devices. This kind of ventilation is required for most surgical procedure under general anesthesia and this can be allowed by using devices such as Double-Lumen Tubes (DLTs) or

*****Address correspondence to Mario Dauri:** Departement of Anesthesiology and Intensive Care, Policlinico Tor Vergata University, Rome, Italy; E-mail: mario.dauri@uniroma2.it

Eugenio Pompeo (Ed)

Bronchial Blockers (BBs). Double-lumen endobronchial tubes have small internal diameters, resulting in a high air flow resistance [5]. Application of the full total lung ventilation minute volume to a single lumen of the DLT results in a 55% increase in peak inspiratory pressure and a 42% increase in plateau pressure [6]. In the literature it is reported that peak ventilation pressures above 40 cm H_2O were associated with lung damage. [7]. OLV causes an extreme challenge to ventilation/perfusion (V/Q) matching [3]. Anesthesia causes a decrease in the Functional Residual Capacity (FRC) of the dependent lung and an improvement in nondependent lung FRC, resulting in preferential ventilation of the upper lung (Fig. **1**). Muscle relaxation and institution of positive pressure ventilation cause a further shift toward upper lung predominance in ventilation. Static displacement of the relaxed diaphragm by abdominal contents and the gravity force of the mediastinum restrict the lower lung, resulting in additional decreases in its compliance. Opening of the chest further deteriorates lower lung ventilation, as the loss of negative intrapleural pressure releases the mediastinal weight onto the lower lung. All these changes result in progressive uncoupling of V/Q matching, as perfusion continues to favor the dependent lung (Fig. **2**). at the beginning of OLV, the upper, nondependent lung with its favorable compliance becomes excluded from the ventilatory circuit and converts to true shunt. Ventilation is now restricted to the noncompliant lower lung [8, 9].Once the operative lung is excluded from the ventilatory circuit, residual oxygen will gradually be absorbed from the nonventilated alveoli until complete absorption atelectasis results. At this point, pulmonary blood flow to the operative lung is wasted perfusion. This right-to-left shunt through the nonventilated lung is in addition to the normal 5% of shunt that exists in the contralateral ventilated lung. Both passive and active mechanisms are at play to decrease the blood flow through the operative lung. Surgical manipulation and, in the lateral position, gravity, passively reduce the blood flow to the nonventilated lung. In addition, Hypoxic Pulmonary Vasoconstriction (HPV) actively increases vascular resistance in the nonventilated lung, resulting in a gradual decrease in blood flow and shunt fraction [3]. Atelectasis formation in the nonoperative lung is highly undesirable during OLV, as it worsens the already high shunt fraction, increasing the potential for hypoxemia. Among the risk factors that predispose to lung de-recruitment during OLV are high FiO2, traditional lack of PEEP, and extrinsic compression by abdominal contents, heart, and mediastinum [11]. Caution is required with the implementation of protective lung ventilation, as low tidal volumes and plateau pressures may promote atelectasis formation and increase FiO_2 and PEEP requirements [10].

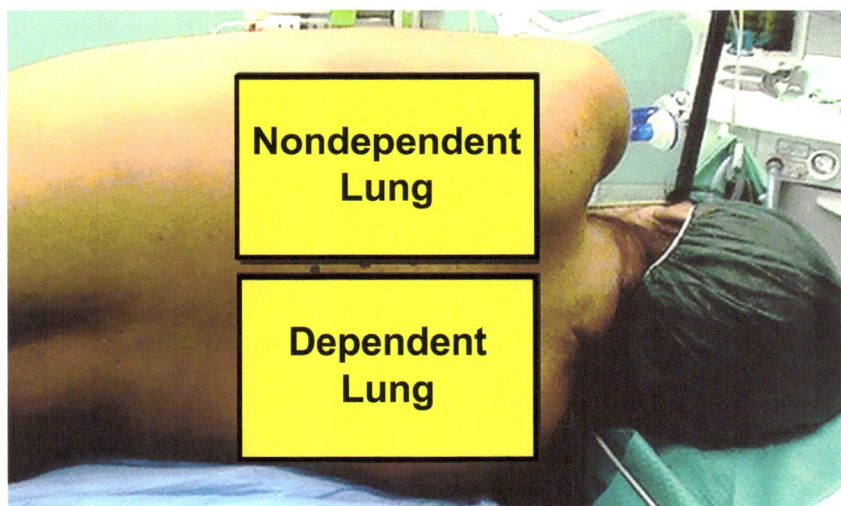

Fig. 1. Dependent and nondependent lung in lateral position.

Anesthetic modifiers of hypoxic pulmonary vasoconstriction (HPV). HPV reduces the shunt flow through the operative lung by roughly 40%, facilitating the safe conduct of OLV. Extremes of HPV may cause harm [12]. The opposite is true in thoracic anesthesia, where inhibition of HPV may result in intraoperative hypoxemia. It must be considered that many agent can modulate the pulmonary vasoconstrictor response to hypoxia such as patient factors, physiologic changes, perioperative interventions, and pharmacologic agents [3].

Inhibition of HPV by inhalational anesthesia is well recognized. Ether, halothane and Nitrous Oxide (NO) clearly inhibit HPV in a dose-dependent fashion [13]. The picture becomes somewhat more confusing, however, when one considers the newer inhalation anesthetics, isoflurane, desflurane, and sevoflurane. For the most part, they appear to be neutral toward HPV or at least do not cause significant depression in clinically relevant doses [14, 15]. Intravenous anesthesia with propofol has been proposed as a means of avoiding HPV modulation [14, 16]. Endogenous Nitric Oxide causes vasodilation and thereby inhibits HPV; however, if given by the inhalational route to the ventilated lung during OLV, NO causes localized vasodilation and thereby decreases shunt fraction [17, 18].

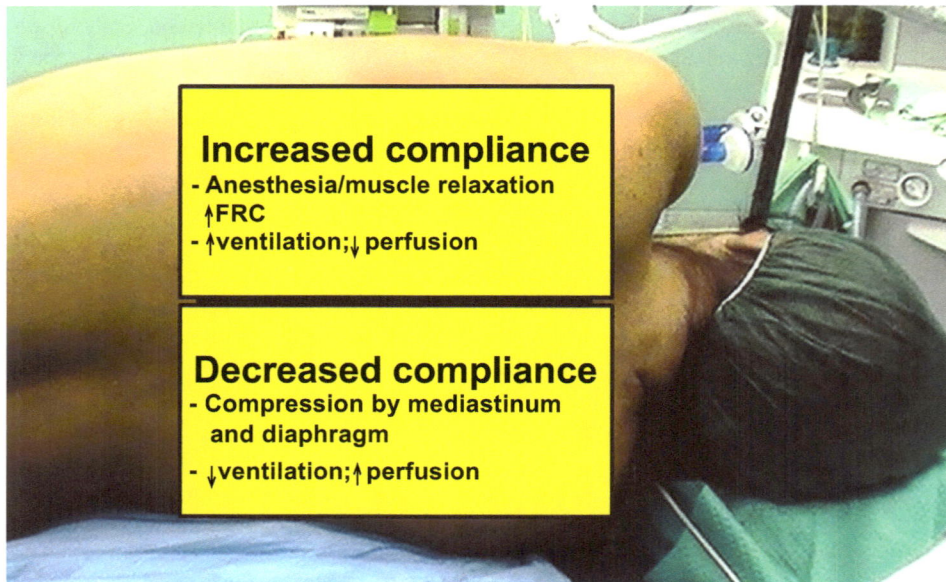

Fig. 2. Dependent and nondependent lung: differences in compliance and V/Q matching.

Oxygen toxicity, hypoxia and PEEP. Oxygen toxicity is a well-recognized complication with prolonged exposure to high FiO_2, characterized by histopathologic changes similar to Acute Lung Injury (ALI). Oxygen toxicity occurs during OLV and involves ischemia–reperfusion injury and oxidative stress [19]. Collapse of the operative lung and surgical manipulation result in relative organ ischemia, which leads to the production of radical oxygen species on re-ventilation-induced reperfusion. Lung re-expansion should likely occur at a lower fraction of inspired oxygen (FiO_2), as hypoxemic reperfusion has been shown to attenuate the reperfusion syndrome [20]. However, there is evidence that the lowest possible FiO_2 should be delivered to the thoracic patient to prevent oxidative damage and postoperative ALI [21].

Hypoxia, however, has become less frequent because of more effective lung isolation, particularly the use of fiberoptic bronchoscopy for confirmation of bronchial blocker or double-lumen tube position, and the use of anesthetic agents with less or no detrimental effects on HPV [3]. Success using PEEP to improve oxygenation during OLV has been documented [22, 23], but excessive total PEEP and dynamic hyperinflation are clearly undesirable, as they may cause cardiovascular depression and may necessitate fluid loading and/or inotropic support [10]. The use of PEEP is thus exceedingly important to treat and prevent hypoxemia, but its use can lead to lung overdistention, variable response depending on the patient and, when used excessively, it may cause or contribute to ALI [3].

Acute lung injury. Acute lung injury (ALI) has replaced hypoxia as the chief concern associated with OLV.

Lung injury after lung resection has long been recognized in the form of Postpneumonectomy Pulmonary Edema (PPPE) [24]. PPPE is part of a spectrum of lung injury, from the milder ALI to the severe Acute Respiratory Distress Syndrome (ARDS).

Diagnosis relies on the oxygenation index of PaO_2/FiO_2 ratio. Critical care consensus definitions specify a PaO_2/FiO_2 ratio of less than 300 for ALI and less than 200 for Acute Respiratory Distress Syndrome ARDS [25].

Causative factors of lung injury after lung resection have remained elusive. Initially, risk factors were felt to be right-sided surgery and large perioperative fluid loads. Over the years, impaired lymphatic drainage, surgical technique, ventilatory trauma, transfusion, aspiration, infection, oxidative stress, and ischemia–reperfusion were added to the list of potential contributors [19]. It has long been recognized that ventilation may have detrimental effects in the critically ill patient in the form of ventilator-induced lung injury (Fig. **3**) [4, 26].

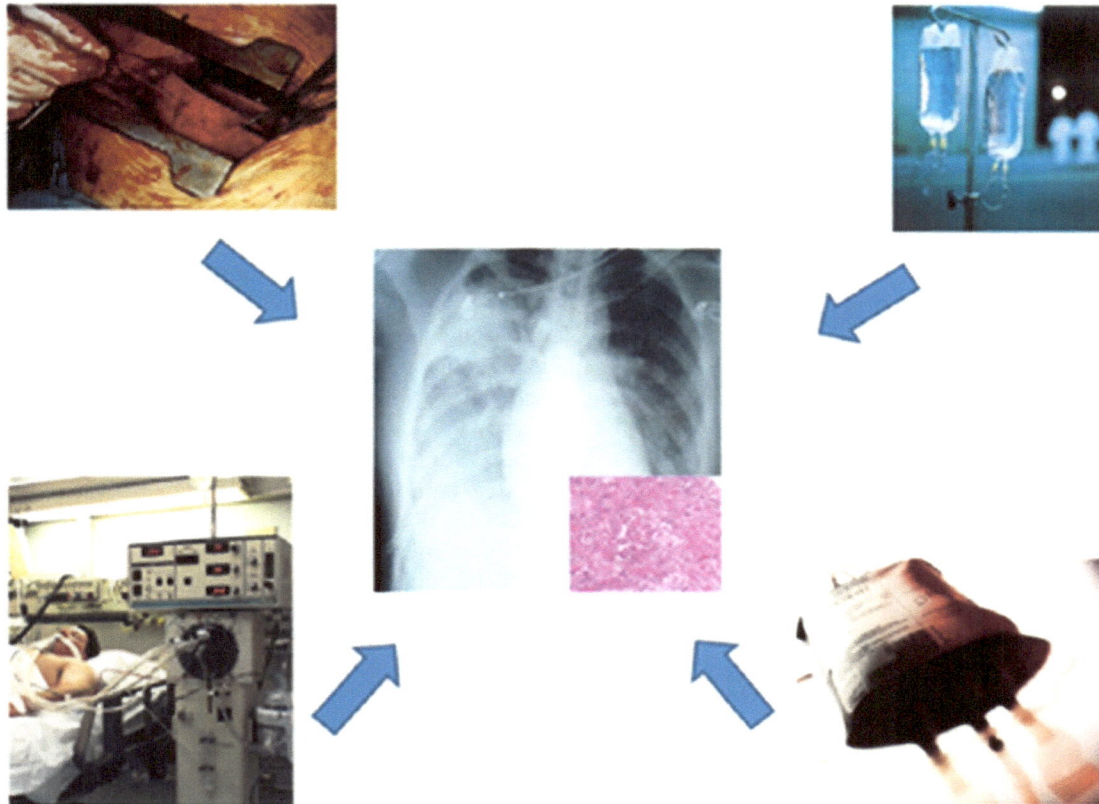

Fig. 3. Some causative factors of lung injury.

Excessive tidal volume or mechanical stress may form the primary hit or create a second hit in a susceptible patient. This leads to the primary recommendations for Protective Lung Ventilation (PLV): tidal volume reduction to a maximum of 6 ml/kg predicted body weight (and ideally less) and limiting the plateau airway pressures to less than $20 cmH_2O$. Further, most PLV protocols also rely on 5-10 cmH_2O PEEP to preserve dependent lung unit aeration, prevent atelectasis and reduce injury from mechanical stress [3]. Many studies provide strong support for the use of a PLV strategy for patients undergoing OLV for thoracic operative procedures and thus at risk for ALI (see chapter "effect of mechanical ventilation") [27-34]. The causal role of OLV in the establishment of lung injury is becoming clearer. Radiologic changes in patients who have ALI after thoracic surgery are worse in the nonoperative, ventilated lung [35]. A retrospective analysis of risk factors for ALI after lung resections showed that an increased duration of OLV in itself is a risk factor for the development of ALI [36, 37].

Lung inflammation and cytokine release. The literature reports that mechanical ventilation (MV) may aggravate pulmonary inflammation, which may be a factor in the additional morbidity/mortality associated with non-protective forms of MV [38, 39]. This so-called "ventilator-associated lung injury" can be characterized by local attraction of inflammatory cells, which produce inflammatory mediators [40].

Even 'physiological' low Tidal Volume VT (4-8 mL/kg) delivered over several hours in healthy lungs may produce subtle lung injuries: neutrophil infiltration, rupture of alveolar–bronchial attachment and chondroitin-sulfate proteoglycan fragmentation in the Endothelial Cell Membrane (ECM) [41]. With larger VT, there is further macromolecular fragmentation, activation of matrix metalloprotease and upregulation of collagen synthesis in the ECM that represent an autoregulatory response to maintain low pulmonary compliance while protecting the ECM against fluid overload [42-44].

For this reason many clinical trial began to compare MV with high tidal volume (10-12 mL/kg) with MV with lower tidal volumes (6-5 mL/kg); the last one has been demonstrated to improve survival of patients with acute lung injury or Acute Respiratory Distress Syndrome (ARDS) [31], to reduce the number of polymorphonuclear cells and proinflammatory mediators in Bronchoalveolar Lavage Fluid (BALF), and to attenuate systemic levels of inflammatory mediators [31, 32], which may be important for clinical outcome: in fact, higher systemic levels of these mediators were associated with higher multiorgan failure scores [33]. It has also been demonstrated that the use of protective ventilation strategies is one of the main reasons for the reduction of mortality from ARDS after pulmunary resection in the last 10 years [34].

The effect of lower tidal volume ventilation and PEEP in patients without preexisting lung injury is controversial; it may in fact limit pulmonary inflammation in mechanically ventilated patients; it attenuated the increase of pulmonary levels of interleukin (IL)-8, myeloperoxidase, and elastase as seen with higher tidal volumes and no PEEP [45]. On the other hand, some authors have demonstrated that when comparing ventilation with high tidal volumes and no PEEP and lower tidal volume and PEEP there are no changes in plasma level of inflammatory mediators in patients without previous lung injury and for surgery lasting from 1 to 3h. Previous lunge damage seems to be mandatory to cause an increase in plasma cytokines after 1 h of high VT mechanical ventilation. [46, 47] Ventilation with large VT is not sufficient per se to induce ALI in healthy lungs, as defense and repair mechanisms (*e.g.* antioxidant, heat-shock protein, p75 receptor for tumor necrosis factor (TNF-α) counteract the initial inflammatory and oxidative responses [48, 49]. The increased permeability of the alveolar–capillary barrier along with a decreased lung compliance initially results from the disruption of intercellular endothelial cell junction, cytoskeleton contraction and alveolar cell death consequent to activation of endothelial/epithelial cell receptors by systemic/alveolar inflammatory mediators (*e.g.* thrombin, Vascular Endothelial Growth Factor [VEGF], transforming growth factor-beta [TGF-β] and thromboxane A2 [TXA2]) [50-52].

During OLV, data from the literature suggest that hyperoxic/mechanical injuries predominate in the nonoperated lung, whereas the operated lung is prone to atelectasis formation due to impaired surfactant and direct surgical manipulation. An imbalance between antioxidants and excess production of RNIs/ROIs has been incriminated in perpetuating the inflammatory process and causing cellular damage by oxidizing nucleic acids, proteins and membrane lipids [53].

Interestingly, a recent prospective, randomized clinical study suggests an immunomodulatory role for the volatile anesthetic sevoflurane in patients undergoing OLV for thoracic surgery with significant reduction of inflammatory mediators (tumor necrosis factor alpha, interleukin 1-beta, interleukin-6, interleukin-8, monocyte chemoattractant protein 1) and a significantly better clinical outcome (defined by postoperative adverse events) during sevoflurane anesthesia [54].

In conclusion, mechanical ventilation can produce injuries, which include airway pressure-induced injury (barotrauma), lung inflation-induced injury (volotrauma), injury due to cyclic opening and closing of small airways/lung units (atelectrauma), and release of a variety of proinflammatory mediators (biotrauma) [4]. In addition, atelectasis in the dependent lung is a frequent finding during one-lung ventilation with muscle paralysis [26], and prolonged collapse of the nondependent lung can delay its complete re-expansion after weaning, leading to the development of further atelectasic areas. Awake anesthesia avoids endotracheal intubation, complications such as hypoxia due to double lumen endotracheal tube malposition, hyperinflation of the dependent lung, re-expansion pulmonary edema, and unilateral ventilator-induced lung injury [55-58].

OTHER COMPLICATIONS OF GENERAL ANESTHESIA

Despite the indisputable and well-known advantages of general anesthesia, this can trigger some adverse effects including an increased risk of pneumonia, impaired cardiac performance, and neuromuscular problems [59-64].

There is enough evidence to show that prolonged mechanical ventilation is a risk factor for pulmonary infections and morbidity [59]. In 1997, the first meta-analysis on pulmonary outcome depending on analgesic regimen showed that an epidural analgesia with local anesthetics reduced pulmonary infections to a third, and overall pulmonary complications to about a half, of the infections and complications under systemic analgesia [65]. In 2000 another meta-analysis confirmed a reduction in postoperative pneumonia of 39% of the rate under epidural anesthesia compared with a systemic analgesic regimen, and a reduction in mortality of about one third [66]. The evidence thus shows that epidural anesthesia reduces the rate of postoperative pulmonary complications [59, 67].

Patients with asthma or chronic Obstructive Pulmonary Disease (COPD) share a high incidence of bronchial hyperreactivity [68, 69]. General anesthesia with tracheal intubation can elicit bronchospasm, which, in some cases, can be life-threatening in these patients [70, 71]. In these patients, TEA, mildly decreasing FEV1 and VC can be used as the primary anesthesia technique for chest wall surgery and is well-tolerated [72].

A hemodynamic compromise related to narcotic medication before intubation can occur, which carries the risk of preoperative myocardial ischemia or infarction in patients with severe coronary artery disease [60-62]. Conversely, cardiovascular effects of epidural anesthesia include decreased determinants of myocardial oxygen demand [73], improved myocardial blood flow [74, 75] and left ventricular function [76], and reduced thrombotic-related complications [77].

Avoiding general anesthesia leads to a reduction of postoperative hospital stay, minimization of intensive care unit admission and cost reduction [1].

Furthermore, the literature reports that general anesthesia in non-malignant surgical procedures leads to an upregulation of the Hypo-Thalamic–Pituitary–Adrenal Axis (HPA) and sympathetic system activity sampling in blood, cortisol, epinephrine, norepinephrine, and glucose, 3 h postoperatively (T1), and on postoperative mornings 2 (T2) and 3 (T3). These preliminary findings thus suggest an attenuated stress response after awake VATS in comparison with an equivalent procedure performed under general anesthesia and one-lung ventilation [78].

Choosing awake anaesthesia makes it possible to avoid the use of muscle relaxants in patients with myasthenia gravis which has an unpredictable response to the action of such drugs [79]. Avoiding muscle relaxants in patients with myasthenia gravis can potentially lower the risk of postoperative muscle weakness and respiratory insufficiency thus leading to faster patient recovery [63, 64, 80, 81].

REFERENCES

[1]   Al-Abdullatief M, Wahood A, Al-Shirawi N, *et al.* Awake anaesthesia for major thoracic surgical procedures: an observational study. Eur J Cardiothorac Surg 2007;32:346-50.

[2]   Mineo TC. Epidural anesthesia in awake thoracic surgery. Eur J Cardiothorac Surg 2007;32:13-9.

[3]   Lohser J. Evidence-based management of one-lung ventilation. Anesthesiology Clin 2008;26:241-72.

[4]   Whitehead T, Slutsky AS. The pulmonary physician in critical care. 7: ventilator induced lung injury. Thorax 2002;57:635-42.

[5]   Slinger PD, Lesiuk L. Flow resistances of disposable double-lumen, single-lumen, and univent tubes. J Cardiothorac Vasc Anesth 1998;12:142-4.

[6]   Szegedi LL, Bardoczky GI, Engelman EE, *et al.* Airway pressure changes during one-lung ventilation. Anesth Analg 1997;84:1034-7.

[7]   Van der Werff YD, Van der Houwen HK, Heijmans PJ, *et al.* Postpneumonectomy pulmonary edema. A retrospective analysis of incidence and possible risk factors. Chest 1997;111:1278-84.

[8]   Grichnik KP, Clark JA. Pathophysiology and management of one-lung ventilation. Thorac Surg Clin 2005;15:85-103.

[9]   Benumof J, Ed. Anesthesia for thoracic surgery. 2nd edition. Philadelphia: Elsevier Health Sciences 1987; pp. 406-31.

[10]   Putensen C, Wrigge H. Tidal volumes in patients with normal lungs: one for all or the less, the better? Anesthesiology 2007;106:1085-7.

[11]   Tusman G, Bohm SH, Sipmann FS, *et al.* Lung recruitment improves the efficiency of ventilation and gas exchange during one-lung ventilation anesthesia. Anesth Analg 2004;98: 1604-9.

[12]   Nagendran J, Stewart K, Hoskinson M, *et al.* An anesthesiologist's guide to hypoxic pulmonary vasoconstriction: implications for managing single-lung anesthesia and atelectasis. Curr Opin Anaesthesiol 2006;19:34-43.

[13]   Gurney AM, Osipenko ON, MacMillan D, *et al.* Two-pore domain K channel, TASK-1, in pulmonary artery smooth muscle cells. Circ Res 2003;93:957-64.

[14]   Bz Nagendran J, Stewart K, Hoskinson M, *et al.* An anesthesiologist's guide to hypoxic pulmonary vasoconstriction: implications for managing single-lung anesthesia and atelectasis. Curr Opin Anaesthesiol 2006;19:34-43.

[15]   Kerbaul F, Guidon C, Stephanazzi J, *et al.* Sub-MAC concentrations of desflurane do not inhibit hypoxic pulmonary vasoconstriction in anesthetized piglets. Can J Anaesth 2001;48: 760-7.

[16]   Pruszkowski O, Dalibon N, Moutafis M, *et al.* Effects of propofol vs sevoflurane on arterial oxygenation during one-lung ventilation. Br J Anaesth 2007;98:539-44.

[17]   Conacher ID. 2000-time to apply occam's razor to failure of hypoxic pulmonary vasoconstriction during one-lung ventilation. Br J Anaesth 2000;84:434-6.

[18]   Bindslev L, Cannon D, Sykes MK. Effect of lignocaine and nitrous oxide on hypoxic pulmonary vasoconstriction in the dog constant-flow perfused left lower lobe preparation. Br J Anaesth 1986;58:315-20.

[19]   Jordan S, Mitchell JA, Quinlan GJ, *et al.* The pathogenesis of lung injury following pulmonary resection. Eur Respir J 2000;15:790-9.

[20]   Douzinas EE, Kollias S, Tiniakos D, *et al.* Hypoxemic reperfusion after 120 mins of intestinal ischemia attenuates the histopathologic and inflammatory response. Crit Care Med 2004;32:2279-83.

[21]   Williams EA, Quinlan GJ, Goldstraw P, *et al.* Postoperative lung injury and oxidative damage in patients undergoing pulmonary resection. Eur Respir J 1998; 11:1028-34.

[22]   Cinnella G, Grasso S, Natale C, *et al.* Physiological effects of a lung-recruiting strategy applied during one-lung ventilation. Acta Anaesthesiol Scand 2008; 52:766-75.

[23]   Alonso-Iñigo JM, Beltran R, Garcia-Covisa NL, *et al.* Effects of alveolar recruitment strategy in gas exchange during one-lung ventilation. Anesthesiology 2007;107:A1827.

[24]   Zeldin RA, Normandin D, Landtwing D, *et al.* Postpneumonectomy pulmonary edema. J Thorac Cardiovasc Surg 1984;87:359-65.

[25]   Bernard GR, Artigas A, Brigham KL, *et al.* The American-European Consensus Conference on ARDS. Definitions, mechanisms, relevant outcomes, and clinical trial coordination. Am J Respir Crit Care Med 1994,149:818-24.

[26]   Tokics L, Hedenstierna G, Svensson L, *et al.* V/Q distribution and correlation to atelectasis in anesthetize paralyzed humans. J Appl Physiol 1996;81:1822-33.

[27]   Amato MB, Barbas CS, Medeiros DM, *et al.* Effect of a protective ventilation strategy on mortality in the acute respiratory distress syndrome. N Engl J Med 1998;338:347-54.

[28]   Schultz MJ, Haitsma JJ, Slutsky AS, *et al.* What tidal volumes should be used in patients without acute lung injury? Anesthesiology 2007;106:1226-31.

[29]   Putensen C, Wrigge H. Tidal volumes in patients with normal lungs: one for all or the less, the better? Anesthesiology 2007;106:1085-7.

[30]   Tremblay LN, Slutsky AS. Ventilator-induced lung injury: from the bench to the bedside. Intensive Care Med 2006;32:24-33.

[31]   No authors listed. Ventilation with lower tidal volumes as compared with traditional tidal volumes for acute lung injury and the acute respiratory distress syndrome. The Acute Respiratory Distress Syndrome Network. N Engl J Med 2000; 342:1301-8.

[32]   Ranieri VM, Suter PM, Tortorella C, *et al.* Effect of mechanical ventilation on inflammatory mediators in patients with acute respiratory distress syndrome: A randomized controlled trial. JAMA 1999; 282:54-61.

[33]   Ranieri VM, Giunta F, Suter PM, *et al.* Mechanical ventilation as a mediator of multisystem organ failure in acute respiratory distress syndrome. JAMA 2000;284:43-4.

[34]   Tang SK, Redmond K, Griffiths M, *et al.* The mortality from acute respiratory distress syndrome after pulmonary resection is reducing: a 10-year single institutional experience. Europ J Cardio-thorac Surg 2008;34:898-902.

[35]   Padley SP, Jordan SJ, Goldstraw P, *et al.* Asymmetric ARDS following pulmonary resection: CT findings initial observations. Radiology 2002;223:468-73.

[36]   Licker M, De Perrot M, Spiliopoulos A, *et al*. Risk factors for acute lung injury after thoracic surgery for lung cancer. Anesth Analg 2003;97:1558-65.

[37]   Misthos P, Katsaragakis S, Milingos N, *et al*. Postresectional pulmonary oxidative stress in lung cancer patients: the role of one-lung ventilation. Eur J Cardiothorac Surg 2005; 27:379-83.

[38]   Pinhu L, Whitehead T, Evans T, *et al*.Ventilator-associated lung injury. Lancet 2003; 361:332-40.

[39]   Slutsky AS: Lung injury caused by mechanical ventilation. Chest 1999; 116:S9-S15.

[40]   Oeckler RA, Hubmayr RD. Ventilator-associated lung injury: a search for better therapeutic targets. Eur Respir J 2007;30:1216-26.

[41]   D'Angelo E, Koutsoukou A, Della Valle P, *et al*. Cytokine release, small airway injury, and parenchymal damage during mechanical ventilation in normal openchest rats. J Appl Physiol 2008;104:41-9.

[42]   Demoule A, Decailliot F, Jonson B, *et al*. Relationship between pressure volume curve and markers for collagen turn-over in early acute respiratory distress syndrome. Intensive Care Med 2006;32:413-20.

[43]   Pavone LA, Albert S, Carney D, *et al*. Injurious mechanical ventilation in the normal lung causes a progressive pathologic change in dynamic alveolar mechanics. Crit Care 2007; 11:R64.

[44]   Musch G, Venegas JG, Bellani G, *et al*. Regional gas exchange and cellular metabolic activity in ventilator-induced lung injury. Anesthesiology 2007;106:723-35.

[45]   Wolthuis EK, Choi G, Dessinget MC, *et al*. Mechanical ventilation with lower tidal volumes and positive end-expiratory pressure prevents pulmonary inflammation in patients without preexisting lung injury. Anesthesiology 2008;108:46-54.

[46]   Wrigge H, Zinserling J, Stüber F, *et al*. Effects of mechanical ventilation on release of cytokines into systemic circulation in patients with normal pulmonary function. Anesthesiology 2000;93:1413-7.

[47]   Wrigge H, Uhlig U, Zinserling J, *et al*. The effects of different ventilatory settings on pulmonary and systemic inflammatory responses during major surgery. Anesth Analg 2004;98:775-81.

[48]   Wilson MR, Goddard ME, O'Dea KP, *et al*. Differential roles of p55 and p75 tumor necrosis factor receptors on stretch-induced pulmonary edema in mice. Am J Physiol Lung Cell Mol Physiol 2007;293:L60-L68.

[49]   Ogawa EN, Ishizaka A, Tasaka S, *et al*. Contribution of high-mobility group box-1 to the development of ventilator-induced lung injury. Am J Respir Crit Care Med 2006;174:400-7.

[50]   Frank JA, Wray CM, McAuley DF, *et al*. Alveolar macrophages contribute to alveolar barrier dysfunction in ventilator-induced lung injury. Am J Physiol Lung Cell Mol Physiol 2006;291:L1191-8.

[51]   Ware LB, Matthay MA, Parsons PE, *et al*. Pathogenetic and prognostic significance of altered coagulation and fibrinolysis in acute lung injury/acute respiratory distress syndrome. Crit Care Med 2007;35:1821-8.

[52]   Lowe K, Alvarez D, King J, Stevens T. Phenotypic heterogeneity in lung capillary and extra-alveolar endothelial cells. Increased extra-alveolar endothelial permeability is sufficient to decrease compliance. J Surg Res 2007;143:70-7.

[53]   Tasaka S, Amaya F, Hashimoto S, Ishizaka A. Roles of oxidants and redox signaling in the pathogenesis of acute respiratory distress syndrome. Antioxid Redox Signal 2008;10:739-53.

[54]   De Conno E, Steurer MP, Wittlinger M *et al*. Anesthetic-induced improvement of the inflammatory response to one-lung ventilation. Anesthesiology 2009;110:1316-26.

[55]   Inoue S, Nishimine N, Kitaguchi K, *et al*. Double lumen tube location predict tube malposition and hypoxemia during one lung ventilation. Br J Anaesth 2004;92:195-201.

[56]   Yusim Y, Berkenstadt H, Keidan I, *et al*. Malignant hyperinflation of the non-dependent lung during chest surgery. Eur J Anaesthesiol 2001;18:774-7.

[57]   Murat A, Arslan A, Balci AE. Re-expansion pulmonary edema. Acta Rediol 2004;45:431-3.

[58]   Farre R, Granell S, Rotger M, *et al*. Animal model of unilateral ventilator-induced lung injury. Intensive Care Med 2005;31:487-90.

[59]   Groeben H. Epidural anesthesia and pulmonary function. J Anesth 2006;20:290-9.

[60]   Tarhan S, Moffitt EA, Taylor WF, Giuliani ER. Myocardial infarction after general anesthesia. JAMA 1972;220:1451-4.

[61]   Seegobin RD, Goodland FC, Wilmshurst TH, *et al*. Postoperative myocardial damage in patients with coronary artery disease undergoing major noncardiac surgery. Can J Anaesth 1991;38:1005-11.

[62]   Blomberg S, Emanuelsson H, Kvist H, *et al*. Effects of thoracic epidural anesthesia on coronary arteries and arterioles in patients with coronary artery disease. Anesthesiology 1990;73:840-7.

[63]   Kiran U, Choudhury M, Saxena N, Kapoor P. Sevoflurane as a sole anesthetic for thymectomy in myasthenia gravis. Acta Anesthesiol Scand 2000;44:351-3.

[64] Chevalley C, Spiliopoulos A, De Perrot M, *et al.* Perioperative medical management and outcome following thymectomy for myasthenia gravis. Can J Anaesth 2001;48:446-51.

[65] Ballantyne JC, Carr DB, De Ferranti S, Suarez T. The comparative effect of postoperative analgesic therapies on pulmonary outcome: cumulative meta-analyses of randomized, controlled trials. Anesth Analg 1998;86:598-612.

[66] Rodgers A, Walker N, Schug S, *et al.* Reduction of postoperative mortality and morbidity with epidural or spinal anaesthesia: results from overview of randomised trials. Br Med J 2000;321:1-12.

[67] Pöpping DM, Elia N, Marret E, *et al.* Protective Effects of Epidural Analgesia on Pulmonary Complications After Abdominal and Thoracic Surgery. Arch Surg. 2008;143:990-9.

[68] Boushey HA, Holtzman MJ, Sheller JR, Nadel JA. Bronchial hyperreactivity. Am Rev Respir Dis 1980; 121:389-413.

[69] Ramsdell JW, Nachtwey FJ, Moser KM. Bronchial hyperreactivity in chronic obstructive bronchitis. Am Rev Respir Dis 1982;126:829-32.

[70] Caplan RA, Posner KL, Ward RJ, Cheney FW. Adverse respiratory events in anesthesia: A closed claims analysis. Anesthesiology 1990;72:828-33.

[71] Warner DO, Warner MA, Offord KP, *et al.* Airway obstruction and perioperative complications in smokers undergoing abdominal surgery. Anesthesiology 1999;90:372-9.

[72] Groeben H, Schäfer B, Pavlakovic G, *et al.* Lung function under high thoracic segmental epidural anesthesia with ropivacaine or bupivacaine in patients with severe obstructive pulmonary disease undergoing breast surgery. Anesthesiology 2002;96:536-41.

[73] Blomberg S, Emanuelsson H, Ricksten SE. Thoracic epidural anesthesia and central hemodynamics in patients with unstable angina pectoris. Anesth Analg 1989;69:558-62.

[74] Davis RF, DeBoer LWV, Maroko PR. Thoracic epidural anesthesia reduces myocardial infarct size after coronary occlusion in dogs. Anesth Analg 1986;65:711-7.

[75] Klassen GA, Bramwell RS, Bromage PR, Zborowska-Sluis DT. Effect on acute sympathectomy by epidural anesthesia on the canine coronary circulation. Anesthesiology 1980;52:8-15.

[76] Kock M, Blomberg S, Emanuelsson H, *et al.* Thoracic epidural anesthesia improves global and regional left ventricular function during stress-induced myocardial ischemia in patients with coronary artery disease. Anesth Analg 1990;71:625-30.

[77] Williams JP, Sullivan EA, Ramakrishna H. Effects of thoracic epidural anesthesia on the coagulation system. Clin Anesth 1999;13:31-56.

[78] Tacconi F, Pompeo E, Sellitri F, Mineo TC. Surgical stress hormones response is reduced after awake videothoracoscopy. Interact CardioVasc Thorac Surg 2010;10:666-71.

[79] Baraka AS, Taha SK, Kawkabbani NI. Neuromuscular interaction of sevoflurane- cisatracurium in a myasthenic patient. Can J Anaesth 2000;47:562-5.

[80] Della Rocca G, Coccia C, Diana L, *et al.* Propofol or sevoflurane anaesthesia without muscle relaxants allow the early extubation of myasthenic patients. Can J Anaesth 2003;50:547-52.

[81] O'Flaherty D, Pennant JH, Rao K, Giesecke AH. Total intravenous anaesthesia with propofol for transsternal thymectomy in myasthenia gravis. J Clin Anesth 1992;4:241-4.

CHAPTER 5

Anesthesia Techniques in Awake Thoracic Surgery

CHAPTER 5

Anesthesia Techniques in Awake Thoracic Surgery

Mario Dauri[*], Sarit Nahmias, Ludovica Celidonio, Elisabetta Sabato, Maria Beatrice Silvi and Eleonora Fabbi.

Department of Anesthesiology and Intensive Care, Policlinico Tor Vergata University, Rome, Italy

Abstract: In order to avoid the adverse effects of general anesthesia in patients undergoing thoracic surgery procedures and to allow surgical treatment for those patients considered at high-risk for general anesthesia because of their compromised medical conditions, some anesthesiological techniques can be employed to perform awake thoracic surgery.

In this chapter we describe three different anesthesiological techniques which can be performed successfully in this setting.

Our favourite technique is Thoracic Epidural Anesthesia (TEA), which can be chosen for most awake thoracic procedures. This technique offers a sympathetic block that decreases stress response to surgery, positively affecting the cardiovascular system, gastrointestinal function and postoperative pulmonary function. Furthermore, it provides excellent postoperative analgesia.

Thoracic paravertebral block is another technique that can offer effective intraoperative and postoperative management of surgical pain. It has a better side-effects profile and lower complication rate compared with TEA, but so far, it has not often been used as a sole anesthetic method for thoracic surgery.

Local anesthesia as a sole technique can also represent a valid method for minor thoracic surgery procedures.

Keywords: Thoracic epidural anesthesia, local anesthesia, paravertebral anesthesia, thoracic surgery.

THORACIC EPIDURAL ANESTHESIA (TEA)

Epidural anesthesia is a neuraxial block in which local anesthetic drugs are injected into the epidural space surrounding the dural sac. It has been demonstrated that the use of epidural blockade can result in a decrease in mortality, reduction in risk of venous thromboembolism, myocardial infarction, bleeding complications, pneumonia, respiratory depression, and renal failure [1]. In 1921 the Spaniard Fidel Pagés described the injection of anesthetics into the epidural space in the lumbar and thoracic level, and this markedly increased the possibilities of the epidural block. The subsequent improvements in needles, catheters and new drugs, as well as a better understanding of physiology and pharmacology, contributed to the development of the epidural block, which nowadays is an essential technique in anesthesiology [2].Thoracic Epidural Anesthesia (TEA), first described by Crawford *et al.* in 1952 [3], has often been used as an adjunct to general anesthesia [4] to achieve ideal postoperative analgesia [5], and can also be utilized as a sole method to provide anesthesia for some thoracic procedures [6-18]. TEA has been consistently shown to provide excellent pain relief and facilitate early extubation (when associated with general anesthesia), oral intake of food, and gastrointestinal function; other advantages include attenuation of the stress response and improvement of postoperative pulmonary function [19].

ANATOMICAL ASPECTS [20, 21]

Special care has to be taken when approaching the thoracic region to perform TEA due to the particular characteristics of the thoracic column:

---

*Address correspondence to Mario Dauri: Departement of Anesthesiology and Intensive Care, Policlinico Tor Vergata University, Rome, Italy; E-mail: mario.dauri@uniroma2.it

Eugenio Pompeo (Ed)

- Vertebral column - the spinous processes of the vertebrae vary in their angulation in the cervical, thoracic, and lumbar regions. The spinous processes are almost horizontal in the cervical, lower thoracic, and lumbar regions but become significantly more sharply angled in the mid-thoracic region. The greatest degree of angulation is found between the T3 and T7 vertebrae.

- Ligamentous tissues - Ligamentun flavum is thinner in the thoracic spine.

- Nerve roots - the upper thoracic and lower cervical roots are larger in size.

- As the others – the epidural space in the thoracic region is usually smaller.

PHYSIOLOGICAL EFFECTS OF TEA

The primary site of action of local anesthetic solutions injected into the epidural space is the spinal nerve roots. The segmental nerve roots in the thoracic region are mixed nerves, containing somatic sensory, motor, and autonomic nerve fibers. Sensory blockade interrupts the transmission of both somatic and visceral painful stimuli, whereas motor blockade provides muscle relaxation with a varying degree of sympathetic blockade [22].

The physiologic effects of epidural blockade depend on the spinal level and the number of spinal segments blocked. In general, high thoracic epidural blocks and extensive epidural blocks are associated with a deeper sympathetic block, resulting in a greater physiologic effect on the cardiovascular system [22].

Cardiovascular effects. Surgical stress provokes excessive sympathetic activation, causing an increased myocardial oxygen demand while inducing coronary arterial vasoconstriction [23]. Clinical features of myocardial ischemia such as ST segment electrocardiographic changes, angina and dysrhythmias may be seen throughout the perioperative period. Postoperative hypercoagulable state, another component of stress response, can also contribute to cause coronary artery thrombosis [24].

TEA provokes sympathetic blockade, interrupting cardiac afferent and efferent fibers, originating from the first to the fourth thoracic levels.

Cardiovascular effects of epidural anesthesia include decreased determinants of myocardial oxygen demand [25], improved myocardial blood flow [25-27] and left ventricular function [28], and reduced thrombotic-related complications [29, 30]. Furthermore, it has been shown that epidural anesthesia can reduce heart rate and occurrence of arrhythmias during manipulation of the heart [31, 32].

Blomberg *et al.* [25] investigated coronary blood flow after TEA in patients with ischemic heart disease. Endocardial to epicardial blood flow was improved, so that regional distribution of perfusion was optimized. By decreasing heart rate, TEA also decreased myocardial oxygen demand.

The same authors concluded that TEA could effectively treat pain and stabilize patients with unstable angina pectoris refractory to medical treatment and, furthermore, that TEA attenuated stress-induced myocardial ischemia. Olausson *et al.* [33] compared occurrence of ischemic periods measured by Holter electrocardiogram (ECG) in patients undergoing TEA vs standard intravenous anesthesia. They found that in the TEA group ischemic periods were reduced both in number and duration.

Berendes *et al.* [34] reported an improved myocardial structure and left ventricular function with lower troponin T and I levels, in patients undergoing Coronary Bypass Grafting (CABG) through high TEA combined with general anesthesia.

Atrial fibrillation and tachycardia are common after cardiac and thoracic surgery [35, 36]. Since TEA reduces overall sympathetic tone and blocks cardiac accelerator fibers, the risk of dysrhythmia is decreased with general anesthesia-TEA combination [34]. In addition, TEA significantly reduced the incidence of supraventricular tachycardia after both cardiac surgery and pulmonary resection [37, 38].

A common physiological effect of epidural anesthesia is hypotension. This is primarily due to blockade of the sympathetic nervous system causing arterial and venous vasodilation with subsequent functional hypovolemia. The range of depressant effects generated by high epidural blockade can be quite broad depending on the extant of spinal segment deafferentation.

TEA produces functional hypovolemia by inhibiting vasoconstrictor sympathetic outflow and by interfering with the integrity of the renin-angiotensin system, but it increases the plasma concentration of vasopressin.

Intravascular volume resuscitation and vasopressors can be preferred in the treatment of TEA-induced hypotension. On the other hand, fluid overload must be avoided in major pulmonary resections such as pneumonectomies.

In a study preformed by Holte *et al.* [39], plasma volume was assessed before as well as 90 minutes after TEA in 12 volunteers. They observed a significant reduction of both systolic and diastolic blood pressure and heart rate after epidural anesthesia. They then administered either 7 ml/kg Hydroxyethyl Starch (HES) or 0.2 mg/kg ephedrine. The authors' conclusion was that epidural anesthesia per se does not lead to any change in intravascular volume whereas both ephedrine and fluids have comparable hemodynamic effects. For this reason, vasopressors might be preferred in the treatment of hypotension after epidural anesthesia, especially for patients with cardiopulmonary diseases in which perioperative fluid overload is undesirable. A study conducted by Neal *et al.* [40], investigating the effects of TEA on outcome in esophageal surgery, suggested that utilization of vasopressors was not needed despite fluid restriction.

Despite its hypotensive effect, TEA shows therapeutic benefits during hemorrhagic shock. The response to hypoxemia but not hypercapnia is blunted by TEA [19].

Respiratory effects. Changes in respiratory mechanism after major thoracic surgery consist of alteration in diaphragm movements [41] and thorax shape, development of atelectasis and redistribution of intathoracic blood volume [42]. General anesthesia with one-lung ventilation causes increased intrapulmonary shunt and ventilation–perfusion mismatch, atelectasis [43] and a reduction in functional residual capacity. Furthermore, spontaneous ventilation can be reduced due to postoperative pain [44, 45].

The physiological effects of TEA on lung function are determined by the extension of the motor blockade, depending on the height of the insertion of the catheter, the choice of local anesthetic and its concentration.

Segmental block can impair the activity of respiratory muscles in the rib cage due to the paralysis of intercostal muscles. However, if the diaphragm maintains a normal function, adequate ventilation should be assured even with a reduction of the thoracic component of ventilation [19].

There is concern, however, in patients with severe chronic lung disease who are dependent on accessory muscle function to maintain adequate ventilation, because paralysis of respiratory muscles and changes in bronchial tone can occur. TEA can also induce hypercapnia, particularly in patients with severe emphysema [19]. Gruber *et al.* [46] evaluated the effects of TEA in patients with end-stage chronic obstructive pulmonary disease. The authors demonstrated that TEA in these patients results in better ventilatory mechanics and does not adversely affect gas exchange or inspiratory muscle force generation.

TEA can induce some modification in lung volume depending on the extent of the neural blockade.

Static and dynamic pulmonary measurements may be reduced by TEA in healthy subjects but when anesthesia is restricted to the first five thoracic segments, lung volumes are less affected [19]. It has been reported that TEA decreases inspiratory capacity by approximately 11%, Vital Capacity (VC) by 13%, total lung capacity by 9% and FRC by 6%. Moreover, both FEV1 and FVC were decreased by 12%. PaO2 decreased significantly 25 min after the block although not to a degree that would have clinical consequences [47].

TEA provides better postoperative analgesia than patient-controlled intravenous administration of opioids [48]. During the intra- and postoperative periods of thoracotomy and major abdominal surgery, TEA results in pain-free ventilation, increases abdominal ventilation [9, 49], eventually resulting in a lower incidence of postoperative complications [50].

TEA-induced analgesia exerts an indirect action on vital capacity, permitting better spontaneous ventilation. Analgesia without sedation facilitates a faster mobilization and an active rehabilitation. In the immediate postoperative period, the ability to cough seems to be one of the most important factors affecting lung function and depends on the efficacy of diaphragmatic contraction and pain relief [51].

Studies have suggested that TEA combined with general anesthesia improves arterial oxygenation during one-lung ventilation, results in a better cardiac output stability and reduces the time before extubation [52]. Huchenberg *et al.* [53] demonstrated that the addition of TEA to general anesthesia does not generate additional impairment of the ventilation-perfusion ratio (V/Q) distribution and gas exchange in patients undergoing major abdominal surgery.

Postoperative pulmonary complications such as infections and atelectasis can be improved by epidural anesthetic treatment [54].

The impact of epidural anesthesia on lung function can be ambiguous. On one hand, effective analgesia, avoidance of mechanical irritation by airway instrumentation, and no need for mechanical ventilation represent theoretical advantages of this anesthesia technique. On the other, a possible impairment of lung function can be induced by the epidural motor blockade of respiratory muscles as well as by the potentially detrimental effects of sympathicolysis, due to an unopposed vagal tone with a potentially increased bronchial tone and reactivity [54].

Gastrointestinal effects. Perioperative stressors, such as surgical trauma or hypovolemia, impair perfusion and oxygenation of the gastrointestinal tract due to the activation of the sympathetic nervous system [55] causing redistribution of perfusion from the splanchnic region to more vital organs.

The gastrointestinal effects of epidural anesthesia are mainly attributable to the blockage of the sympathetic splanchnic fibers from T5 through L1 level. As splanchnic vessels present a dense sympathetic innervation, an extended sympathetic block should promote splanchnic vasodilation [56] perfusion and ultimately, tissue oxygenation.

TEA sympatholysis and mesenteric vasodilatation are dose-dependent and related to the extent of the block.

In animal models [57], TEA increased gastrointestinal blood flow, improved microcirculation and delayed the progression of intestinal ischemia. However, an increase of sympathetic activity in segments below the block, leading to impaired splanchnic blood flow, can also occur.

Several studies have demonstrated the positive effect of TEA on visceral perfusion. In particular, Meissner *et al.* [57], in a study comparing awake and anesthetized dogs, suggested that an upper thoracic epidural block had no compromising effect on gastrointestinal perfusion. Christopherson *et al.* [58], employed intramucosal pH (pHi) measurements as an indicator of stable visceral perfusion during abdominal surgery. They suggested that TEA prevented the decrease of pHi as an effect of a more stable visceral perfusion. Schwarte *et al.* [59] performed a study on the effects of TEA on gastric mucosal microvascular hemoglobin oxygenation (μHbO$_2$) in anaesthetized and ventilated dogs. They suggested that TEA maintains μHbO2 under physiological conditions, but worsened the reduction of μHbO$_2$ induced by cardiocirculatory depression, thereby preserving the relationship between gastric mucosal- and systemic oxygenation.

TEA affects gastrointestinal motility by accelerating colon transit after postischemic or postoperative ileus without affecting colon anastomotic healing [60]. Postoperatively, gastrointestinal motility returns more quickly when epidural analgesia with a local anesthetic is instituted [61]. In patients undergoing major abdominal surgery, TEA has been shown not only to hasten the recovery of gastrointestinal function, but also to positively affect food intake and out-of-bed mobilization [19].

Effects on stress response. Many physiological and metabolic events occur due to surgical stress. They start during general anesthesia and can last for several postoperative days [23].

Established components of the recovery process are fever, the release of cytokines and euroendocrine mediators, catabolic state, immuncompromise, increased oxygen consumption, hypermetabolism, and altered carbohydrate metabolism to name but a few.

Further attention should be paid to the possibility of long-lasting and inadequate perioperative stress that may easily increase postoperative cardiac, vascular and infectious complications.

In order to decrease morbidity in high-risk patients, modulation of neurohumoral response is essential [62].

Major initiation of the endocrine activation comes from afferent stimuli. Therefore, blocking these impulses may modify endocrine responses.

During epidural or spinal anesthesia, an introperative single-dose of anesthetic results only in a transient stress-reducing effect without prolonged endocrine or metabolic changes. Therefore, continuous epidural blockade for 24-48 hours postoperatively [63] is considered a more appropriate approach.

Lumbar epidural block is usually sufficient during lower body surgical procedures since it practically eliminates stress response.

In abdominal surgery, the advantages of TEA are well recognized whereas with regard to upper body procedures it is partially effective in neutralizing other reflexes (usually phrenic nerve) or concomitant hypothalamic stimulation [64].

TEA has also been shown to numb stress response through a suppressive effect on whole-body lipolysis after colorectal surgery [65].

In a meta-analysis performed by Ballantyne *et al.* [66], patients who had neuroaxial blockade were found to have lower maximal catecholamine and cortisol levels. Maximal blood glucose levels were similarly well controlled, resulting in a successful modulation of neurohumoral response.

Coagulation. Primary contributors to the pro-thrombotic state, starting with surgical stress, include a reduction in venous blood flow secondary to positive pressure ventilation, neuromuscular blockade and activation of the sympathetic system. This produces significant increases in factors VIII and von Willebrand factor, inhibits fibrinolysis through PAI-1, decreases antithrombin III, and initiates platelet aggregation [67]. It has been demonstrated that epidural anesthesia can modify the hypercoagulable perioperative state, thus decreasing thromboembolic complications by blunting the neurohunoral response and improving lower extremity blood flow [68]. In addition, the analgesic effect of TEA allows early mobilization that decreases the incidence of clot formation. Moreover, acting on the sympathetic response, TEA is associated with demonstrable effects on the coagulation cascade.

It normalizes both factors VIII and von Willebrand factor, decreases PAI-1 and increases antithrombin III [69]. This hypercoagulable process is more dangerous for patients with coronary artery disease. Sympathetic stimulation causes paradoxical vasoconstriction in the atherosclerotic coronary bed instead of the physiologic vasodilatation in the normal arterial smooth muscle. In addition to the loss of endothelial cell integrity, the vasodilatatory capacity and abnormal release of mediators have a role in pathogenesis pathway. However, TEA induces a successful ablation of sympathetic constriction in this setting [29].

In a recent meta-analysis entailing a very large population, neuroaxial blockade was found to improve patients survival [1]. Coagulation effect was accepted as one of the major benefits of central neural blocks, reducing deep vein thrombosis, pulmonary embolism and myocardial infarction [70].

USE OF TEA IN THORACIC SURGERY

Many thoracic surgical procedures can be accomplished with satisfactory anesthesia and analgesia by epidural administration of local anesthetics. Reported procedures that have been carried out through TEA alone include:

- Coronary artery bypass [6-10].

- Management of pneumothorax [11-13].

- Resection of pulmonary nodules and solitary metastases [14, 15].

- Lung volume reduction [16].

- Thymectomy [17].

- Sympathectomy [71].

- Lung biopsy and mediastinal lymph node biopsy [18].

- Bronchopleural fistula closure [18].

- Pleural decortication [18].

- Talc pleurodesis [18].

CONTRAINDICATIONS OF TEA [72]

Absolute Contraindications

- Patient refusal.

- Coagulopathy. Insertion of an epidural needle or catheter may cause traumatic bleeding into the epidural space. Clotting abnormalities may lead to the development of a large hematoma leading to spinal cord compression.

- Therapeutic anticoagulation: full oral anticoagulation with warfarin or Standard Heparin (SH) are absolute contraindications to epidural blockade.

- Uncorrected hypovolemia: the sympathetic blockade produced by epidural anesthesia, in combination with uncorrected hypovolemia, may cause profound circulatory collapse.

- Skin infection at insertion site: insertion of the epidural needle through an area of skin infection may introduce pathogenic bacteria into the epidural space, leading to serious complications such as meningitis or epidural abscess.

- Increased intracranial pressure: accidental dural puncture in a patient with raised intracranial pressure may lead to brainstem herniation (coning).

- Thrombocytopenia (platelet count below $50.000/mm^3$).

Relative Contraindications

- Sepsis [72].

- Anatomical abnormalities of the vertebral column (*e.g.* spinal stenosis). May make the placement of an epidural needle/catheter technically impossible [73].

- Previous surgery of the cervical or upper thoracic spine [73].

- Neurological disease (*e.g.* multiple sclerosis). Any new neurological symptoms may be ascribed to the epidural [73].

- Uncooperative patient. May render insertion and/or positioning of the epidural catheter difficult if not impossible [73].

DRUGS USED FOR TEA

When choosing drugs for thoracic epidural blockade, many factors have to be considered: potency and duration of the drugs, their ability to preferentially block sensory and motor fibers, as well as the anticipated duration of surgery or the need for postoperative analgesia. Local anesthetics and opioids are still the pharmacological agents most widely used epidurally; nevertheless, other drugs from different pharmacological classes are administered as adjuvants to local anesthetics and opioids, some of them are still being investigated [74].

Local anesthetics. Thoracic surgical anesthesia *via* the epidural route requires dense sensory block and usually moderate to dense motor block. The most commonly used agents to achieve surgical anesthesia in thoracic surgery are the long-acting local anesthetics bupivacaine, ropivacaine and levobupivacaine.

Levobupivacaine and ropivacaine are two relatively new long-acting local anesthetics introduced into the market in the last few years, and developed after reports of simultaneous seizure and cardiac arrest following accidental intravascular injection of bupivacaine [74].

The molecules of local anesthetics have a three-dimensional structure, and possess an asymmetric carbon atom which is bound to four different substitutes (Fig. **1**). The structures of these compounds are defined as chiral. Enantiomers are optically active, and can be differentiated by their effects on the rotation of the plane of a polarized light into dextrorotatory [(R+)] or levorotatory [(S-)] stereoisomers. A solution of bupivacaine contains equal amounts of the two enantiomerics and is called racemic solution, while technological advances have allowed the production of solutions containing only one enantiomer of a chiral molecule, which is optically pure. R- and S- enantiomers of local anesthetics have been demonstrated to have a different affinity for the different ion channels of sodium, potassium, and calcium [75]. This results in a significant reduction of both central nervous system and cardiac toxicity of the S enantiomer as compared with the R-enantiomer [76]. Ropivacaine and levobupivacaine are available as optically pure solutions.

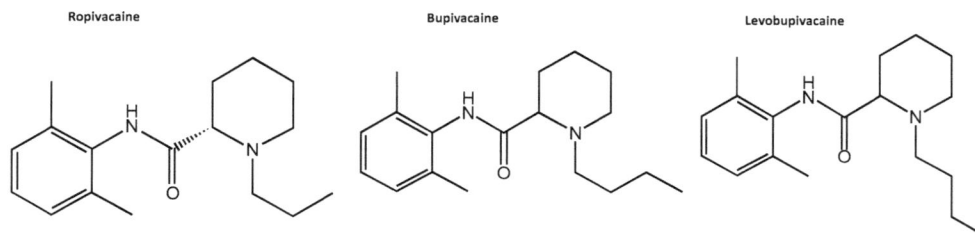

Fig. 1. Structure of the three local anesthetics.

Pharmacology and toxicology. Bupivacaine is an amino-amide local anesthetic which belongs to the family of the n-alkylsubstituted pipecoloxylidides, which were first synthesized by Ekenstam in 1957 [77]. Its molecular structure is highly lipid-soluble, and contains a chiral center on the piperidine ring, resulting in two optically active stereoisomers. Ropivacaine also belongs to the same pipecoloxylidide group , but whereas ropivacaine has a propyl group, bupivacaine has a butyl group on the amine portion of pipecoloxylidide (Fig. **1**). The pKa of the three agents is similar, as well as their protein binding, while ropivacaine is much less lipophilic than the two other molecules because of the substitution of the pipecoloxylidine with a 3-carbon side-chain instead of a 4-carbon side-chain [78].

Central nervous system toxicity. Systemic toxicity of local anesthetics may occur as a consequence of unwanted intravascular or intrathecal injection, or after the administration of an excessive dose of these drugs. Systemic toxicity of local anesthetic drugs initially involves the Central Nervous System (CNS) and subsequently the cardiovascular system. The CNS is usually more susceptible to the actions of local anesthetics than the cardiovascular system; thus signs of CNS intoxication are usually evident before the appearance of cardiovascular toxicity. Initial signs of CNS toxicity are usually excitatory and include shivering, muscle twitching, and tremors, which are produced by a preferential block of inhibitory central pathways. With the increase of the local anesthetic plasma concentrations, the excitatory pathway of CNS toxicity is blocked and signs of CNS excitation are followed by a generalized CNS depression with hypoventilation and respiratory arrest, and, finally, generalized convulsions [79]. A recent study has confirmed a better neurotoxic profile of levobupivacaine when compared to racemic bupivacaine, and this is indicative of a safer profile of levobupivacaine in clinical practice [80]. The absolute dose of local anesthetic inducing toxic effects is affected by several factors, including the method and rate of administration, the rapidity with which a certain plasma level is achieved, and whether the patient is under the influence of anesthesia. This often makes it difficult to compare and extrapolate the results of animal studies to human patients. Based on animal and volunteer studies, it can be concluded that both levobupivacaine and ropivacaine seem to be less neurotoxic than bupivacaine. They had a higher convulsive threshold in different animal models, fewer CNS symptoms after intravenous administration in human volunteers, and fewer excitatory changes in the electroencephalography (EEG) than bupivacaine [79].

Cardiovascular toxicity. The first signs of cardiac toxicity are related to the CNS excitatory phase with the activation of the sympathetic nervous system, which can mask direct myocardial depression. However, with increasing plasma concentrations of the local anesthetic this stage is followed by arrhythmias and deep cardiac depression, resulting in cardiovascular collapse [81].

All three long-acting local anesthetics show a dose-dependent prolongation of cardiac conduction, with an increase in the PR interval and QRS duration on the ECG. These effects are explained by the persisting block of sodium channels into diastole, predisposing to re-entrant arrhythmias [81]. Since the dissociation caused by bupivacaine is nearly 10 times longer than that of lidocaine, bupivacaine-induced block can accumulate, resulting in a more marked cardiac depression [82, 83]. Local anesthetics also affect the conductivity of potassium channels, increasing the QTc interval and enhancing the block of the inactivated state of the sodium channel [84]. The levorotatory isomer of bupivacaine is seven-fold less potent in blocking the potassium channel than the dextrorotatory one [85]. Local anesthetics block adenosine triphosphate-sensitive potassium (KATP) channels, with an approximately eight-fold higher potency than vascular KATP channels, and bupivacaine is more potent than both levobupivacaine and ropivacaine in blocking cardiac KATP channels [86]. The inhibition of cardiac contractility is also proportional to the lipid solubility and nerve-blocking potency of the local anesthetics, suggesting a rank order (from lowest to highest) of the cardiotoxic potency of the three local anesthetics with ropivacaine <(S-) bupivacaine <racemic bupivacaine <(R+) bupivacaine [87]. When the cardiovascular effects of levobupivacaine and ropivacaine were compared after intravascular injection in healthy volunteers, no differences in mean percentage changes from baseline to the end of infusion were reported for stroke index, cardiac index, acceleration index, as well as for PR interval, QRS duration, QT interval and heart rate [88]. Depression of conduction and contractility appeared at lower doses and plasma concentration with bupivacaine compared with ropivacaine [89, 90] or levobupivacaine [91].

It has been suggested that lipid emulsion (Intralipid) may reverse local anesthetic toxicity by extracting lipophilic local anesthetics from aqueous plasma or tissues or by counteracting local anesthetic inhibition of myocardial fatty acid oxygenation. Studies in animal models have shown that lipid emulsion is effective in resuscitating animals who are asystolic after the administration of intravenous bupivacaine. Few case reports support the use of lipid emulsion to reverse systemic toxicity, including seizures, electrocardiogram abnormalities, and cardiac arrest, resulting from the administration of levobupivacaine, ropivacaine, bupivacaine, or mepivacaine. The regimens used in these cases consisted of bolus doses of 1.2-2 mL/kg followed by continuous infusions of 0.25-0.5 mL/kg/min. All of the patients recovered fully with no neurologic sequelae [227].

Relative potency. Local anesthetics bind directly to the intracellular voltage-dependent sodium channels. They block primarily open and inactive sodium channels, at specific within-channel sites. Lipid solubility appears to be the primary determinant of intrinsic anesthetic potency. Chemical compounds which are highly lipophilic tend to penetrate the nerve membrane more easily, so that less molecules are required for conduction blockade, resulting in enhanced potency. For this reason, a strict correlation between the lipid solubility of the local anesthetic and its potency and toxicity does exist [79].

The relative potency of these three long-acting local anesthetics has been evaluated in patients by determining the Minimum Local Anesthetic Concentration (MLAC) producing adequate pain control in 50% of patients receiving an epidural block for labor pain with an up-and-down sequential allocation technique. No differences in the MLAC were shown between levobupivacaine (0.083%) and bupivacaine (0.081%) [91] whereas ropivacaine had a nearly 50% higher MLAC value [92, 93].

Opioids. Compared with administration of either component alone, the combination of epidural local anesthetic and opioid reduces dynamic pain after abdominal, orthopedic and thoracic surgery [104, 105]. Epidural opioids can provide analgesia *via* three mechanisms: transport to supraspinal receptors by cerebrospinal fluid, blood-borne transport to supraspinal receptors after systemic absorption, and direct stimulation of spinal opioid receptors. Epidural or spinal administration of sufentanil produces concentration gradients within the cerebrospinal fluid, with the largest concentrations being near the drug administration site [106-110].

There is nonetheless, significant cephalad spread to supraspinal opioid receptors after epidural administration [107].

These studies, however, involved large doses of sufentanil (10–50 mg) given as a bolus—far more than given in other studies [111]. In contrast, small doses of lipid-soluble opioids are poorly transmitted to the spinal fluid. Morphine, a poorly lipid-soluble opioid, produces analgesia by a spinal mechanism whether administered epidurally or intrathecally [112, 113]. In contrast, highly soluble opioids, including fentanyl [114-116] and sufentanil [117-119], apparently produce analgesia mostly *via* systemic uptake and redistribution to the brain. This suggests that sufentanil given epidurally with small concentrations of local anesthetic produces analgesia primarily by a spinal effect rather than systemic absorption [111].

Lipophilic opioids such as fentanyl have a more rapid onset and a shorter duration of action than hydrophilic opioids such as morphine when administered either intrathecally or epidurally. Their ring also shows a narrower band of segmental analgesia because of rapid uptake by neural (and fatty) tissue, and equally rapid systemic absorption. This rapid and sustained systemic uptake from fatty tissue also increases the systemic contribution to their analgesic and adverse effects [109, 120, 121].

Hydrophilic opioids such as morphine penetrate neural tissue more slowly, resulting in a slower onset, and their elimination from the neuraxis is delayed, allowing widespread CSF distribution. Thus, analgesia can be achieved at sites relatively distant from the spinal cord level at which the injection has taken place [109, 120, 121].

For this reason the most commonly used agents are the liposoluble opioids fentanyl and sufentanil.

Fentanyl appears to be one of the most commonly administered neuraxial opioids and is registered for such use in many countries [122]. Its relatively high lipid solubility results in more restricted segmental activity and rapid onset of action than with other opioids, but also mandates administration close to the site of the desired effect.

There is ongoing debate about whether the main effect of epidural fentanyl is by systemic uptake; however, a well designed study showed significantly increased analgesic potency of epidural over intravenous fentanyl by a factor of 1.9, indicating an epidural effect [123]. Sufentanil is another widely used and highly lipophilic neuraxial opioid.

Owing to its high potency early respiratory depression is an adverse effect of concern, even after small epidural doses such as 5µg [124].

Adverse effects of neuraxial opioids. As with systemic administration, respiratory depression is the most serious and potentially life-threatening adverse effect of neuraxial opioid use. It can occur as a consequence of systemic absorption due to the uptake of the opioid into the epidural veins. Rostral spread with the cerebrospinal fluid, particularly with hydrophilic opioids and after intrathecal administration can represent an alternative mechanism [125]. The elderly appear to display increased sensitivity to opioid-induced CNS depression and are at higher risk for this adverse effect. It can occur when opioids are used *via* the epidural route. A reduction in the bolus dose and infusion rates of up to 50% have thus been suggested in older patients [126]. Pruritus is a characteristic adverse effect of neuraxial opioid use. Although dose-related, it is very common, with reported rates of 30% up to 100% [127]. Postulated causative mechanisms include itch-specific neural pathways with reduced tonic inhibition induced by opioids and activation of the medullary dorsal horn with antagonism of inhibitory transmitters [117].

Nausea and vomiting continue to be disturbing adverse effects of opioids, even after neuraxial administration [125] although dose requirements are much lower than with systemic administration.

ADJUVANT DRUGS

A variety of other classes of drugs have been studied to try to improve the quality of epidural and subarachnoid blockade. Alpha-adrenergic agonists, cholinesterase inhibitors, semisynthetic opioid agonist–antagonists, ketamine, and midazolam have been studied in this setting [105].

Clonidine. Clonidine, the prototypical α2-adrenoceptor agonist used in neuraxial blocks, has been studied extensively in combination with local anesthetics, as a primary agent, and in combination with a variety of other drugs. It has been demonstrated that clonidine prolongs and intensifies the effects of epidural local anesthetics [105] without increasing the degree of hypotension for epidural anesthesia and analgesia [128]. It also produces analgesia without motor impairment and prolongs the duration of the local anesthetic analgesic effect [128, 129]. It also has a synergist effect when combined with opioids and opioid agonist–antagonists, allowing reduced doses and therefore side effects of both [129, 130]. Finally, clonidine, modulates the immune stress response to thoracic surgery [131].

Clonidine is a lipophilic drug with similar lipophilicity to fentanyl. Its systemic absorption with subsequent redistribution to peripheral sites of action may also play a role in its mode of action. However, clonidine has higher neuraxial rather than systemic potency, thereby reducing systemic adverse effects such as sedation [128]. Sedation mainly reflects systemic drug absorption, tends to be dose related [128] and does not potentiate opioid-induced respiratory depression [132].

Ketamine. The combination of epidural ketamine with local anesthetic and/or opioid infusions results in improved analgesia without significantly increasing adverse effects [130, 133]. The nature of specific spinal versus systemic effects remains to be elucidated and the neuraxial use of ketamine is currently experimental only [105].

Midazolam. Midazolam is a neuraxial analgesic because of its effect on GABA receptors, which are thought to be involved in anti-nociception by reducing spinal cord hyperexcitability [134]. There has been extensive recent discussion related to its potential neurotoxicity [135] and a thoughtful review supports "the assertion of a degree of safety" for its intrathecal use [136]. Some studies support the analgesic efficacy of intrathecal midazolam at doses below 2mg and in concentrations below 1 mg/ml [136, 137].

CLINICAL APPLICATIONS AND DOSING REGIMEN

Despite the potency ratio issue discussed above, there are a large number of clinical studies showing that, when used at clinically relevant concentrations (0.5-0.75%), epidural ropivacaine produces an epidural blockade, which is substantially similar to that produced by equivalent concentrations and doses of racemic bupivacaine [94-99].

Ropivacaine for intraoperative anaesthesia is usually used at a concentration of 0.5% in combination or not with sufentanil 0.5-1.6 µg/ml [14, 100]. Bupivacaine [18] and levobupivacaine [101] are used at the same concentration.

After catheter positioning, a test dose (2-3 ml) of local anesthetic (usually lidocaine with epinephrine) is given in order to exclude intrathecal or intravascular placement of the catheter.

In order to achieve surgical anesthesia with TEA, drugs can be administrated in different ways:

- Injection of an initial dose that provides the level of anesthesia necessary for the surgical procedure followed by intermittent bolus [138].

- Injection of an initial dose that provides the level of anesthesia necessary for the surgical procedure followed by continuous infusion. During surgical procedure anesthesia level is maintained with a continuous infusion into the epidural space of bupivacaine or ropivacaine 0.5% and sufentanil 1.66 µg/ml at an hourly rate of 2-5 ml [102].

- Continuous infusion solely. If the anesthetic level is achieved with a continuous infusion alone, the drug concentration is the same but the infusion rate has to be increased to an hourly rate of 20-30 ml until the desired anesthetic level is established [103].

The initial activating dose of local anesthetics and opioids given to achieve surgical anesthesia depends on the age and size of the patient. As a general guideline, 0.7 ml of local anesthetic per segment to be blocked is required for a thoracic epidural.

In total, a range of 30–40 mg of bupivacaine 0.5% or ropivacaine 0.5%, and 20 µg of sufentanil or 50 µg of fentanil is given before the surgical incision.

During wound closure, the anesthetic regimen is changed in order to provide postoperative analgesia [103].

TECHNICAL ASPECTS [139]

Patient preparation. Intravenous access with a catheter large enough to administer fluids or emergency drugs should be in place. Drugs and equipment for life support, including airway management, must be readily available. Standard non-invasive monitoring is routinely applied. Adequate premedication should be administered in order to reduce patient stress before placing the patient in the lateral position.

Morphological Landmarks for Thoracic Region.

- C7 - protuberant cervical process.

- T3 - origin of the spine of the scapula.

- T7 - tip of the scapula.

- L1 - tip of the 12th rib.

Equipment. A disposable epidural sterile kit containing an epidural needle (the Tuohy needle with the Huber tip is most commonly used), a plastic syringe, an epidural catheter and a filter is usually used.

Approaches to the thoracic epidural space. There are 2 approaches for thoracic epidural space localization:

- Mid-line (median) approach.

- Paramedian approach.

The difference between the 2 approaches lies in the insertion sites of the needle with regard to the interspinous processes.

The mid-line approach is commonly used to perform lumbar or lower thoracic epidural block. A Tuohy needle is introduced in the mid-line and directed slightly cephalad between the two spinous processes of the desired interspinous space. The needle passes through the skin and supraspinous ligaments, into the interspinous ligament. At this point the Tuohy needle stylet is removed and the loss-of-resistance syringe is attached to detect loss of resistance as the needle traverses the ligamentum flavum and enters the epidural space, which is usually 3–5 cm from the skin in the mid-line. A sudden 'give' may be felt as the needle tip exits the ligamentum flavum and the loss-of-resistance indicator (air or saline) is expelled into the epidural space.

The paramedian approach is more commonly used in the upper thoracic region because of the long, sloping spinous processes and narrow interspinous spaces. The Tuohy needle is inserted at about 1.0–1.5 cm laterally from mid-point of the spinous process immediately above the level of the desired intervertebral space. The needle is then moved forward, perpendicular to the skin, through the underlying subcutaneous tissue and muscle, until it strikes the vertebral lamina. The needle is then withdrawn slightly. The loss-of-resistance syringe is then attached and redirected cephalad and medially so that the needle is walked off the lamina until it pierces the ligamentum flavum and enters the epidural space (Fig. **2**).

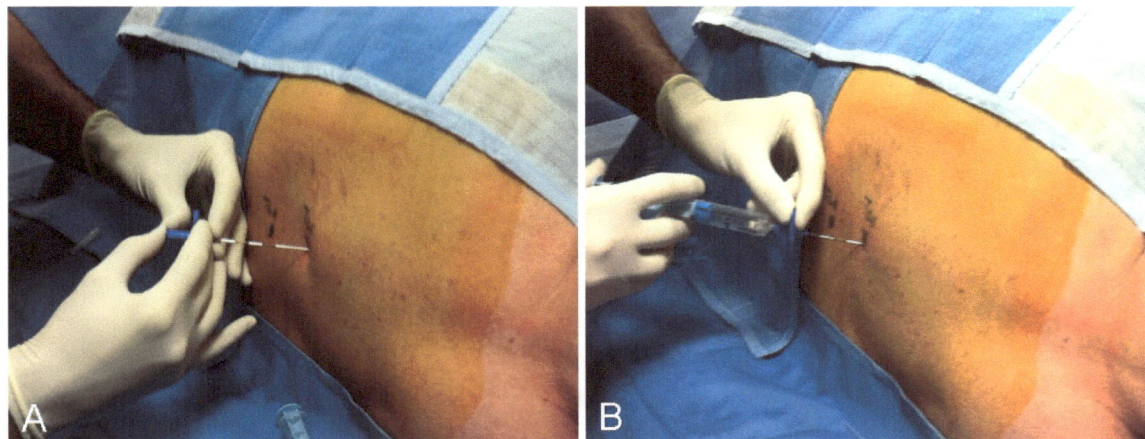

Fig. 2. Insertion of the Thuoy needle (A) and loss of resistance technique (B).

Because of the greater incidence of false loss of resistance in the midline thoracic approach, the paramedian approach is preferred for catheter placement. Moreover the sharp angulation of the spinous processes especially in the midthoracic area can make the midline approach difficult even for the most experienced clinicians.

Identification of loss of resistance. The pressure in the epidural space is usually sub-atmospheric. The two methods currently used rely on the loss of resistance to the injection of saline or air as the needle penetrates the ligamentum flavum and enters the epidural space. Each technique has its own benefits and drawbacks. To minimize bubble formation, dilution of local anesthetic and the difficulty in discerning saline and cerebrospinal fluid, a maximum of 3 ml of air or saline can be used.

Placement of the catheter. An epidural block provides the most intense block at the insertion site, so the tip of the catheter should be placed at mid-incision level. The objective of TEA in most thoracic procedures is to achieve somatosensory and motor block between T1 and T8 level, providing motor block of the intercostal muscles while preserving diaphragmatic motion. The thoracic epidural catheter is usually inserted at the level of the T3–T4 intervertebral spaces. For symphatectomy and thymectomy, the epidural catheter has to be inserted between C7—T1 and T1—T2 to achieve sensory and motor block between C5 and C6. At this level of block, the cervical horn of the thymus is included. The catheter is inserted through the Tuohy needle about 4–5 cm into the epidural space, and the depth of insertion is noted by counting the markers on the catheter. It is normal practice for the catheter to be inserted to a depth of between 15 and 20 cm. The needle is then carefully withdrawn from the epidural space, ensuring that the catheter is not withdrawn with it. When the needle has been removed, the catheter is gently withdrawn until the desired depth marker is just visible at the skin-puncture site (Fig. **3**).

Test dose. The volume and concentration of local anesthetic needed for epidural anesthesia is larger than that required for spinal anesthesia. Therefore, the catheter should be tested for evidence of proper placement in the epidural space. The purpose of the "test dose" of 2 ml of 2% lidocaine is to make sure that the catheter is not in the subarachnoid, intravascular, or subdural space.

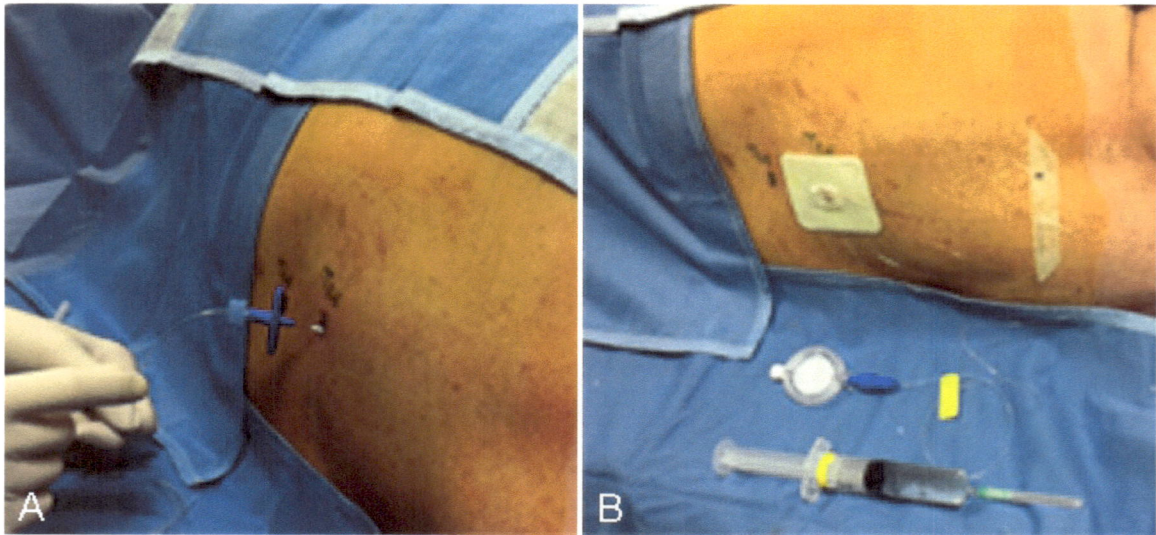

Fig. 3. Catheter insertion (A); test dose (B).

Monitoring the onset of block. The effects of local anesthetics act primarily on the segmental spinal nerve roots, although limited diffusion through the dura allows some of these effects to act on the spinal cord directly.

Differential blockade of motor and sensory modalities is related to the size and therefore the sensitivity of different neurons to local anesthetics. The small sympathetic preganglionic fibers and sensory fibers are more easily blocked than the large motor fibers. Vasodilatation is an early sign of the onset of the block, which usually manifests first in the veins of the feet, with flushing and increased warmth. The level of sympathetic block is normally two segments higher than sensory block level, whilst motor block is up to two segments lower than the sensory block.

Because of the differing segmental height for the sympathetic, sensory and motor blocks, it is important to formally monitor and record the sensory and motor block as the epidural begins to work, to ensure the sensory block is high enough for the planned surgery, and that the degree of motor block is appropriate. As the block develops, physiological changes occur due to the relative effects of motor, sensory and autonomic blockade.

Mid-to-Low Thoracic Block (T6–T12)

- Sensory blockade of abdominal organs and skin of anterior abdominal wall.

- Motor block of anterior abdominal wall muscles and lower intercostal muscles.

- Block of sympathetic chain, including coeliac ganglion, causing marked hypotension with compensatory tachycardia, loss of sweating and unopposed parasympathetic activity that maintains gut tone and motility.

High Thoracic Block (T1–T5)

- Sensory block of chest wall, thoracic viscera and medial aspect of upper arm.

- Motor block of upper intercostal muscles and some arm weakness.

- Block of sympathetic cardiac accelerator fibers, causing unopposed vagal tone with bradycardia, hypotension and potential risk of cardiovascular collapse.

The anesthesia level is usually monitored by warm—cold discrimination or by loss of pinprick sensation 15 to 20 minutes after the injection of the bolus dose.

POSTOPERATIVE ANALGESIA

Pain following thoracic procedures can occur in >70% of patients and it is considered to be one of the most severe types of postoperative pain [140]. Pain can last up to 2 months or even persist longer, becoming chronic in 30% of patients. Multiple factors are involved in the pathogenesis of thoracotomy pain. Surgical incision, stretch of ligaments and the placement of rib retractors in the intercostal space are traumatic events that provoke sympathetic and inflammatory responses. The inflammatory response activates peripheral nociceptors that transmit nociceptive signals centrally and initiate larger inflammatory process, amplifying pain transmission and altering pain sensation through central sensitization. When postoperative nociceptive and inflammatory pain disappear, pain can persist in the absence of peripheral noxious stimuli. Central sensitization can be maintained by continued peripheral nociceptive input, contributing to the development of chronic pain. Chronic pain is mostly related to nerve injury and myofascial involvement [140]. Factors hypothesized to decrease the chance of developing chronic pain include analgesic regimen, gender and type of incision. Female patients may be at higher risk for the development of painful conditions following thoracotomy. Intercostal nerve damage during a muscle-sparing thoracotomy occurs less likely compared with a classic posterolateral incision [141]. Mediansternotomy and VATS seem to be less acutely painful approaches than thoracotomy for thoracic surgery [142].

VATS techniques seem not only to improve patient comfort, but also to reduce early postoperative depression of pulmonary function [143].

Pain due to thoracotomy, combined with the loss of parenchyma, drastically reduces respiratory function for the first postoperative days [108, 144, 145]. It produces a reversible restrictive pattern of ventilation with a decrease of VC and FRC [146]. Incomplete pain treatment results in reduced pulmonary compliance, inability to breath deeply or cough forcefully and retention of secretions, atelectasis and pneumonia [147].

The initiation of an early and aggressive analgesia regimen is therefore important to reduce pulmonary complications as well as the risk of developing long-term pain [146].

Although several methods described in the literature are used for post-thoracotomy pain management, including systemic opioids, non-steroid anti-inflammatory drugs, ketamine, regional techniques such as paravertebral, intercostal and interpleural blocks, thoracic epidural analgesia remains the most beneficial approach [148, 149].

TEA enables a significant increase in pulmonary function by allowing deep breathing and coughing with adequate pain relief [146]. Patients treated with TEA have better preservation of lung volume, no increase in airway resistance and lower pain score (Visual Analogue Scale, VAS) at rest and on coughing than patients treated with intravenous morphine [48].

Such effective pain management improves postoperative mobilization and recovery, reduces overall morbidity and thus shortens hospitalization time, eventually reducing costs [150].

Adequate pain control could be well maintained throughout the postoperative period by continuous epidural application of analgesic agents through an epidural catheter. Another possible approach could be Patient Controlled Epidural Analgesia (PCEA) [151].

Drugs used for analgesia and dosing regimen. Many analgesic protocols are described in the literature, including the use of local anesthetics alone, an opioid alone or either a combination of both.

The mixture of both local anesthetic and liposoluble opioid produces better results than the individual drugs used alone [152]. Their infusion into the thoracic epidural space allows a reduction in the use of both drugs and a reduction of i.v. analgesic drugs. Reduction of local anesthetic concentration also reduces motor blockade and other undesired effects of local anesthetics [108, 153].

The most used local anesthetics are bupivacaine and ropivacaine while fentanyl and sufentanil are the most used opiods. Results of comparative studies of postoperative epidural analgesia infusions of ropivacaine versus bupivacaine for pain relief in labor [154] and after abdominal [155] or orthopedic surgery are conflicting. Some studies reported equipotency [156], others equal analgesic potency but decreased motor-block with ropivacaine [157]. A comparative study of epidural after thoracotomy reported that a continuous epidural infusion of ropivacaine/fentanyl provided similar analgesia to bupivacaine/fentanyl during the first two postoperative days after posterolateral thoracotomy [158].

Moreover, administration of large-volume/small-concentration solutions of drugs could produce more extensive sensory block and increased spread of a dilute opioid to allow interaction with a larger surface area of opioid receptors [160].

The most commonly used regimen consists of the administration of ropivacaine 0.15-0.2% or bupivacaine 0.1%, and sufentanil 0.5-1 μg /ml or fentanyl 5 μg /ml at an hourly continuous infusion rate of 2-5 ml according to the patient's height [157, 160, 161].

Complications of TEA. They include:

- Spinal cord injury associated with neuroaxial hematoma: The epidural space is filled with a rich network of venous plexuses, and puncture of these veins with bleeding into the confined epidural space may lead to the rapid development of a hematoma with compression of the spinal cord, which can have disastrous consequences for the patient including paraplegia [162].

- Epidural infection including epidural and paraspinal abscesses, as well as meningitis [162].

- Hypotension secondary to sympatholysis induced by anesthetic blockade [163].

- Transient neurological side effects, such as paresis, paresthesias in the upper limb and Horner syndrome [164].

- High epidural block: an excessively large dose of local anesthetic in the epidural space may cause hypotension, nausea, sensory loss or paresthesia of high thoracic or even cervical nerve roots (arms); difficult breathing due to blockade of nerve supply to the intercostal muscles; difficulty in talking (small tidal volumes due to phrenic block) and drowsiness indicate that the block is becoming excessively high and should be managed as an emergency [165].

- Total spinal: a rare complication occurring when the epidural needle, or epidural catheter, is inadvertently advanced into the subarachnoid space and an "epidural dose" of local anesthetic is injected directly into the cerebrospinal fluid. The result is profound hypotension, apnea, unconsciousness and dilated pupils as a result of the action of local anesthetic on the brainstem [166].

- Accidental dural puncture: usually easily recognized by the immediate loss of cerebrospinal fluid through the epidural needle. This complication occurs in 1-2% of epidural blocks, although it is more common in inexperienced hands. It leads to a high incidence of post dural puncture headache, which is severe and associated with a number of characteristic features [167].

- Drug-related complications:
  - Local anesthetic-related - When an excessive dose of local anesthetics is injected into the epidural space or when a moderate dose is accidentally injected into an epidural vein, systemic toxicity can occur. The central nervous system is the first affected system. Symptoms include lightheadedness, tinnitus, circumoral numbness and tingling, numbness of the tongue, and blurred vision. Signs include muscle twitching, confusion, tremors of the facial muscles and extremities, and shivering. Cardiovascular effects of local anesthetics range from mild changes in blood pressure and pulse to complete cardiovascular collapse. At low doses, a slight increase in blood pressure may be noted secondarily to an increase in cardiac output. At higher doses, a marked increase in blood pressure and heart rate will precede severe hypotension and cardiovascular collapse [168].

- Opioid-related pruritus, nausea and vomiting, urinary retention, and respiratory depression [125].

Advantages. Various benefits can be obtained by using TEA as the sole anesthetic technique for awake thoracic surgery procedures:

- Avoidance of general anesthesia and one-lung mechanical ventilation (less pronounced postoperative impairment of oxygenation) [13].

- Adequate postoperative analgesia [148, 149].

- Faster recovery with immediate return to many daily life activities including drinking, eating and walking [51].

- Better patient satisfaction [13, 14, 18].

- Shorter anesthesia time, operative time, and global time spent in the operating room [16].

- Shorter hospital stay [13, 18].

- Potential decrease of cost and improved resource utilization [150].

- Avoidance of muscle relaxants in patients with myasthenia gravis since they can have an unpredictable response to their action. Avoiding muscle relaxants in such patients can potentially lower the risk of postoperative muscle weakness and respiratory insufficiency thus leading to faster recovery [228-232].

- Interactive cooperation between the surgeon and the conscious patient is allowed.

- Whenever TEA is combined with general anesthesia, arterial oxygenation is improved during one-lung ventilation, which results in better cardiac output and earlier tracheal extubation [52].

Disadvantages. Some inconveniences may be related to the use of TEA:

- The open pneumothorax created to perform an awake lung resection can determine a mediastinal shifting with compression of the dependent lung, potentially resulting in a functional compromise [14].

- Bleeding and/or neuroaxial hematoma, especially in patients using concomitant anticoagulant therapy [51].

- Limited space for surgical maneuvering particularly in patients with emphysema [16].

- Loss of an immobile surgical field such as that achieved by one-lung ventilation due to maintained spontaneous ventilation and diaphragmatic motion.

- Risk of phrenic nerve palsy with high epidural anesthesia [16].

PARAVERTEBRAL BLOCK

Paravertebral blockade is a safe and effective technique for intraoperative and postoperative management of acute surgical pain [169, 170]. Thoracic Paravertebral Block (PVB) has been shown to provide superior post-thoracotomy analgesia and lung function, compared with systemic opioids or intrapleural Local Anesthetics (LA) [171, 172].

In contrast to epidural technique, this mode of analgesia is not considered to be a stand-alone technique and most patients will require additional analgesia, usually parenteral patient-controlled analgesia [173].

Compared to epidural analgesia, the paravertebral block has a better side-effect profile and a lower complication rate than epidural analgesia [174].

ANATOMY

The Thoracic Paravertebral Space (TPVS), when viewed in transverse cross-section, is triangular-shaped. The base is formed by the posterolateral aspect of the vertebral body/intervertebral discs/intervertebral foramina/articular processes. The anterolateral border is formed by the parietal pleura, whilst the posterior border is formed by the superior costotransverse ligament. This ligament extends from the inferior aspect of the transverse process above to the superior aspect of the rib tubercle below. Lateral to this ligament (and continuous with it) is the internal intercostal membrane, which is the aponeurotic continuation of the internal intercostal muscle, and this runs between the upper and lower border of adjacent ribs [175]. The apex of the triangular TPVS communicates with the intercostal space laterally. The TPVS contains mainly fatty tissue and is traversed by the intercostal or spinal nerves, intercostal vessels, dorsal rami, rami communicantes, and the sympathetic chain.

The spinal nerves do not have a fascial sheath in the TPVS, which explains their susceptibility to local anesthetic blockade. The endothoracic fascia is the deep investing fascia of the thoracic cavity. It blends medially with the periosteum of the vertebral body and laterally is closely applied to the ribs. Caudally, it is continuous with the transversalis fascia of the abdominal cavity and this may explain why solutions injected in the TPVS may spread to the lumbar region. The spinal nerves have been described as running through the compartment posterior to the endothoracic fascia [176].

TECHNIQUE

In the original description, a 10 cm needle was inserted three fingerbreadths from the midline at a 45° angle to the skin, and advanced into the TPVS until the tip contacted the thoracic vertebral body [177]. The technique was eventually abandoned because of the risk of needle penetration through the intervertebral foramen, and thus inadvertent dural puncture and spinal cord injury [178, 179]. However, ultrasonographic visualization of in-plane needle advancement reduces the risk of pleural puncture as well as entry of the needle into the intervertebral foramen [180]. Nevertheless, the practitioner should be aware that there is a risk of epidural local anesthetic spread with paravertebral injection [181, 182].

Thoracic paravertebral block using real-time ultrasound guidance [180]. The thoracic vertebral level is identified by palpating and counting down from vertebra prominens (C7) and using a 38-mm broadband (5–10 MHz) linear array transducer placed initially at a point 2.5 cm lateral to the tip of the spinous process in a vertical orientation, obtaining a sagittal paramedian view of the transverse process, superior costotransverse ligament, and underlying pleura. The parietal pleura is identified as a bright structure running deep to the adjacent transverse processes, distinct from the deeper lung tissue, which could be seen to shimmer and move with patient breathing. The superior costotransverse ligament, less distinct, can be seen as a collection of homogeneous linear echogenic bands alternating with echo poor areas running from 1 transverse ligament to the next.

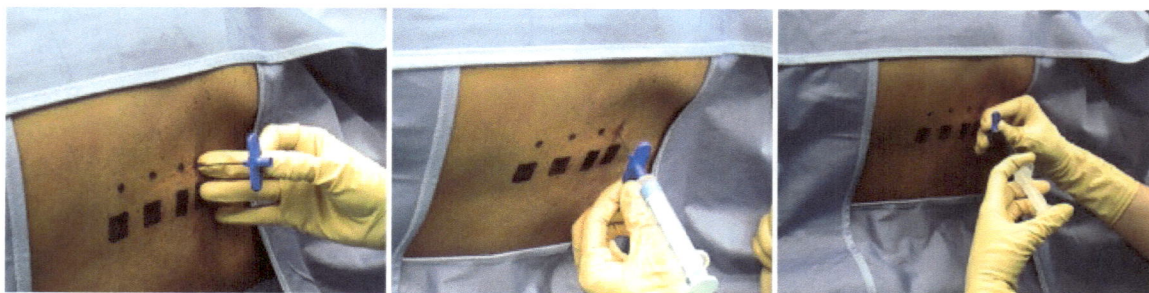

Fig. 4. Main landmarks and steps of thoracic paravertebral block.

The midpoint of the transducer is aligned midway between the 2 adjacent transverse processes, local anesthesia infiltrated at its lower border, and an 18-gauge Tuohy needle introduced in a needle-in-plane approach in a cephalad orientation. The paravertebral space is entered midway between the 2 transverse processes avoiding bony contact. The tip of the needle is advanced under direct vision to puncture the costotransverse ligament (Fig. **4**).

Saline (3 mL) is then injected deep into the superior costotransverse ligament in order to demonstrate the position of injectate deep into the ligament, and allow easier passage of the catheter to a distance of 2–3 cm beyond the needle tip.

A technical difficulty with this technique is potential loss of image of the needle tip as it is advanced. This is due to the acute angle the needle must take to enter between adjacent transverse processes. Tissue disturbance may facilitate tracking of the needle tip in these circumstances.

Mechanism and spread of anesthesia. A thoracic paravertebral injection may remain localized at the injected level [183], or it may spread to the contiguous levels above and below [181, 184], the intercostal space laterally, the epidural space medially [181, 182], or a combination of the above to affect ipsilateral somatic and sympathetic nerves [185], including the posterior primary ramus in multiple contiguous thoracic dermatomes. Thoracic paravertebral anesthesia does not appear to be gravity-dependent, but there is a tendency for preferential caudal spread of somatic and sympathetic blockade [186]. There is controversy regarding epidural spread and its contribution to the extension of TPVB. Radio-opaque contrast medium infused postoperatively through an extrapleural paravertebral catheter placed intraoperatively under direct vision, remains confined to the paravertebral space [187]. In contrast, varying degrees of epidural spread have been shown to occur after 70% of percutaneous paravertebral injections, which is mostly unilateral [182], and the volume involved is considered too small to produce clinically significant epidural block [188]. The vertebral attachment of the endothoracic fascia attenuates prevertebral spread [189] and may also influence epidural spread or mass movement of drug after an extrapleural paravertebral compartment injection. Clinically, sensory anesthesia is predominantly ipsilateral and greater after epidural spread than after paravertebral spread only [182].

INDICATIONS

TPBV offers several technical and clinical advantages and is indicated for anesthesia and analgesia when the afferent pain input is predominantly unilateral from the chest and/or abdomen. Common indications are:

Postoperative Analgesia

- Thoracic surgery [173, 174]: There is good evidence that paravertebral block can provide acceptable pain relief compared with thoracic epidural analgesia for thoracotomy. Important side-effects such as hypotension, urinary retention, nausea, and vomiting appear to be less frequent with paravertebral block than with TEA.

- Paravertebral block is associated with better pulmonary function and fewer pulmonary complications than TEA. Importantly, contraindications to thoracic epidural analgesia do not preclude paravertebral block, which can also be safely performed in anesthetized patients without an apparent increased risk of neurological injury [190].

- Breast surgery [191]. Paravertebral block improves the quality of recovery after breast cancer surgery and provides the patient with the option of ambulatory discharge [192].

- Video-assisted thoracoscopic surgery [191]. Perioperative multiple-injection thoracic paravertebral blocks with bupivacaine provide effective pain relief and a significant reduction in opioid requirements. This approach may also contribute to earlier postoperative ambulation after video-assisted thoracic surgery [193].

- Traumatic rib fracture: thoracic paravertebral infusion of bupivacaine is a simple and effective method of providing continuous pain relief in patients with unilateral multiple fractured ribs. It also produced a sustained improvement in respiratory parameters and oxygenation [194].

Surgical Anesthesia

- Breast surgery: Paravertebral block can be used to perform major operations for breast cancer with minimal complications and a low rate of conversion to general anesthesia. Paravertebral block markedly improves the quality of recovery after breast cancer surgery and provides the patient with the option of ambulatory discharge [170].

- VATS: Thoracic paravertebral block has proven to provide excellent surgical conditions and postoperative pain relief in two oncology patients with severe respiratory disease. It has allowed an optimal assessment of the anesthetic impact on respiratory function [234].

In a recent review it has been demonstrated that PVB can be at least as effective as epidural analgesia. It also has a better side-effect profile and a lower complication rate than epidural analgesia [174]. Other authors have shown that epidural analgesia is more efficient than paravertebral continuous block in reducing pain after thoracic surgery [173]. Quantitative meta-analyses were limited by heterogeneity in study design, and subject numbers were small. Further well designed studies are required to investigate the optimum components of the epidural solution and to rigorously evaluate the risks/benefits of continuous infusion paravertebral and intercostal techniques compared with TEA [159]. It must be underlined that this technique is used above all for postoperative analgesia but can reach a good level of anesthesia only for small surgical procedures [170].

Management of paravertebral block. The strongest predictor of improved analgesia and hence a lower failure rate after thoracotomy is the use of a higher dose of local anesthetic [195]. Postoperative pain appears to be decreased by around 50% with higher dose regimens, which is both clinically and statistically significant [195]. Perhaps even more importantly, the improved analgesia from higher dose regimes also translated into better recovery in pulmonary function [195]. The improvement in analgesia and pulmonary mechanics with the use of higher doses of paravertebral local anesthetics shown above must be balanced against the risk of possible local anesthetic toxicity. The absorption of bupivacaine from the paravertebral space has been shown to be rapid, with accumulation to toxic levels after prolonged infusion at 0.5 mg/kg/h [196-199], but not when dosage is reduced to 0.25 mg/kg/h after 24 h [200].

The incidence of serious local anesthetic toxicity with higher dose regimes is likely to be low regardless of the agent, especially where high doses are administered for 24h or less. Ropivacaine does not appear to accumulate in the same linear manner as bupivacaine, and is seen by some authors as a safer choice for PVB [201-203].

Considering the use of pre-emptive PVB and the use of an additive to LA , the authors found a modest improvement in perceived pain [195]. Adjuvant clonidine increased the risk of sedation [204].

TECHNICAL AND CLINICAL ADVANTAGES

Thoracic paravertebral block is technically easy to learn, has a high success rate regardless of the number of blocks performed, and does not appear to be operator-dependent [170, 205].

PVB provides comparable analgesia with epidural blockade after surgery but has a better side-effect profile. It is associated with less urinary retention, less postoperative nausea and vomiting, less hypotension and a reduction in pulmonary complications [206].

PVB offers an attractive alternative to epidural technique with few contraindications [200, 207].

Placement of the paravertebral catheter by the surgeon during thoracotomy further avoids some of the concerns regarding epidural placement in the presence of difficult anatomy, local sepsis or impaired coagulation [206]. For thoracic surgery, surgical placement of the catheter under direct vision would seem to be the most logical solution to avoid complications and guarantee drug delivery to the desired location [206]. It appears that PVB is advantageous and can be recommended for major thoracic and upper abdominal surgery [206].

CONTRAINDICATIONS

This technique is contraindicated in the case of infection at the site of needle insertion, empyema, allergy to local anesthetic drugs, and tumor occupying the TPVS [169, 170].

Relative contraindications involve coagulopathy, bleeding disorders or therapeutic anticoagulation [208]. One must be cautious with patients with kyphoscoliosis and those who had previous thoracotomy [169, 170]. Chest deformity in the former may predispose to thecal or pleural puncture, whereas obliteration of the TPVS by scar tissue and adhesion of the lung to the chest wall [206] in the latter, may predispose to pleural and pulmonary puncture.

COMPLICATIONS

- Possible local anesthetic toxicity manifested by confusion that resolved after its interruption, convulsions or cardiac dysrhythmias were the only complications reported in the majority of studies [199, 209-213].

- Vascular puncture [188].

- Hypotension [188]. This is uncommon after TPVB in normovolemic patients because of unilateral sympathetic blockade [185] but TPVB may unmask hypovolemia and result in hypotension [169, 170, 188]. Interestingly, hypotension does not appear to be a problem even after bilateral TPVB [188].

- Pleural puncture [188].

- Pneumothorax. Inadvertent pleural puncture is uncommon and may or may not result in a pneumothorax [188]. A unique case of clicking pneumothorax is also described [214].

- Pulmonary hemorrhage has been reported after percutaneous TPVB in a patient who had undergone previous thoracic surgery [215].

- Dural puncture–related complications: intrathecal injection, spinal anesthesia, and postural headache appear to be exclusive to the medial approach to the TPVS [178] and are probably related to the closer proximity of the needle to the dural cuff and intervertebral foramen. Transient ipsilateral [182, 216] or bilateral [182] Horner syndrome can also develop. The former is likely to be caused by spread of local anesthetic to the ipsilateral stellate ganglion or the preganglionic fibers originating from the first few segments of the thoracic spinal cord, whereas the latter may be caused by contralateral paravertebral spread *via* the prevertebral or epidural route [183, 216].

- Ipsilateral sensory changes in the arm [216] may also develop as a result of spread of local anesthetic to the T1 component of the brachial plexus in the thorax or the C8 component where it originates between C7 and T1, although further spread to the brachial plexus in the neck cannot be excluded [169].

- Bilateral symmetrical anesthesia [217] and ipsilateral thoracolumbar anesthesia [218].

LOCAL ANESTHESIA

Simple surgical procedures in thoracic surgery can be performed with the sole use of local anesthesia. For example, endobronchial electrocautery for tumor ablation and the treatment of hemoptysis can be performed under local anesthesia during a "routine" outpatient bronchoscopy [219].

Local anesthesia and sedation can represent a valid method to achieve anesthesia and analgesia in minor procedures performed in VATS and needlescopic VATS, especially when diagnosis and management of pleural disease are involved [220].

Minor procedures that can be carried out successfully using local anesthetic and sedation, as described in the literature, are:

- Drainage of empyema [220].

- Pleural biopsy [220].

- Pleural effusion with talc pleurodesis [220, 221].

- Lung biopsy (in VATS or minithoracotomy) [220, 222].

- Evacuate hemothorax [220].

- Pericardial window [220].

- Biopsy of chest wall mass [220].

- Mediastinal biopsy [233].

Local anesthesia can be performed in patients who are at high risk for general anesthesia because of sever pulmonary or underling disease when the intrathoracic pathology does not necessarily require the use of a double-lumen tube or need for intrathoracic or mediastinal dissection and in the absence of coagulopathy or cardiac dysfunction [220] (Fig. **5**).

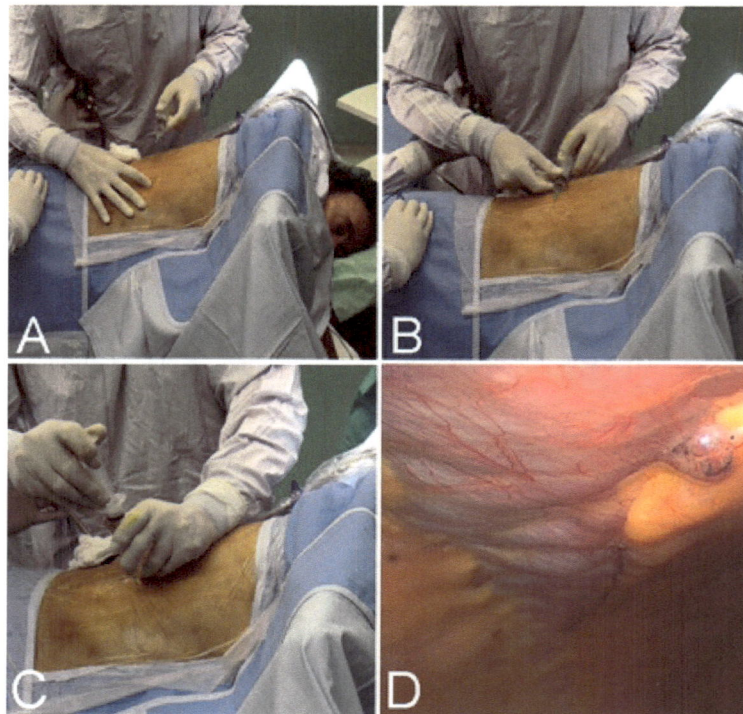

Fig. 5. Local anesthesia for awake thoracoscopic procedures. Subcutaneous puncture (A, B) is followed by infiltration of the intercostals (C) and subpleural space. After insertion of the camera, the proper position of the needle during subpleural infiltration can be carried out under thoracoscopic vision (D).

It can not be performed in patients who are not cooperative, in children, in obese patient or patients with thick muscles.

For a variety of diagnostic and therapeutic operations, VATS compared with thoracotomy results in reduced postoperative pain. However, some degree of pain may still afflict up to 63% of patients after VATS procedures [223-225].

Local anesthesia can also be used in order to achieve effective analgesia. It can be performed as a pre-emptive local anesthesia prior to surgery in the incision area [226] or by infiltration of local anesthetic in the wound at the end of surgery.

REFERENCES

[1]   Rodgers A, Walker N, Schug S, *et al.* Reduction of postoperative mortality and morbidity with epidural or spinal anaesthesia: results from overview of randomized trials. Br Med J. 2000;321:1493-497.

[2]   Franco A, Diz J.C. The history of the epidural block. Curr Anaesth Crit Care 2000;11:274-6.

[3]   Crawford OB, Springfield M. Peridural anaesthesia for thoracic surgery. NY State J Med 1952;52:2637-41.

[4]   Tenling A, Joachimsson P.O, Tydén H, Hedenstierna G. Thoracic epidural analgesia as an adjunct to general anaesthesia for cardiac surgery. Acta Anaesthesiol Scand 2001;44:1071-6.

[5]   Ali M, Winter D.C, Hanly A.M, *et al.* Prospective, randomized, controlled trial of thoracic epidural or patient-controlled opiate analgesia on perioperative quality of life. Br J Anaesth 2010;104:292-7.

[6]   Karagoz HY, Sonmez B, Bakkaloglu B, *et al.* Coronary artery bypass grafting in the conscious patient without endotracheal general anesthesia. Ann Thorac Surg 2000;70:91-6.

[7]   Karagoz HY, Kurtoglu M, Bakkaloglu B, *et al.* Coronary artery bypass grafting in the awake patient: three years' experience in 137 patients. J Thorac Cardiovasc Surg 2003;125:1401-4.

[8]   Paiste J, Bjerke R, Williams JP, *et al.* Minimally invasive direct coronary artery bypass surgery under high thoracic epidural. Anesth Analg 2001;93:1486-8.

[9]   Anderson MB, Kwong KF, Furst AJ, Salerna TA. Thoracic epidural anesthesia for coronary bypass *via* left anterior thoracotomy in the conscious patient. Eur J Cardiothorac Surg 2001;20:415-7.

[10]   Meininger D, Neidhart G, Bremerich DH, *et al.* Coronary artery bypass grafting *via* sternotomy in conscious patients. World J Surg 2003;27:534-8.

[11]   Mukaida T, Andou A, Date H, Aoe M, Shimizu N. Thoracoscopic operation for secondary pneumothorax under local and epidural anesthesia in highrisk patients. Ann Thorac Surg 1998;65:924-6.

[12]   Sugimoto S, Date H, Sugimoto R, *et al.* Thoracoscopic operation with local and epidural anesthesia in the treatment of penumothorax after lung transplantation. J Thorac Cardiovasc Surg 2005;130:1219-20.

[13]   Pompeo E, Tacconi F, Mineo D, Mineo TC. The role of awake video-assisted thoracoscopic surgery in spontaneous pneumothorax. J Thorac Cardiovasc Surg 2007;133:786-90.

[14]   Pompeo E, Mineo D, Rogliani P, Sabato AF, Mineo TC. Feasibility and results of awake thoracoscopic resection of solitary pulmonary nodules. Ann Thorac Surg 2004;78:1761-8.

[15]   Pompeo E, Mineo TC. Awake pulmonary metastasectomy. J Thorac Cardiovasc Surg 2007;133:960-6.

[16]   Mineo TC, Pompeo E, Mineo D, *et al.* Awake nonresectional lung volume reduction surgery. Ann Surg 2006;243:131-6.

[17]   Tsunezuka Y, Oda M, Matsumoto I, Tamura M, Watanabe G. Extended thymectomy in patients with myasthenia gravis with high thoracic epidural anesthesia alone. World J Surg 2004;28:962-5.

[18]   Al-Abdullatief M, Wahood A, Al-Shirawi N, *et al.* Awake anaesthesia for major thoracic surgical procedures: an observational study. Eur J Cardiothorac Surg 2007;32:346-50.

[19]   Clemente A, Carli F. The physiological effects of thoracic epidural anesthesia and analgesia on the cardiovascular, respiratory and gastrointestinal systems. Minerva Anestesiol 2008;74:549-63.

[20]   Quinn HH. Anatomy of the neuraxis. In: Cousins MJ, Bridenbaugh PO, Eds. Neural blockade in clinical anaesthesia and management of pain. Philadelphia, Lippincott, Williams & Wilkins, 1988; pp.181-212.

[21]   Maiman DJ, Pintar FA. Anatomy and clinical biomechanics of the thoracic spine. Clin Neurosurg 1992;38:296-324.

[22]   Bromage PR. Physiology and pharmacology of epidural analgesia. Anesthesiology 1967;28:592-622.

[23]   Tsigos C, Chrousos GP. Hypothalamic-pituitary-adrenal axis, neuroendocrine factors and stress . J Psychosom Res 2002;53:865-71.

[24]   Wilmore DW, Long JM, Mason AD, Pruitt BA Jr. Stress in surgical patients as a neurophysiologic reflex response. Surg Gynecol Obstet 1976;142:257-69.

[25]   Blomberg S, Emanuelsson H, Ricksten SE. Thoracic epidural anesthesia and central hemodynamics in patients with unstable angina pectoris. Anesth Analg 1989;69:558-62.

[26]   Davis RF, DeBoer LWV, Maroko PR. Thoracic epidural anesthesia reduces myocardial infarct size after coronary occlusion in dogs. Anesth Analg 1986;65:711-7.

[27]   Klassen GA, Bramwell RS, Bromage PR, Zborowska-Sluis DT. Effect on acute sympathectomy by epidural anesthesia on the canine coronary circulation. Anesthesiology 1980;52:8-15.

[28]   Kock M, Blomberg S, Emanuelsson H, *et al.* Thoracic epidural anesthesia improves global and regional left ventricular function during stress-induced myocardial ischemia in patients with coronary artery disease. Anesth Analg 1990;71:625-30.

[29] Williams JP, Sullivan EA, Ramakrishna H. Effects of thoracic epidural anesthesia on the coagulation system. Clin Anesth 1999;13:31-56.

[30] Jacobaeus H. The practical importance of thoracoscopy in surgery of the chest. Surg Gynecol Obstet 1922;34:289-96.

[31] Mark DB, Lam LC, Lee KI, *et al.* Effects of coronary angioplasty, coronary bypass surgery, and medical therapy on employment in patients with coronary artery disease. A prospective comparison study. Ann Intern Med 1994;120:111-7.

[32] Ribakove GH, Miller JS, Anderson RV, *et al.* Minimally invasive port-access coronary artery bypass grafting with early angiographic follow-up: initial clinical experience. J Thorac Cardiovasc Surg 1998;115:1101-10.

[33] Olausson K, Magnusdottir H, Lurje L *et al.* Anti-ischemic and anti-anginal effects of thoracic epidural anesthesia versus those of conventional medical therapy in the treatment of severe refractory unstable angina pectoris. Circulation 1997;96:2178-82.

[34] Berendes E, Schmidt C, Van Aken H *et al.* Reversible cardiac sympathectomy by high thoracic epidural anesthesia improves regional left ventricular function in patients undergoing coronary artery bypass grafting. Arch Surg 2003;138:1283-90.

[35] Fuller JA, Adams GG, Buxton B. Atrial fibrillation after coronary artery bypass grafting: is it a disorder of the elderly? J Thorac Cardiovasc Surg 1989;97:821-5.

[36] Hobbs WJC, Fitchet A, Cotter L, *et al.* Atrial Arrhythmias after Cardiac Surgery. N Engl J Med 1997;337:860-86.

[37] Liu SS, Block BM, Wu CL. Effects of perioperative central neuroaxial analgesia on outcome after coronary artery bypass surgery: a meta-analysis. Anesthesiology 2004;101:153-61.

[38] Oka T, Ozawa Y, Ohkubo Y. Thoracic epidural bupivacaine attenuates supraventricular tachyarrhythmias after pulmonary resection. Anesth Analg 2001;93:253-9.

[39] Holte K, Foss N, Svense'n C *et al.* Epidural anesthesia, hypotension, and changes in intravascular volume Anesthesiology 2004;100:281-6.

[40] Neal JM, Wilcox RT, Allen HW, Low DE. Near-total esophagectomy: the influence of standardized multimodal management and intaoperative fluid restriction. Reg Anesth Pain Med 2003;28:328-34.

[41] Ford GT, Whitelaw WA, Rosenal TW, *et al.* Diaphragm function after upper abdominal surgery in humans. Am Rev Respir Dis 1983;127:431-6.

[42] Brooks-Brunn JA. Postoperative atelectasis and pneumonia. Heart Lung 1995;24:94-115.

[43] Tokics L, Hedenstierna G, Svensson L, *et al.* V/Q distribution and correlation to atelectasis in anesthetize paralyzed humans. J Appl Physiol 1996;81:1822-33.

[44] Grichnik KP, Clark JA. Pathophysiology and management of one-lung ventilation. Thorac Surg Clin 2005;15:85-103.

[45] Benumof J. Anesthesia for thoracic surgery: recent advances. Can Anaesth Soc J 1986;33:528-37.

[46] Gruber EM, Tschernko EM, Kritzinger M *et al.* The effects of thoracic epidural analgesia with bupivacaine 0.25% on ventilatory mechanics in patients with severe chronic obstructive pulmonary disease. Anesth Analg 2001;92:1015-9.

[47] Takasaki M, Takahashi T. Respiratory function during cervical and thoracic extradural analgesia in patients with normal lungs. Br J Anaesth 1980;52:1271-6.

[48] Bauer C, Hentz J.G, Ducrocq X *et al.* Lung function after lobectomy: a randomized, double-blinded trial comparing thoracic epidural Ropivacaine/Sufentanil and intravenous Morphine for patient-controlled analgesia. Anesth Analg 2007;105:238-44.

[49] Mankikian B, Cantineau JP, Bertrand M *et al.* Improvement of diaphragmatic function by a thoracic extradural block after upper abdominal surgery. Anesthesiolgy 1988;68:379-86.

[50] Park WY, Thompson JS & Lee KK. Effect of epidural anesthesia and analgesia on perioperative outcome: randomized, controlled Veterans Affairs Cooperative Study. Ann Surg 2001;234:560-9.

[51] Mineo T.C. Epidural anesthesia in awake thoracic surgery. Eur J Cardiothorac Surg 2007;32:13-19.

[52] Von Dossow V, Welte M, Zaune U, *et al.* Thoracic epidural anesthesia combined with general anesthesia: the preferred anesthetic technique for thoracic surgery. Anesth Analg 2001;92:848-54.

[53] Hachenberg T, Holst D, Ebel C, *et al.* Effect of thoracic epidural anaesthesia on ventilation-perfusion distribution and intrathoracic blood volume before and after induction of general anaesthesia. Acta Anaesthesiol Scand 1997;41:1142-8.

[54] Groeben H. Epidural anesthesia and pulmonary function. J Anesth 2006;20:290-9.

[55]   Jordan DA, Miller ED jr. Subarachnoid blockade alters homeostasis by modifying compensatory splanchnic responses to hemorrhagic hypotension. Anesthesiology 1991;75:654-61.

[56]   Sielenkämper AW, Van Aken H. Thoracic epidural anesthesia: more than just anesthesia/analgesia. Anesthesiology 2003;99:523-5.

[57]   Meissner A, Weber T, Van Aken H, *et al*. Limited upper thoracic epidural block and splanchnic perfusion in dogs. Anesth Analg 1999;89:1378-81.

[58]   Christopherson R, Beattie C, Frank SM, *et al*. Perioperative morbidity in patients randomized to epidural or general anesthesia for lower extremity vascular surgery. Anesthesiology 1993;79:422-34.

[59]   Schwarte L.A., Picker O, Höhne C, *et al*. Effects of thoracic epidural anaesthesia on microvascular gastric mucosal oxygenation in physiological and compromised circulatory conditions in dogs. Br J Anaesth 2004;93:552-9.

[60]   Freise H, Fischer LG. Intestinal effects of thoracic epidural anesthesia. Curr Opin Anaesthesiol 2009;22:644-8.

[61]   Carli F, Phil.M, Mayo N, *et al*. Epidural analgesia enhances functional exercise capacity and health-related quality of life after colonic surgery. Results of a randomized trial. Anesthesiology 2002;97:540-9.

[62]   Waurick R, Van Aken H. Update in thoracic epidural anaesthesia. Best Pract Res Clin Anaesthesiol. 2005;19:201-13.

[63]   Holte K , Kehlet H: Epidural anaesthesia and analgesia - effects on surgical stress responses and implications for postoperative nutrition.Clin Nutr 2002;21:199-206.

[64]   Segawa H, Mor K, Kasai K, *et al*. The role of the phrenic nerves in stress response in upper abdominal surgery. Anesth Analg 1996;82:1215-24.

[65]   Lattermann R, Carli F, Wykes L, Schricker T. Epidural blockade modifies perioperative glucose production without affecting protein catabolism. Anesthesiology 2002;97:374-81.

[66]   Ballantyne JC, Carr DB, De Ferranti S, *et al*. The comparative effects of postoperative analgesic therapies on pulmonary outcome: cumulative meta-analyses of randomized, controlled trials. Anesth Analg 1998;86:598-612.

[67]   Bredbacka S, Blomback M, Hagnevik K, *et al*. Peri- and postoperative changes in coagulation and fibrinolytic variables during abdominal hysterectomy under epidural or general anaesthesia. Acta Anaesthesiol Scand 1986;30:204-1.

[68]   Modig J, Borg T, Bagge L, Saldeen T. Role of extradural and of general anaesthesia in fibrinolysis and coagulation after total hip replacement. Br J Anaesth 1983;55:625-9.

[69]   Moraca RJ, Sheldon DG, Thirlby RC. The role of epidural anesthesia and analgesia in surgical practice. Ann Surg 2003,238:663-73.

[70]   Kehlet H, Holte K. Effect of postoperative analgesia on surgical outcome. Br J Anaesth 2001;87:62-72.

[71]   Elia S, Guggino G, Mineo D, *et al*. Awake one stage bilateral thoracoscopic sympathectomy for palmar hyperhidrosis: a safe outpatient procedure. Eur J Cardiothorac Surg 2005;28:312-7.

[72]   Visser L. Epidural Anesthesia. Update in Anesthesia [serial on the Internet]. 2001. Available from: http://www.nda.ox.ac.uk/wfsa/htlm/u13/u1311_01.htm

[73]   Beaudroit L, Ripart J. Nerve blocks of the trunk: indications, techniques, advantages and complications. Ann Fr Anesth Reanim 2009;28:79-83.

[74]   Congedo E, Sgreccia M, De Cosmo G. New drugs for epidural analgesia. Curr Drug Targets 2009;10:696-706.

[75]   Albright GA. Cardiac arrest following regional anesthesia with etidocaine and bupivacaine. Anesthesiology 1979;51:285-7.

[76]   Buyse I, Stockman W, Columb M, *et al*. Effect of sufentanil on minimum local analgesic concentrations of epidural bupivacaine, ropivacaine and levobupivacaine in nullipara in early labour. Intern J Obst Anest 2007;16:22-8.

[77]   Ekenstam BAF, Egner B, Petterson GN. N-alkyl pyrrolidine and N-alkyl piperidine carboxylic acid amines. Acta Chem Scand 1957;11:1183-90.

[78]   Aberg G. Toxicological and local anesthetic effects of optically active isomers of two local anesthetic compounds. Acta Pharmacol Toxicol Scand 1972;31:273-86.

[79]   Leone S, Di Cianni S, Casati A, Fanelli G. Pharmacology, toxicology, and clinical use of new long acting local anesthetics, ropivacaine and levobupivacaine. Acta Biomed 2008;79:92-105.

[80]   Marganella C, Bruno V, Matrisciano F, *et al*.Comparative effects of levobupivacaine and racemic bupivacaine on excitotoxic neuronal death in culture and N-methyl-D-aspartate-induced seizures in mice. Eur J Pharmacol 2005;518:111-5.

[81]   Gristwood RW. Cardiac and CNS toxicity of levobupivacaine: strengths of evidence for advantage over bupivacaine. Drug Saf 2002;25:153-63.

[82]   Clarkson CW, Hondeghem LM. Mechanism for bupivacaine depression of cardiac conduction: fast block of sodium channels during the action potential with slow recovery from block during diastole. Anesthesiology 1985;62:396-405.

[83]   Arlock P. Actions of three local anesthetics: lidocaine, bupivacaine and ropivacaine on guinea pig papillary muscle sodium channels (Vmax). Pharmacol Toxicol 1988;63:96-104.

[84]   Avery P, Redon D, Schaenzer G, Rusy B. The influence of serum potassium on cerebral and cardiac toxicity of bupivacaine and lidocaine. Anesthesiology 1984;61:134-8.

[85]   Valenzuela C, Delpon E, Tamkun MM, *et al.* Stereoselective block of a human cardiac potassium channel (Kv 1.5) by bupivacaine enantiomers. Biophys J 1995;69:418-2.

[86]   Kawano T, Oshita S,Takahashi A, *et al.* Molecular mechanisms of the inhibitory effects of bupivacaine, levobupivacaine, and ropivacaine on sarcolemmal adenosine triphosphate-sensitive potassium channels in the cardiovascular system. Anesthesiology 2004;101:390-8.

[87]   Heavner JE. Cardiac toxicity of local anesthetics in the intact isolated heart model: a review. Reg Anesth Pain Med 2002;27:545-5.

[88]   Stewart J, Kellett N, Castro D. The central nervous system and cardiovascular effects of levobupivacaine and ropivacaine in healthy volunteers. Anesth Analg 2003; 97:412-6.

[89]   Knudsen K, Suurkula MB, Blomberg S, *et al.* Central nervous and cardiovascular effects of i.v. infusion. Br J Anaesth 1997;78:507-14.

[90]   Scott DB, Lee A, Fagan D, *et al.* Acute toxicity of ropivacaine compared with that of bupivacaine. Anesth Analg 1989;69:563-9.

[91]   Bardsley H, Gristwood R, Baker H, *et al.* A comparison of the cardiovascular effects of levobupivacaine and rac-bupivacaine following intravenous administration to healthy volunteers. Br J Clin Pharmacol 1998;46:245-9.

[92]   Polley LS, Columb MO, Naughton NN, *et al.* Relative analgesic potencies of ropivacaine and bupivacaine for epidural analgesia in labor. Anesthesiology 1999;90:944-50.

[93]   Capogna G, Celleno D, Fusco P, *et al.* Relative potencies of bupivacaine and ropivacaine for analgesia in labour. Br J Anaesth 1999;82:371-3.

[94]   Katz JA, Knarr D, Bridenbaugh PO. A double-blind comparison of 0.5% bupivacaine and 0.75% ropivacaine administered epidurally in humans. Reg Anesth 1990;15:250-2.

[95]   Kerkkamp HE, Gielen MJ, Edstrom HH. Comparison of 0.75% ropivacaine with epinephrine and 0.75% bupivacaine with epinephrine in lumbar epidural anesthesia. Reg Anesth 1990;15:204-7.

[96]   Wolff AP, Hasselstrom L, Kerkkamp HE *et al.* Extradural ropivacaine and bupivacaine in hip surgery. Br J Anaesth 1995;74:458-60.

[97]   McGlade DP, Kalpokas MV, Mooney PH, *et al.* Comparison of 0.5% ropivacaine and 0.5% bupivacaine in lumbar epidural anaesthesia for lower limb orthopaedic surgery. Anaesth Intensive Care 1997;25:262-6.

[98]   Crosby E, Sandler A, Finucane B, *et al.* Comparison of epidural anaesthesia with ropivacaine 0.5% and bupivacaine 0.5% for caesarean section. Can J Anaesth 1998;45:1066-71.

[99]   Kampe S,Tausch B, Paul M, *et al.* Epidural block with ropivacaine and bupivacaine for elective cesarean section: maternal cardiovascular parameters, comfort and neonatal well-being. Curr Med Res Opin 2004;20:7-12.

[100] Tacconi F, Pompeo E, Fabbi E, Mineo TC. Awake video-assisted pleural decortication for empyema thoracis. Eur J Cardiothorac Surg 2010;37:594-61.

[101] Casati A, Santorsola R, Aldegheri G, *et al.* Intraoperative epidural anesthesia and postoperative analgesia with levobupivacaine for major orthopedic surgery: a double-blind, randomized comparison of racemic bupivacaine and ropivacaine. J Clin Anesth 2003;15:126-31.

[102] Aybek T, Kessle Pr, Dogan S, *et al.* Awake coronary artery bypass grafting: utopia or reality? Ann Thorac Surg 2003;75:1165-70.

[103] Kessle Pr, Neidhar Gt, Bremerich DH, *et al.* High thoracic epidural anesthesia for coronary artery bypass grafting using two different surgical approaches in conscious patients. Anesth Analg 2002;95:791-7.

[104] Wheatley RG, Schug SA, Watson D. Safety and efficacy of postoperative epidural analgesia. Br J Anaesth 2001;87:47-61.

[105] Schug SA, Saunders D, Kurowski I, *et al.* Neuraxial drug administration. Review article. CNS Drugs 2006;20:917-33.

[106] Hansdottir V, Woestenborghs R, Nordberg G. The cerebrospinal fluid and plasma pharmacokinetics of sufentanil after thoracic or lumbar epidural administration. Anesth Analg 1995;80:724-9.

[107]   Stevens RA, Petty RH, Hill HF, *et al*. Redistribution of sufentanil to cerebrospinal fluid and systemic circulation after epidural administration in dogs. Anesth Analg 1993;76:323-7.

[108]   Hansdottir V, Bake B, Nordberg G. The analgesic efficacy and adverse effects of continuous epidural sufentanil and bupivacaine infusion after thoracotomy. Anesth Analg 1996;83:394-400.

[109]   Ummenhofer WC, Arends RH, Shen DD, *et al*. Comparative spinal distribution and clearance kinetics of intrathecally administered morphine, fentanyl, alfentanil, and sufentanil. Anesthesiology 2000;92:739-53.

[110]   Swenson JD, Owen J, Lamoreaux W, *et al*. The effect of distance from injection site to the brainstem using spinal sufentanil. Reg Anesth Pain Med 2001;26:306-9.

[111]   Joris JL, Jacob EA, Sessler DI, *et al*. Spinal mechanisms contribute to analgesia produced by epidural sufentanil combined with bupivacaine for postoperative analgesia. Anesth Analg 2003;97:1446-51.

[112]   Kilbride MJ, Senagore AJ, Mazier WP, *et al*. Epidural analgesia. Surg Gynecol Obstet 1992;174:137-40.

[113]   Bernards CM. Epidural and intrathecal opioids: which drugs should we choose and how should they be used? In: Schwartz AJ, Ed. Refresher courses of anesthesiology. Baltimore, Lippincott, Williams & Wilkins, 1999; pp. 13-30.

[114]   Ellis DJ, Millar WL, Reisner LS. A randomized double-blind comparison of epidural versus intravenous fentanyl infusion for analgesia after cesarean section. Anesthesiology 1990;72:981-6.

[115]   Loper KA, Ready LB, Downey M, *et al*. Epidural and intravenous fentanyl infusions are clinically equivalent after knee surgery. Anesth Analg 1990;70:72-5.

[116]   Guinard JP, Mavrocordatos P, Chiolero R, Carpenter RL. A randomized comparison of intravenous versus lumbar and thoracic epidural fentanyl for analgesia after thoracotomy. Anesthesiology 1992;77:1108-15.

[117]   Geller E, Chrubasik J, Graf R, *et al*. A randomized double-blind comparison of epidural sufentanil versus intravenous sufentanil or epidural fentanyl analgesia after major abdominal surgery. Anesth Analg 1993;76:1243-50.

[118]   Lubenow TR, Tanck EN, Hopkins EM, *et al*. Comparison of patient-assisted epidural analgesia with continuous-infusion epidural analgesia for postoperative patients. Reg Anesth 1994;19:206-11.

[119]   Miguel R, Barlow I, Morrell M, *et al*. A prospective, randomized, double-blind comparison of epidural and intravenous sufentanil infusions. Anesthesiology 1994;81:346-52

[120]   Bernards CM. Understanding the physiology and pharmacology of epidural and intrathecal opioids. Best Pract Res Clin Anaesthesiol 2002;16:489-505.

[121]   Bernards CM, Shen DD, Sterling ES, *et al*. Epidural, cerebrospinal fluid, and plasma pharmacokinetics of epidural opiods (part 1): differences among opiods. Anesthesiology 2003;99:455-65.

[122]   Hamber EA, Viscomi CM. Intrathecal lipophilic opioids as adjuncts to surgical spinal anesthesia. Reg Anesth Pain Med 1999;24:255-63.

[123]   Polley L, Columb M, Naughton N, *et al*. Effect of intravenous versus epidural fentanyl on the minimum local analgesic concentration of epidural bupivacaine in labor. Anesthesiology 2000;93:122-8.

[124]   Fournier R, Gamulin Z, Van Gessel E. Respiratory depression after 5 micrograms of intrathecal sufentanil. Anesth Analg 1998;87:1377-8.

[125]   Chaney MA. Side effects of intrathecal and epidural opioids. Can J Anaesth 1995;42: 891-903.

[126]   Tsui BC, Wagner A, Finucane B. Regional anaesthesia in the elderly: a clinical guide. Drugs Aging 2004;21:895-910.

[127]   Szarvas S, Harmon D, Murphy D. Neuraxial opioid-induced pruritus: a review. J Clin Anesth 2003;15:234-9.

[128]   Eisenach JC, De Kock M, Klimscha W. Alpha (2)-adrenergic agonists for regional anesthesia: a clinical review of clonidine (1984-1995). Anesthesiology 1996;85:655-74.

[129]   Bouguet D: Caudal clonidine added to local anesthetics enhances post-operative analgesia after anal surgery in adults.Anesthesiology 1994;81:A942.

[130]   Walker SM, Goudas LC, Cousins MJ, *et al*. Combination spinal analgesic chemotherapy: a systematic review. Anesth Analg 2002;95:674-715.

[131]   Novak-Jankovic V, Paver E, Iban A, *et al*: Effect of epidural and intravenous clonidine on the neuro-endocrine and immune stress response in patients undergoing lung surgery. Eur J Anaesthesiol 2000;17:50-6.

[132]   Bailey PL, Sperry RJ, Johnson GK, *et al*. Respiratory effects of clonidine alone and combined with morphine, in humans Anesthesiology 1991;74:43-8.

[133]   Subramaniam K, Subramaniam B, Steinbrook RA. Ketamine as adjuvant analgesic to opioids: a quantitative and qualitative systematic review. Anesth Analg 2004;99:482-95.

[134]   Kohno T, Wakai A, Ataka T, *et al*. Actions of midazolam on excitatory transmission in dorsal horn neurons of adult rat spinal cord. Anesthesiology 2006;104:338-43.

[135] Yaksh TL, Allen JW. Preclinical insights into the implementation of intrathecal midazolam: a cautionary tale. Anesth Analg 2004;98:1509-11.

[136] Yaksh TL, Allen JW. The use of intrathecal midazolam in humans: a case study of process. Anesth Analg 2004;98:1536-45.

[137] Tucker AP, Mezzatesta J, Nadeson R, *et al.* Intrathecal midazolam II: combination with intrathecal fentanyl for labor pain. Anesth Analg 2004;98:1521-7.

[138] Wilson W, Benumof J. Anesthesia for thoracic surgery. In Miller RD, Ed. Miller's Anesthesia, 6th edition. Oxford, Churchill Livingstone, 2005; pp. 1907-8 .

[139] Fischer B, Chaudhari M. Techniques of epidural block. Anaesth Intens Care Med 2006;7:422-6.

[140] De Cosmo G, Aceto P, Gualtieri E, Congedo E. Analgesia in thoracic surgery: review. Minerva Anestesiol 2009;75:393-400.

[141] Ochroch EA, Gottschalk A, Augostides J, *et al.* Long-term pain and activity during recovery from major thoracotomy using thoracic epidural analgesia. Anesthesiology 2002;97:1234-44.

[142] Hazelrigg SR, Cetindag IB, Fullerton J. Acute and chronic pain syndromes after thoracic surgery. Surg Clin North Am 2002;82:849-65.

[143] Wailer DA, Forty J, Morritt G. Video-assisted thoracoscopic surgery versus thoracotomy for spontaneous pneumothorax. Ann Thorac Surg 1994;58:372-7.

[144] Schulman M, Sandler AN, Bradley JW, *et al.* Post-thoracotomy pain and pulmonary function following epidural and systemic morphine. Anesthesiology 1984;61:569-71.

[145] Slinger P, Shennib H, Wilson S. Postthoracotomy pulmonary function: a comparison of epidural versus intravenous meperidine infusions. J Cardiothorac Vasc Anesth 1995;9:128-34.

[146] Guai J. The benefit of adding epidural analgesia to general anaesthesia: a meta-analysis. Br. J Anaesth 2006;20:290-9.

[147] Perttunen K, Nilsson E, Heinonen J. Exradural paravertebral and intercostal nerve blocks for postthoracotomy pain. Br J Anaesth 1995;75:541-7.

[148] Peeters-Asdourian C, Gupta S. Choices in pain management following thoracotomy. Chest 1999;115:S122-S124.

[149] Debrecini G, Molnar Z, Szelig L, Molnar TF. Continuous epidural or intercostal analgesia following thoracotomy: a prospective randomised double-blind clinical trial. Acta Anaesthesiol Scand 2003;47:1091-5.

[150] Carli F, Klubien K. Thoracic epidurals: is analgesia all we want? Can J Anaesth 1999;46:409-14.

[151] Liu SS, Allen HW, Olsson GL. Patient controlled epidural analgesia with bupivacaine and fentanyl on hospital wards: prospective experience with 1,030 surgical patients. Anesthesiology 1998;88:688-95.

[152] Azad SC. Perioperative pain management in patients undergoing thoracic surgery. Curr Opin Anaesthesiol 2001;14:87-91.

[153] Mourisse J, Hasenbos MAWM, Gielen MJM, *et al.* Epidural bupivacaine, sufentanil or the combination for postthoracotomy pain. Acta Anaesthesiol Scand 1992;36:70-4.

[154] Gautier P, De Kock M, Van Steenberge A, *et al.* A double-blind comparison of 0.125% ropivacaine with sufentanil and 0.125% bupivacaine with sufentanil for epidural labor analgesia. Anesthesiology 1999;90:772-8.

[155] Berti M, Fanelli G, Casati A, *et al.* Patient supplemented epidural analgesia after major abdominal surgery with bupivacaine/fentanyl or ropivacaine/fentanyl. Can J Anaesth 2000;47:27-32.

[156] Hodgson PS, Liu SS. A comparison of ropivacaine with fentanyl to bupivacaine with fentanyl for postoperative patientcontrolled epidural analgesia. Anesth Analg 2001;92:1024-8.

[157] Muldoon T, Milligan K, Quinn P, *et al.* Comparison between extradural infusion of ropivacaine or bupivacaine for the prevention of postoperative pain after total knee arthroplasty. Br J Anaesth 1998;80:680-1.

[158] Macias A, Monedero P, Adame M, *et al.* A randomized, double-blinded comparison of thoracic epidural ropivacaine, ropivacaine/fentanyl, or bupivacaine/fentanyl for postthoracotomy analgesia. Anesth Analg 2002;95:1344-50.

[159] Joshi GP, Bonnet F, Shah R. A systematic review of randomized trials evaluating regional techniques for postthoracotomy analgesia. Anesth Analg 2008;107:1026-40.

[160] Liu SS, Moore JM, Luo AM, *et al.* Comparison of three solutions of ropivacaine/fentanyl for postoperative patient-controlled epidural analgesia. Anesthesiology 1999;90:727-33.

[161] Wang SC, Chang YY, Chang KY, *et al.* Comparison of three different concentrations of ropivacaine for postoperative patient-controlled thoracic epidural analgesia after upper abdominal surgery. Acta Anaesthesiol Taiwan 2008;46:100-5.

[162] Cook TM, Counsell D, Wildsmith JA; Royal College of Anaesthetists Third National Audit Project. Major complications of central neuraxial block: report on the Third National Audit Project of the Royal College of Anaesthetists. Br J Anaesth 2009;102:179-90.

[163] Curatolo M, Scaramozzino P, Venuti FS, *et al.* Factors associated with hypotension and bradycardia after epidural blockade. Anesth Analg 1996;83:1033-40.

[164] Brull R, McCartney CJ, Chan VW, El-Beheiry H. Neurological complications after regional anesthesia: contemporary estimates of risk. Anesth Analg 2007;104:965-74.

[165] D'agapeyeff A, Crabb IJ. Unexpectedly high block following epidural catheter placement under direct vision: a case report. Anaesth Intensive Care 2005;33:128-30.

[166] Jenkins JG. Some immediate serious complications of obstetric epidural analgesia and anaesthesia: a prospective study of 145,550 epidurals.Int J Obstet Anesth 2005;14:37-42.

[167] Harrington BE, Schmitt AM. Meningeal (postdural) puncture headache, unintentional dural puncture, and the epidural blood patch: a national survey of United States practice. Reg Anesth Pain Med 2009;34:430-7.

[168] Cox B, Durieux ME, Marcus MA. Toxicity of local anaesthetics. Best Pract Res Clin Anaesthesiol 2003;17:111-36.

[169] Karmakar MK. Thoracic paravertebral block. Anesthesiology 2001;95:771.

[170] Coveney E, Weltz CR, *et al.* Use of paravertebral block anesthesia in the surgical management of breast cancer. Ann Surg 1998;227:496-501.

[171] Detterbeck FC. Efficacy of methods of intercostal nerve blockade for pain relief after thoracotomy. Ann Thorac Surg 2005;80:1550-9.

[172] Richardson J, Sabanathan S, Shah R. Post-thoracotomy spirometric lung function: the effect of analgesia. J Cardiovasc Surg 1999;40:445-6.

[173] Messina M, Boroli F, Landoni G, *et al.* A comparison of epidural vs. paravertebral blockade in thoracic surgery. Minerva Anestesiol. 2009;75:616-21.

[174] Scarci M, Joshi A, Attia R. In patients undergoing thoracic surgery is paravertebral block as effective as epidural analgesia for pain management? Interact Cardiovasc Thorac Surg 2010;10:92-96.

[175] Naja MZ, Ziade MF, El Rajab M, *et al.* Varying anatomical injection points within the thoracic paravertebral space: effect on spread of solution and nerve blockade. Anaesthesia 2004;59:459.

[176] Shibata Y, Chin KJ. The costovertebral angle. Thorac Surg Clin 2007;17:503-10.

[177] Eason MJ, Wyatt R. Paravertebral thoracic block-a reappraisal. Anaesthesia 1979;34:638-42.

[178] Sharrock NE. Postural headache following thoracic somatic paravertebral nerve block. Anesthesiology 1980;52:360-2.

[179] Evans PJ, Lloyd JW, Wood GJ. Accidental intrathecal injection of bupivacaine and dextran. Anaesthesia 1981;36:685-7.

[180] Riain SC, Donnell BO, Cuffe T, *et al.* Thoracic paravertebral block using real-time ultrasound guidance. Anesth Analg 2010;110:248-51.

[181] Conacher ID, Kokri M: Postoperative paravertebral blocks for thoracic surgery: A radiological appraisal. Br J Anaesth 1987;59:155-61.

[182] Purcell-Jones G, Pither CE, Justins DM: Paravertebral somatic nerve block: A clinical, radiographic, and computed tomographic study in chronic pain patients. Anesth Analg 1989;68:32-9.

[183] MacIntosh RR, Mushin WW. Observations on the epidural space. Anaesthesia 1947;2:100-4.

[184] Conacher ID. Resin injection of thoracic paravertebral spaces. Br J Anaesth 1988;61:657-61.

[185] McKnight CK, Marshall M. Monoplatythela and paravertebral block (letter). Anaesthesia 1984;39:1147.

[186] Cheema SP, Ilsley D, Richardson J, Sabanathan S. A thermographic study of paravertebral analgesia. Anaesthesia 1995;50:118-21.

[187] Eng J, Sabanathan S. Site of action of continuous extrapleural intercostal nerve block. Ann Thorac Surg 1991;51:387-9.

[188] Lönnqvist PA, MacKenzie J, Soni AK, Conacher ID. Paravertebral blockade: failure rate and complications. Anaesthesia 1995;50:813-5.

[189] Moore DC. Intercostal nerve block: spread of india ink injected to the rib's costal groove. Br J Anaesth 1981;53:325-9.

[190] Daly DJ, Myles PS. Update on the role of paravertebral blocks for thoracic surgery: are they worth it? Curr Opin Anaesthesiol 2009;22:38-43.

[191] Boughey JC, Goravanchi F, Parris RN, *et al.* Improved postoperative pain control using thoracic paravertebral block for breast operations. Breast J 2009;15:483-8.

[192] Naccache N, Jabbour H, Nasser-Ayoub E, *et al.* Regional analgesia and breast cancer surgery. J Med Liban 2009;57:110-4.

[193] Kaya FN, Turker G, Basagan-Mogol E, *et al.* Preoperative multiple-injection thoracic paravertebral blocks reduce postoperative pain and analgesic requirements after video-assisted thoracic surgery. J Cardiothorac Vasc Anesth 2006;20:639-43.

[194] Karmakar MK, Critchley LA, Ho AM, *et al.* Continuous thoracic paravertebral infusion of bupivacaine for pain management in patients with multiple fractured ribs. Chest 2003;123:424-31.

[195] Kotze A, Scally A, Howell S. Efficacy and safety of different techniques of paravertebral block for analgesia after thoracotomy: a systematic review and metaregression. Br J Anaesth 2009;103:626-36.

[196] Berrisford RG, Sabanathan SS. Direct access to the paravertebral space at thoracotomy. Ann Thorac Surg 1990;49:854.

[197] Burlacu CL, Frizelle HP, Moriarty DC, Buggy DJ. Pharmacokinetics of levobupivacaine, fentanyl, and clonidine after administration into the paravertebral space. Reg Anesth Pain Med 2007;32:136-4.

[198] Cheung SLW, Booker PD, Franks R, Pozzi M. Serum concentration of bupivacaine during prolonged continuous paravertebral infusion in young infants. Br J Anaesth 1997;79:9-13.

[199] Dauphin A, Gupta RN, Young AE, Morton WD. Serum bupivicaine concentrations during continuous extrapleural infusion. Can J Anaesth 1997;44:367-70.

[200] Kaiser AM, Zollinger A, De Lorenzi D, *et al.* Prospective, randomized comparison of extrapleural versus epidural analgesia for postthoracotomy pain. Ann Thorac Surg 1998;66:367-72.

[201] Cheema S, Richardson J, McGurgan P. Factors affecting the spread of bupivacaine in the adult thoracic paravertebral space. Anaesthesia 2003;58:684-711.

[202] De Cosmo G, Aceto P, Campanale A, *et al.* Comparison between epidural and paravertebral intercostals nerve block with ropivacaine after thoracotomy: effects on pain relief, pulmonary function and patient satisfaction. Acta Med Rom 2002;40:340-7.

[203] Marrett E, Bazelly B, Taylor G, *et al.* Paravertebral block with ropivacaine 0.5% versus systemic analgesia for pain relief after thoracotomy. Ann Thorac Surg 2005;79:2109-14.

[204] Bhatnagar S, Mishra S, Madhurima S, *et al.* Clonidine as an analgesic adjuvant to continuous paravertebral bupivacaine for post-thoracotomy pain. Anaesth Intensive Care 2006;34:586-9.

[205] Kirvela O, Antila H. Thoracic paravertebral block in chronic postoperative pain. Reg Anesth 1992;17:348-50.

[206] Davies RG, Myles PS, Graham JM. A comparison of the analgesic efficacy and side-effects of paravertebral vs epidural blockade for thoracotomy-a systematic review and meta-analysis of randomized trials. Br J Anaesth 2006;96:418-26.

[207] Perttunen K, Nilsson E, Heinonen J, *et al.* Extradural, paravertebral and intercostal nerve blocks for postthoracotomy pain. Br J Anaesth 1995;75:541-7.

[208] Richardson J, Lönnqvist PA. Thoracic paravertebral block. Br J Anaesth 1998;81:230-8.

[209] Carabine UA, Gilliland H, Johnston JR, McGuigan J. Pain relief after thoracotomy: comparison of morphine requirements using an extrapleural infusion of bupivacaine. Reg Anesth 1995;20:412-7.

[210] Casati A, Alessandrini P, Nuzzi M, *et al.* A prospective, randomized, blinded comparison between continuous thoracic paravertebral and epidural infusion of 0.2% ropivacaine after lung resection surgery. Eur J Anaesthesiol 2006;23:999-1004.

[211] Catala E, Casa JI, Unzueta MC, *et al.* Continuous infusion is superior to bolus doses with thoracic paravertebral blocks after thoracotomies. J Cardiothorac Vasc Anesth 1996;10:586-8.

[212] Deneuville M, Bisserier A, Regnard JF, *et al.* Continuous intercostals analgesia with 0.5% ropivacaine after thoracotomy: a randomized study. Ann Thorac Surg 1993;55:381-5.

[213] Watson DS, Panian S, Kendall V, *et al.* Pain control after thoracotomy: bupivacaine versus lidocaine in continuous extrapleural intercostal nerve blockade. Ann Thorac Surg 1999;67:825-9.

[214] Lall NG, Sharma SR. "Clicking" pneumothorax following thoracic paravertebral block: Case report. Br J Anaesth 1971;43:415-7.

[215] Thomas PW, Sanders DJ, Berrisford RG. Pulmonary haemorrhage after percutaneous paravertebral block. Br J Anaesth 1999;83:668-9.

[216] Tenicela R, Pollan SB. Paravertebral-peridural block technique: a unilateral thoracic block. Clin J Pain 1990;6:227-34.

[217] Bigler D, Dirkes W, Hansen R, *et al.* Effects of thoracic paravertebral block with bupivacaine versus combined thoracic epidural block with bupivacaine and morphine on pain and pulmonary function after cholecystectomy. Acta Anaesthesiol Scand 1989;33:561-4.

[218]   Saito T, Gallagher ET, Yamada K, *et al.* Broad unilateral analgesia. Reg Anesth 1994; 19:360-1.

[219]   Ernst A, Silvestri G A, Johnstone D. Interventional Pulmonary Procedures Guidelines from the American College of Chest Physicians. Chest 2003;123:1693-717.

[220]   Migliore M.Giuliano R.Aziz T. *et al* Four-step local anesthesia and sedation for thoracoscopic diagnosis and management of pleural diseases. Chest 2002;121;2032-5.

[221]   Danby CA, Adebonojo SA, Moritz DM. Video-assisted talc pleurodesis for malignant pleural effusions utilizing local anesthesia and i.v sedation. Chest 1998;113;739-42.

[222]   Mohebbi HA, Mehrvarz SH, Panahi F. Open lung biopsy with local anesthesia. IRCMJ 2007;9:147-9.

[223]   Landreneau RJ, Mack MJ, Hazelrigg SR, *et al.* Prevalence of chronic pain after pulmonary resection by thoracotomy or video-assisted thoracic surgery. J Thorac Cardiovasc Surg 1994;107:1079-86.

[224]   Stammberger U, Steinacher C, Hillinger S, *et al.* Early and long-term complaints following video-assisted thoracoscopic surgery: evaluation in 173 patients. Eur J Cardiothorac Surg 2000;18:7-11.

[225]   Passlick B, Born CH, Sienel W, Thetter O. Incidence of chronic pain after minimal-invasive surgery for spontaneous pneumothorax. Eur J Cardiothorac Surg 2001;19:355-9.

[226]   Sihoe ADL, Manlulu AV, Lee TW, *et al.* Pre-emptive local anesthesia for needlescopic video-assisted thoracic surgery: a randomized controlled trial. Eur J Cardiothorac Surg 2007; 31:103-8.

[227]   Corman SL, Skledar SJ. Use of lipid emulsion to reverse local anesthetic-induced toxicity. Ann Pharmacother 2007;41:1873-17.

[228]   Garcia-Aguado R, Onrubia J, Liagunes J, *et al.* Anaesthesia with continuous infusion of propofol for transsternal thymectomy in myasthenia patients. Rev Esp Anestesiol Reanim 1995;42:283-5.

[229]   Kiran U, Choudhury M, Saxena N, Kapoor P. Sevoflurane as a sole anesthetic for thymectomy in myasthenia gravis. Acta Anesthesiol Scand 2000;44:351-3.

[230]   Della Rocca G, Coccia C, Diana L, *et al.* Propofol or sevoflurane anaesthesia without muscle relaxants allow the early extubation of myasthenic patients. Can J Anaesth 2003;50:547-52.

[231]   O'Flaherty D, Pennant JH, Rao K, Giesecke AH. Total intravenous anaesthesia with propofol for transsternal thymectomy in myasthenia gravis. J Clin Anesth 1992;4:241-4.

[232]   Chevalley C, Spiliopoulos A, de Perrot M, *et al.* Perioperative medical management and outcome following thymectomy for myasthenia gravis. Can J Anaesth 2001;48:446-51.

[233]   Pompeo E, Tacconi F, Mineo TC. Awake video-assisted thoracoscopic biopsy in complex anterior mediastinal masses. Thorac Surg Clin 2010;20:225-33.

[234]   Piccioni F, Langer M, Fumagalli L, *et al.* Thoracic paravertebral anaesthesia for awake video-assisted thoracoscopy. Anaesthesia 2010;65:1221-4.

CHAPTER 6

Awake Resection of Solitary Pulmonary Nodules

Eugenio Pompeo[*], Francesco Sellitri, Benedetto Cristino and Tommaso Claudio Mineo

Department of Thoracic Surgery, Policlinico Tor Vergata University, Rome, Italy

Abstract: The term Solitary Pulmonary Nodule (SPN) refers to a newly developed lung nodular lesion of unknown origin and up to 3 cm in diameter, which is completely surrounded by normal parenchyma without atelectasis or adenopathy.

Video-Assisted Thoracic Surgery (VATS) has been increasingly advocated as an ideal approach for management of peripheral SPN due the satisfactory results and negligible morbidity rates reported with this minimal invasive surgical option. General anesthesia with one-lung ventilation has been considered mandatory to accomplish a safe operation by VATS. However, this type of anesthesia should not be considered strictly necessary to accomplish simple pulmonary resection and can be associated with several adverse effects that can increase the procedure-related morbidity with a potential negative impact on hospital stay and overall costs.

We have employed VATS performed through sole thoracic epidural anesthesia in awake patients to resect undetermined lung nodules, solitary metastases and non-small-cell lung cancer in high-risk patients. Early results have been encouraging although the pros and cons of awake VATS pulmonary resections still need to be fully elucidated.

Keywords: Pulmonary nodule, VATS, awake thoracic surgery, lung resection.

The term Solitary Pulmonary Nodule (SPN) refers to a newly developed lung nodular lesion of unknown origin and up to 3 cm in diameter, which is completely surrounded by normal parenchyma without atelectasis or adenopathy [1]. SPN is observed on 0.09% to 0.20% of all chest radiographs [2, 3] and its malignant potential mandates accurate diagnostic and therapeutic management. Currently, more than 150, 000 patients/year in the United States undergo clinical examination with the diagnostic dilemma of an SPN [4].

Since 1992, Video-Assisted Thoracic Surgery (VATS) has been increasingly advocated as an ideal approach for management of SPN [5] due the satisfactory results and negligible morbidity rates reported with this minimal invasive surgical option. In this setting, general anesthesia with one-lung ventilation has been considered mandatory to accomplish a safe operation. However, this type of anesthesia can be associated with several adverse effects that can increase the procedure-related morbidity [6] with a potential negative impact on hospital stay and overall costs.

In 2004, we first reported on awake VATS resection of SPN by using sole Thoracic Epidural Anesthesia (TEA) in fully awake, spontaneously ventilating patients according to the rationale of combining the minimal invasiveness of the thoracoscopic approach with avoidance of adverse effects of general anesthesia [7, 8].

So far, undetermined nodules [7], solitary metastases [9], and even non-small-cell lung cancer in high-risk patients [8] have been treated by this novel surgical approach.

Early series results have been encouraging although the pros and cons of awake VATS pulmonary resections still need to be fully elucidated. Moreover, only a few surgeons perform awake thoracic surgery procedures as yet and there is still some skepticism regarding their feasibility, particularly in patients with poor pulmonary function.

*Address correspondence to Eugenio Pompeo: Department of Thoracic Surgery, Policlinico Tor Vergata University, Rome, Italy; E-mail: pompeo@med.uniroma2.it

In this chapter we sought to describe indications, surgical techniques and overall results of awake VATS management of SPN.

ETIOLOGY AND DIFFERENTIAL DIAGNOSIS

Although most SPNs are benign, primary malignancy may be found in approximately 35% of them [4]. The definitive diagnosis requires histological analysis although medical history can help identify those patients who are more likely to have malignant lesions. Attention should be paid to those risk factors that have the greatest influence on the likelihood of malignancy [10]. Among these, age, smoking history, nodule size, edge characteristics on Computed Tomography (CT) and prior history of malignancy, have been shown to be the most useful.

History of exposure to carcinogens, travel history to areas endemic for pulmonary mycoses, and prior pulmonary diseases are other important features to be investigated. The relative risk of developing lung carcinoma in smokers is about 10 times that in nonsmokers [11]. Half of all smokers over 50 years of age have at last one lung nodule at the time of an initial screening examination. In addition, approximately 10% of screened subjects develop a new nodule during a 1-year period [12]. The probability that a given nodule is malignant increases in a parallel fashion with nodule size [13, 14]. Even in smokers, amongst nodules smaller than 4-mm, the percentage of lesions eventually evolving into lethal cancers is less than 1% whereas for those in the 8-mm range, this occur in approximately 10%-20% of instances [13, 15-17]. Cigarette smokers are at greater risk for development of cancer and, on average, malignant nodules in smokers grow faster than do those in nonsmokers [11, 18, 19]. In addition, the cancer risk for smokers increases in proportion to the degree and duration of exposure to cigarette smoke [20].

The radiological morphology characteristics of the nodule correlate with likelihood of malignancy, histology and growth rate. For instance, small purely ground-glass opacity (nonsolid) nodules that have malignant histopathological features tend to grow very slowly, with a mean volume doubling time in the order of 2 years [18]. Solid cancers, on the other hand, tend to grow more rapidly, with a mean volume doubling time of about 6 months.

As a general rule the older the patient the highest the likelihood of malignancy. In fact, lung cancer is uncommon in patients under 40 years old and is exceedingly rare in those under 35 years old [21].

Noncalcifield nodules larger than 8mm in diameter can have a substantial risk of malignancy and should be managed accordingly [22]. Management decisions should not be based on nodule size alone. Solid versus nonsolid appearance, spiculated margins, or other characteristics influence the likelihood of malignancy as well as growth rate in any given case. In general, all newly developed SPN should be suspected as being malignant until proven otherwise, particularly in individuals considered at higher risk for cancer development [4].

So far, the only certain diagnosis of the nature of the nodule is obtained by histological examination of the surgical sample [23].

IMAGING

Chest radiography in standard lateral and posteroanterior projections is the most commonly performed first-line radiological investigation and often proves useful in detecting undetermined lung nodules. However, the accuracy of chest roentgenograms in detecting small lesions is limited. They are in fact capable of identifying at least 50% of nodules with diameters ranging from 6 to 10 mm whereas they are rarely able to detect nodules with a diameter less than 6 mm even if their sensitivity reaches 90% when the nodule is calcified.

The diffusion of CT screening programs for lung cancer has increased the incidental discovery of SPN. In this respect, the superiority of CT when compared to conventional radiography is due to the greater contrast resolution between the nodule and the parenchyma and to the ability of CT to scan thin tissue layers, thus avoiding the overlap of anatomical structures. Differential diagnosis through sole imaging alone is very complex because the etiology of the SPN includes malignant tumors, benign tumors, inflammatory diseases, vascular diseases and other less frequent features (Fig. **1**). Radiological characteristics that must be taken into account when assessing SPNs include nodule size, changes in volume over time, logy (edges and contours) and mode of impregnation after administration of contrast medium.

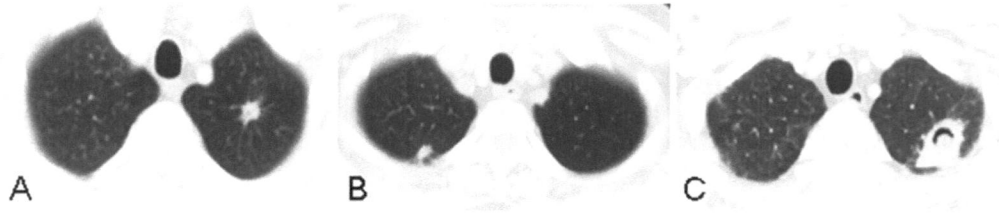

Fig. 1. CT-scan findings of benign nodules. Sarcoidosis (A); calcified nodule (B); mycetoma (C).

Taking size only into account is not reliable. Nodules with diameters between 0.5 and 1 cm are benign in 68% of cases, while this rate falls to 15% for nodules measuring $\geq$ 2 cm. Up to 97%-100% of malignant nodules present spiculated and blurred margins, suggesting radial extension of the tumor along the interlobular septa, lymphatics and small airways.

Nodules with lobulated margins are malignant in 82% of cases whereas those with rounded edges prove benign in 80% instances. Structural characterization analysis of pulmonary nodules entails the presence of calcification, fatty tissue, air bronchogram, excavation, pseudo excavation and sub-solid density. A nodule may be considered benign with 100% accuracy if there is a central calcification or a "popcorn" pattern that is characteristic of hamartoma whereas eccentric and pointed-like calcifications more commonly suggest a malignant lesion. The presence of fatty tissue inside the SPN suggests a benign nature although there are rare metastases with fatty components in patients with liposarcoma or renal cell carcinoma.

Partially solid nodules surrounded by ground-glass opacity are likely to reveal bronchiole-alveolar carcinoma or adenocarcinoma. Quantitative and qualitative differences in vascularization can also contribute to the characterization of the SPN. The absence of significant enhancement ($\leq$ 15 Hunsfield Units, HU) is strongly predictive of benignity. After administration of the contrast medium, an increase in the density of more than 15 HU is an expression of malignancy. This feature has a sensitivity of 98% but a specificity of 58% which is mainly due to granulomas that can also induce a significant enhancement. The dynamic stage of repeated acquisitions during the first 4-5 minutes of infusion of contrast medium has improved the diagnostic accuracy by reducing the number of false positives due to the possibility to assess both wash-in and wash-out phases.

The doubling time, that is the expression of the growth speed of a malignant lesions, can vary considerably between 30 and 400 days. Stability in size of an SPN over a period of two years is an expression of benignity with a positive predictive value of 65% although it is difficult to assess the growth of nodules with diameter <1 cm in size. Volumetric measurement permits an evaluation of the asymmetric growth and recognize the increase in size even when occurring in one dimension only. Nodules larger than 3 cm in size are more properly called "mass"and are mostly malignant in nature.

Positron Emission Tomography (PET) has also considerably added to the diagnostic accuracy of SPN. PET is a nuclear medicine imaging diagnostic method based on the nodule's capacity to concentrate a biologically active molecule. If the chosen molecule is an analogue of glucose, 18F-FDG, a pharmaceutical radioisotope labeled emitting positron, concentration of the imaged radiotracer indicates tissue metabolic activity, in terms of regional glucose uptake, which is conventionally quantified as Standardized Uptake Value (SUV). This diagnostic method can be run in a short time and is becoming increasingly employed for clinical staging of lung cancer. With PET scanning, a nodule is defined as suspicious when it has an SUV>2.5 whereas for SUV below this value a follow-up over time is recommended. When dealing with the differential diagnosis between the malignant and benign nature of nodules between 1 and 3 cm in size, PET has shown a sensitivity of 89-95% and a specificity of 85-89%. Unfortunately, the sensitivity is greatly reduced for nodules of less than 1 cm in size, that may lead to false negatives, as well as for tumors such as bronchioloalveolar carcinoma and carcinoids, which usually have low metabolic activity. On the other hand, both acute and chronic inflammatory diseases can lead to false positives. Finally, some benign tumors such as hamartomas may show some metabolic activity at PET scan [24]. Examples of PET-positive lesions successfully managed by awake VATS are illustrated in Figs. **2** and **3**.

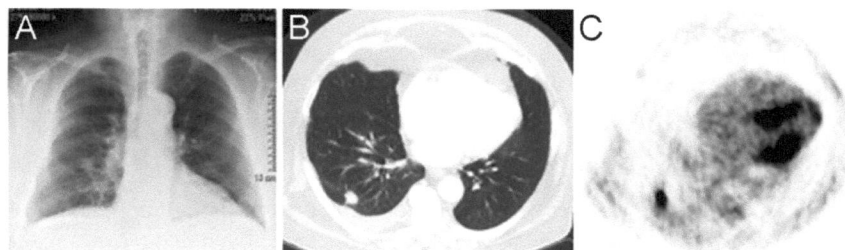

Fig. 2. Roengtenogram (A), CT-scan (B), and PET imaging (C) of a single lung metastasis arising from colorectal cancer, with minimal reactive pleural effusion. The patient was successfully treated by awake VATS metastasectomy.

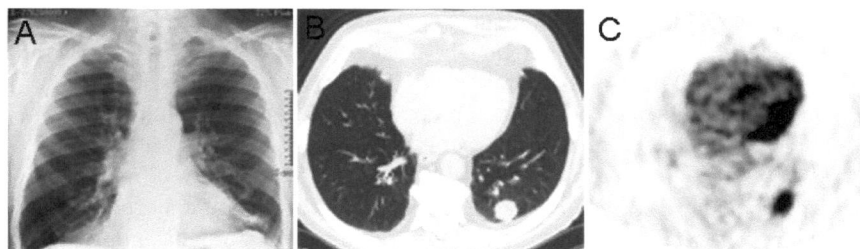

Fig. 3. Roengtenogram (A), CT-scan (B), and PET imaging (C) of a peripheral, stage IA non-small cell lung cancer in a patient with severe chronic obstructive pulmonary disease. Wide wedge resection performed with awake VATS. Disease-free at 36-months follow-up.

AWAKE VATS MANAGEMENT OF SPN

Indications. Criteria of eligibility for awake VATS resection of SPN are listed in Table **1**. As a rule, all candidates for VATS resection of SPN who have no contraindications for epidural catheterization and accept the operation are theoretically eligible for an awake surgical approach. Furthermore, patients with poor pulmonary function due to chronic obstruvtive pulmonary disease who are deemed unfit for general anesthesia can be elected for an awake VATS unless they have an arterial carbon dioxide tension >50 mmHg or a room air oxygen tension <50 mmHg. Additional aspects that must be accurately investigated include the presence of severe anxiety or depression that constitute a contraindication for an awake procedure in general. Furthermore, written informed consent must be obtained after careful description of pros and cons of each type of anesthesia and the clear advice that conversion to general anesthesia and even thoracotomy may prove necessary according to the surgeon and anesthesiologist's judgement.

Table 1. Main indications for awake pulmonary resection of SPN.

Radiologic presence of peripheral undetermined pulmonary nodule < 3cmm in maximal size.
No signs on CT-scan of diffuse pleural adhesions in the involved hemithorax.
No history of previous thoracic surgery on the involved hemithorax.
No advanced interstitial lung disease with restrictive ventilatory pattern.
Absence of severe anxiety or depression.
Absence of coagulation disorders.
Arterial carbon dioxide tension less than 55 mm Hg.
Absence of unfavourable anatomy for thoracic epidural anesthesia.

As far as the nature of the nodule is concerned, the awake VATS approach is indicated for treatment of peripheral pulmonary lesions including undetermined nodules, solitary metastases and early stage NSCLC in patients deemed at high-risk for anatomic lung resection through general anesthesia.

Anesthesia. TEA is performed at T4 level using a loss-of-resistance technique to achieve somatosensory and motor block between T1 and T8 level while preserving diaphragmatic motion. Premedication with oral midazolam 7.5 mg is routinely administered before surgery. Appropriateness and extent of the epidural blockade is evaluated using warm-cold discrimination test about 10-15 min after the injection of the anesthetic drug. Thoracic analgesia is obtained with continuous infusion of ropivacaine 0.5% and sufentanil 1.66 ug/mL into the epidural space. During the procedure, a Venturi mask is used if necessary, to keep oxygen saturation above 90%.

Concerns have been raised as to the patient's participation in operating room conversations and the risk for development of perioperative panic attacks. However, the authors have found that reassuring the patient during the procedure, explaining step-by-step what is being performed, and even showing the ongoing procedure on the operating video can greatly improve the perioperative wellness and expectations of the patient. Panic attacks occur in a minority of patients due to perceived difficulty in breathing that is triggered by the increased inspiratory load generated by the surgical pneumothorax. Nonetheless, in most instances this adverse event does not cause an impairment in oxygenation and can be managed by moderate sedation achieved with further midazolam or sub-hypnotic boluses of propofol while maintaining spontaneous breathing. During wound closure, the TEA anesthetic regimen is changed to ropivacaine 0.16% and sufentanil 1 ug/mL at 2 to 5 mL/hour to assure postoperative analgesia. The epidural catheter is removed 24 hours after surgery.

Surgical techniques. The patient is placed in the lateral decubitus position as for a thoracotomy. Before starting the procedure, a chest drainage system must be kept ready on the nurse's table to allow its immediate insertion in the event of unexpected technical problems requiring conversion to general anesthesia with single-lung ventilation. Surgical instruments that might be needed for an emergency thoracotomy must also be ready in the operating room.

To provide optimal view to all members of the operating team, the video-monitor is placed behind the patient's head [25]. Instrumentation for awake VATS is identical to that normally used for non-awake procedures. We usually use ring forceps, a 30°-angled camera as well as 35mm or 45 mm endoscopic staplers. Whenever adhesiolisis proves necessary standard endoshears, endodissectors and 10-mm cotton swabs are also employed.

Trocars' insertion is accomplished according to the baseball-diamond principle outlined by Landreneau *et al.* [26] with ports placed at the angles of an ideal reversed isosceles triangle and with the camera introduced through the lowest port.

The first 15-mm flexible trocar is introduced along the mid-axillary line between the sixth and eighth intercostal space through 1.5-cm skin incisions. A straight Crile forceps is inserted to bluntly widen the muscular layers, along the superior border of the lower rib, until entering the pleural cavity.

This method allows the camera port to be inserted for exploration of the lung and pleural cavity. The other 2 15-mm flexible trocars are then introduced, one in the third or fourth intercostal space along the anterior axillary line, and another one in the fifth or sixth intercostal spaces along the posterior axillary line [27].

As far as detection of small nodules is concerned, a number of methods including CT-guided percutaneous injection of dyes or radiotracers into the nodule, insertion of CT-guided hookwire, as well as intraoperative sonography, can be employed [28-32] although we have found that accurate instrumental and/or digital palpation of the perilesional area can allow identification of nodules in most instances.

Whenever detection of the lung nodule is difficult due to its small size or deeper localization, we routinely employ an original digital-instrumental palpation method. For this purpose we use custom-shaped ring forceps with an open ring and a closed-in ring that allows the nodule to be pushed forward towards the fingertip thus allowing a fine, bimanual-like palpation of the lung. In this respect, the partially ventilated lung status induced by the maintained spontaneous ventilation contribute to aid identification of the lesion due to the low density of lung tissue surrounding the nodule. This allows even radiologically undetected lesions to be identified, particularly during awake lung metastasectomy.

Once the nodule has been identified, it is removed through excision or staple wedge resection (Video 1, Video 2) depending on the nodule's location and its presumed nature (Figs. **4-6**).

In the case of precise excision, the lung tissue is incised by electrocautery just above the nodule and the lesion is progressively dissected free by combined use of blunt and sharp maneuvers, taking care to coagulate small perilesional vessels. Once the nodule has been almost completely enucleated it is completely excised following application of hemostatic clips on its posterior aspects (Fig. **4**). To avoid potential seeding of neoplastic cells at operating ports [33], the excised nodule is eventually extracted from the pleural cavity through an endoscopic retrieval bag.

Hemostasis is then accurately revised and the clamp is temporarily released to check the presence of bleeding points that are coagulated or clipped. The parenchymal defect is repaired by endo-suture or non-cutting endoscopic stapling (Fig. **5**).

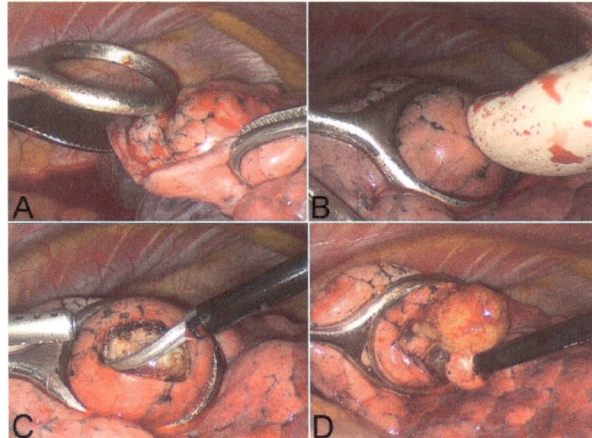

Fig. 4. Awake excision of a SPN. The nodule is grasped by modified ring forceps (A) that allows bimanual-like palpation (B). After incision of the lung surface (C) the nodule is excised by combined sharp and blunt dissection (D).

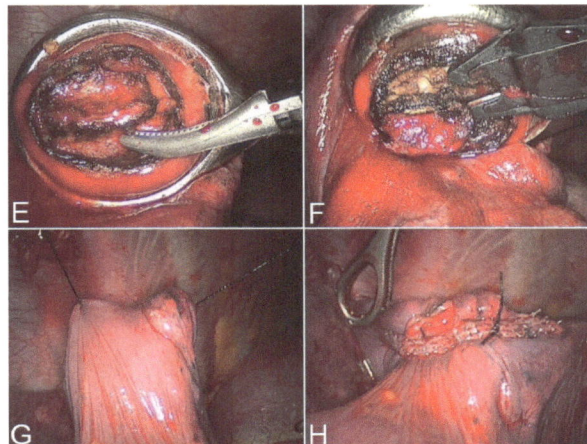

Fig. 5. After excision of the nodule, hemostasis is controlled by cautery (E) and/or endoscopic clips (F). Thereafter, the resulting defect is re-approximated by an untied running suture (G) and eventually sutured by a no-knife endostapler (H).

On completion of the procedure, a single 28Ch chest tube is inserted and connected to a waterseal. The tube is introduced into the chest at the lowest intercostals access site and positioned dorsally under thoracoscopic guidance up to the apex of the pleural cavity. Complete lung re-expansion is achieved by asking the patient to breathe deeply and cough repeatedly, while keeping the operating ports closed with the fingers, and the camera port with gauzes, to restore negative intrapleural pressure (Fig. **7**). Finally, trocar incisions are sutured in a standard manner [8].

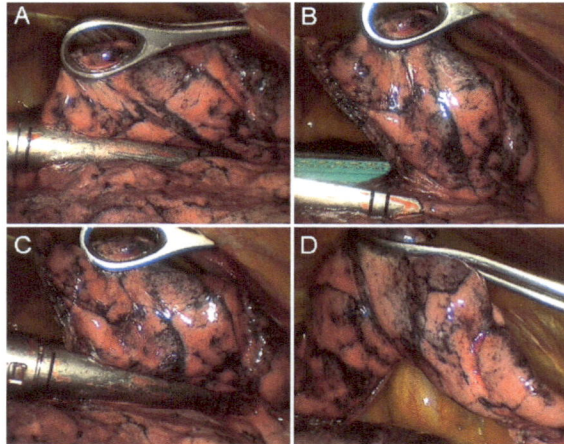

Fig. 6. Awake VATS for stage I NSCLC in a patient with severe emphysema. In this favorable circumstance, the tumor could be resected by firing multiple cartridges along a continuous, "hockey-stick" shaped suture line (A, B, C) as in formal lung-lung volume reduction (D). This allows to combine the advantage of complete tumor removal with the benefit of lung remodeling leading to improvement in clinical and respiratory function measures.

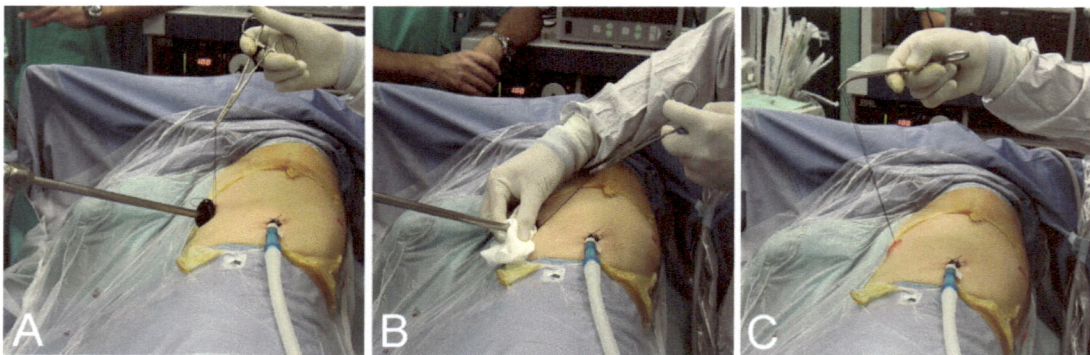

Fig. 7. At end procedure, lung expansion is achieved under thoracoscopic vision (A) asking the patient to cough repeatedly while keeping the last trocar closed with gauzes (B). Rapid extraction of the camera is accomplished while tying a previously passed parietal stitch to assure air-tight closure of the chest (C).

RESULTS

Awake resection of undetermined pulmonary nodules. VATS wedge resection is considered an ideal option in the presence of a SPN, which is peripherally located and less than 3 cm in size. Indeed, complete removal of the nodule is not only diagnostic but has also therapeutic value in most instances [4]. So far, the vast majority of reported series on VATS resection of SPN have entailed use of general anesthesia with one-lung ventilation (Table **2**).

In 2004, we reported the results of the first randomized study comparing VATS wedge resection of SPN carried out either by TEA alone or general anesthesia with double-lumen intubation plus TEA [1]. In this analysis, there was no intergroup difference in technical feasibility although two patients in the awake group required conversion to thoracotomy due to severe adhesions. Two other patients in each group required conversion to thoracotomy due to unexpected lung cancer requiring lobectomy. In addition, anesthesia satisfaction score, postoperative fall in arterial oxygen tension, nursing care calls and median hospital stay were significantly better in the awake group. Finally, in the awake group avoidance of general anesthesia allowed immediate resumption of many daily life activities including drinking, eating and walking. This eventually reflected in a short hospitalization with 50% of the patients being discharged by the second postoperative day.

Table 2. Literature series on VATS wedge resections for SPN performed through general anesthesia.

First Author	Year	Patients	Benign (%)	Malignant (%)	Morbidity (%)	Conversion (%)	Hospital Stay (days)
Swanson[36]	1999	65	42	58	0	NR	3
Jimenez[37]	2001	209	51.1	48.8	9.6	16.3	6.2
Murasugi[38]	2002	81	45	55	1.2	11	9.2
Cardillo[39]	2003	429	86.2	13.8	3.0	NR	4.6
Ciriaco[40]	2004	151	51	49	NR	13.9	3
Ambrogi[32]	2005	183	43.8	56.2	0	4.9	3
Solaini[27]	2007	412	NR	NR	5.7	12.4	3.8
Varoli[23]	2008	276	50	50	0	0	3

NR: not reported.

An interesting issue of awake VATS resection of SPN is the possibility to apply the concept of outpatient or ambulatory thoracic surgery that so far has been anecdotally advocated by Molins *et al.*[34] using general anesthesia. Furthermore, in a very recent case report, Rocco and coworkers [35] described features of a patient undergoing awake uniportal VATS resection of a pulmonary nodule in a complete ambulatory setting.

Awake pulmonary metastasectomy. Surgical metastasectomy has become a standard of care of patients with lung metastases [41]. Complete macroscopic resection proved to be the most important prognostic factor in this setting and aggressive, iterative surgical procedures can also have a rationale [42]. In fact, patients with untreated metastatic lung disease have a median survival of less than 10 months and a 5-year survival rate of less than 5% [43].

Since the majority of pulmonary metastases are located in the outer one third of the lung and are frequently subpleural [44], VATS metastasectomy has been advocated as a viable surgical option, particularly for patients with solitary peripheral lesions (Table **3**).

Table 3. VATS series on pulmonary metastasectomy performed through general anesthesia.

First Author	Period	Patients	Primary Tumor	Hospital Stay (days)	Recurrence Rate (%)	5-ys Survival (%)
De Giacomo[45]	1992-1998	24	Colorectal	4.3	56.5	49.5
Carballo[46]	1986-2006	36	Various	NR	27.7	69.6
Lin[47]	1991-1998	99	Various	4.4	58	53.6
Landreneau[48]	90 months	80	Colorectal	4.5	67	30.8
Nakajima[49]	1987-2005	72	Colorectal	NR	NR	49.3
Gossot[50]	2000-2007	31	Sarcoma	3.7	3.2	52.5

NR: not reported.

Advocated advantages of VATS include the limited surgical trauma with consequent reduction of postoperative morbidity and pain [51, 52]. Additional benefits are thought to be represented by a more rapid postoperative recovery, short length of hospital stay, low medical costs and early resumption of work [52, 53]. Unfortunately, radiologically undetectable lesions have proved to be frequently missed at VATS [54].

For these reasons in 1999 we had proposed the transxiphoid approach which allowed bimanual lung palpation during VATS metastasectomy [55]. More recently, we have reported the results of a novel awake VATS approach developed for lung metastasectomy and entailing a new method of digital-instrumental palpation that allowed bimanual-like palpation of the lung [56](Fig. **4**). Eligibility criteria for awake VATS metastasectomy are listed in Table **4**.

Table 4. Main eligibility criteria for awake metastasectomy.

Lung metastasis located at less than 2 cm from visceral pleura and measuring not more than 3 cm at the helical TC and amenable of VATS rsection.
Complete control of the primary tumor.
Absence of extrapulmonary metastases.
No radiological evidence of pleural scarring.

In our 14-patient series [56], awake pulmonary metastasectomy was easily and safely accomplished under TEA alone.

There was no mortality or major morbidity and the operation resulted in optimal patient acceptance and satisfaction as shown by the high anesthesia satisfaction score which was rated as excellent to good in 86% of the patients.

Global operating room time and hospital stay were also significantly shorter than those of a control group operated under general anesthesia while oncological results and survival were comparable. The rapidity of the procedure together with the significantly reduced anesthesia time and the lack of weaning time improved patient turnover in the operating theatre and offered the double advantage of less risk for the patient and less cost for the institution, thus facilitating our fast-track surgery program.

In this series, nodules as small as 5 mm in size were identified with our lung palpation method and the low rate of ipsilateral lung recurrence suggested that it was as effective as bimanual palpation in detecting all lesions.

Furthermore, despite the use of helical CT scan, which is currently the most accurate tool in detecting metastases, direct lung palpation made it possible to discover some radiologically undetected lesions, a finding which is in line with data from previous studies [57] (Fig. **8**).

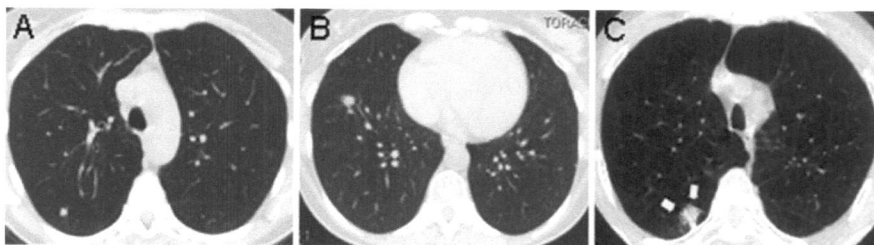

Fig. 8. CT-scans of pulmonary metastases arising from endometrial cancer (A), colo-rectal cancer (B), and renal cancer (C) (Video 2) treated by awake metastasectomy.

Awake resection of non-small-cell lung carcinoma. Lung cancer is the most common cause of cancer-related mortality in the world. For surgical candidates with a nodule that proves to be a Non-Small-Cell-Lung Cancer (NSCLC), lobectomy and systematic mediastinal lymph node dissection is the standard of care to achieve optimal pathologic staging and correct oncological treatment. Five-year survival following complete resection of stage IA or IB NSCLC is 65 to 80% and 50 to 60%, respectively [4].

Patients who are deemed unfit for surgery because of impaired pulmonary function, cardiac status, or general health have been usually treated with radiation therapy with little hope for cure and a 5-year survival rate between 5% and 21% [58]. This low disease-free survival rate had stimulated interest in offering these patients surgery in the form of limited resection. Several uncontrolled studies have suggested a role of limited surgical resection (wedge resection and segmentectomy) alone or with adjuvant radiotherapy in treatment of early-stage NSCLC in patients with compromised cardiopulmonary status [59-61]. These studies have suggested that limited lung resection can be safe and effective and that VATS represents an attractive noninvasive option in this setting (Table **5**).

Table 5. Series on limited resection for NSCLC performed through general anesthesia.

	Year	Patients	Morbidity (%)	Mortality (%)	Follow-Up (months)	Recurrence (%)	5-year Survival (%)
LCSG*[62]	1995	122	NR	0.8	54	6.3	44
Landreneau [63]	1997	102	21	0	26	13.7	62
Koike [64]	2003	74	NR	NR	52	2.7	89.1
Okada [65]	2004	262	6.6	0.4	72	4.9	89.6
El-Sherif [66]	2006	207	NR	1.4	31	7.2	40
Sienel [67]	2008	87	17.2	0	45	26.4	63

*NR: not reported. *: Lung Cancer Study Group.*

VATS resection of NSCLC represents the most provocative indication for an awake surgical approach although it is worth noting that already in 1950 that Buckingham *et al.* [68] reported on 617 major awake thoracic surgery procedures including 64 pneumonectomies and 58 lobectomies that were performed through TEA with additional general anesthesia employed only in a minority of cases.

Much more recently, Abdullatief *et al.* [69] reported on an 11-patients experience of awake open anatomic lung resections including 2 pneumonectomies that were performed through just TEA in fully awake patients.

Although concerns can arise in advocating awake VATS resection of lung cancer, this approach might entail some beneficial effects including a more limited postoperative impairment in stress hormone and lymphocyte responses [70, 71], which might play a role in assuring a more effective immunologic surveillance in the early postoperative period.

We have started to perform awake VATS limited resection of peripheral stage I NSCLC in selected patients who were deemed at high-risk for standard surgery through general anesthesia (Table **6**). The most frequent clinical feature that we have encountered has been that of a peripheral tumor associated with severe emphysema and impaired pulmonary function not amenable to lobectomy due to the prevalence of emphysematous destruction in a lobe other than that containing the cancer lesion, or in patients with severe and yet homogeneous emphysema. Additional indications might be those of medically inoperable patients with peripheral early stage NSCLC that have already been treated with unsuccessful non-surgical local therapies [72, 73].

Table 6. Main indications for awake resection of Stage I NSCLC.

Main surgical prerequisites
Lesion of less than 3 cm in maximal size.
Peripheral location.
No history of pleural-pulmonary infections or previous surgery on the affected side.

Medical conditions associated with increased risk for general anesthesia and OLV
Age > 80 years.
Severe emphysema documented at high-resolution CT.

FEV₁ less than 40% predicted.

Arterial oxygen tension less than 65 mmHg.

Diffusion capacity for carbon monoxide less than 40% predicted.

Exercise oxygen consumption less than 50% predicted.

American Society of Anesthesiology (ASA) score: 2-3.

Our initial results have been encouraging and we had no mortality nor major morbidity with a satisfactory 3-year survival rate of 66%, which compare favourably with results of stereotactic irradiation [74, 75] and radiofrequency ablation [76, 77].

In a recent analysis, Grills *et al.* [78] compared outcomes between stereotactic radiotherapy and wedge resection for stage I NSCLC in medically inoperable patients. In this nonrandomized population overall survival was better in the surgical group although cause-specific survival was identical amongst study groups.

The authors concluded that both treatments are reasonable options for patients ineligible for anatomic lobectomy.

CONCLUSION

So far, despite relevant technological advances in radiologic imaging and noninvasive diagnostic methods, correct preoperative characterization of undetermined SPN remains an inexact science and newly discovered nodules constitute a diagnostic and therapeutic dilemma. Many of these lesions eventually prove to be benign, but the possibility of a malignant etiology makes it mandatory to obtain a rapid and definitive diagnosis, particularly in patients considered at increased risk for cancer development.

Radiological dimension and morphology of the nodule, contrast enhancement at CT as well as positivity of PET scan can all contribute to increase the likelihood of malignancy although none of them either alone or in combination can permit a definitive diagnosis, which can be ascertained only by cyto-histological assessment. In this respect, there is little role for bronchoscopy, because the parenchymal site of the nodule is difficult to reach endobronchially.

On the other hand, the introduction of Transthoracic Needle Aspiration (TTNA) has changed the diagnostic work-up of pulmonary nodules. The sensitivity for malignancy is 64 to 100%. Unfortunately, the sensitivity of TTNA for a specific benign diagnosis is 12 to 68% [10]. The diagnosis of "absence of malignant tumor cells" in the sample is always interlocutory and not definitive [24]. In addition, TTNA is not a complication-free option since pneumothorax can occur in up to 25%-30% of patients and this rate increases considerably when dealing with patients with emphysema.

For NSCLC, early surgical excision is the only therapy currently offering a reasonable chance of cure. Furthermore, in patients with a history of successfully treated extrapulmonary tumors who develop pulmonary metastases, surgical metastasectomy is a standard of care and for all these reasons, the possibility to resecting SPNs without general anesthesia can undoubtedly represent an attractive option.

In conclusion, awake VATS resection of SPN proved safe and feasible, particularly in patients with undetermined nodules, solitary metastases and those with early stage, peripheral NSCLC who were deemed unfit for an anatomic resection and nonetheless, potential applications of this promising surgical approach are still evolving and further investigation is needed to better elucidate advantages, indications and limits.

REFERENCES

[1]   Tuddenham WI. Glossary of terms of thoracic radiology: recommendations of the Nomenclature Committee of the Fleisher Society. Am J Roentgenol 1984;43:509-17.

[2] Holin SN, Dwork RE, Glaser S, *et al.* Solitary pulmonary nodules found in a community-wide chest roentgenographic survey. Am Tuberc Pulm Dis 1959;79:427-39.

[3] Swensen SJ, Silverstein MD, Edell ES, *et al.* Solitary pulmonary nodules: clinical prediction model versus physicians. Mayo Clin Proc 1999;74:319-29.

[4] Tan BB, Flaherty KR, Kazerooni EA, Iannettoni MD, American College of Chest Physicians. The solitary pulmonary nodule. Chest 2003;123:89-96.

[5] Miller DL, Allen MS, Deschamps C, Trastek VF, Pairolero PC. Video-assisted thoracic surgical procedure: management of a solitary pulmonary nodule. Mayo Clin Proc 1992;67:462-4.

[6] Whitehead T, Slutsky AS. The pulmonary physician in critical care. 7: ventilator induced lung injury. Thorax 2002;57:635-42.

[7] Pompeo E, Mineo D, Rogliani P, Sabato AF, Mineo TC. Feasibility and results of awake thoracoscopic resection of solitary pulmonary nodules. Ann Thorac Surg 2004;78:1761-8.

[8] Pompeo E, Mineo TC. Awake operative videothoracoscopic pulmonary resections. Thorac Surg Clin 2008;18:311-20.

[9] Pompeo E, Mineo TC. Awake pulmonary metastasectomy. J Thorac Cardiovasc Surg 2007;133:960-6.

[10] Gurney JW. Determining the likelihood of malignancy in solitary pulmonary nodules with Bayesian analysis. Part I: theory. Radiology 1993;186:405-13.

[11] MacMahon H, Austin JHM, Gasmu G, *et al.* Guidelines for Management of small pulmonary nodules detected on CT scans: a statement from the Fleischner Society. Radiology 2005;237:395-400.

[12] Swensen SJ. CT screening for lung cancer. AJR Am J Roentgenol 2002;179:833-6.

[13] Midthun DE, Swensen SJ, Jett JR, *et al.* Evaluation of nodules detected by screening for lung cancer with low dose spiral computed tomography. Lung Cancer 2003;41:S40.

[14] Henschke CI, Yankelevitz DF, Naidich DP, *et al.* CT screening for lung cancer: suspiciousness of nodules according to size on baseline scans. Radiology 2004;231:164-8.

[15] Swensen SJ, Jett JR, Hartman T, *et al.* Lung cancer screening with CT: Mayo Clinic experience. Radiology 2003;226:756-61.

[16] Henschke CI, Naidich DP, Yankelevitz DF, *et al.* Early Lung Cancer Project: initial findings on repeat screening. Cancer 2001;92:153-9.

[17] Pastorino U, Bellomi M, Landoni C, *et al.* Early lung-cancer detection with spiral CT and positron emission tomography in heavy smokers: 2-year results. Lancet 2003;362:593-7.

[18] Hasegawa M, Some S, Takashima S, *et al.* Growth rate of small lung cancers detected on mass CT screening. Br J Radiol 2000;73:1252-9.

[19] Guyatt GH, Newhouse MD. Are active and passive smoking harmful? determination of causation. Chest 1985;88:445-51.

[20] Bach PB, Kattan M, Thornquist MD, *et al.* Variations in lung cancer risk among smokers. J Natl Cancer Inst 2003;95:470-8.

[21] Gadgeel SM, Ramalingam S, Cummings G, *et al.* Lung cancer in patients < 50 years of age: the experience of an academic multidisciplinary program. Chest 1999;115:1232-6.

[22] Henschke CI, Yankelevitz DF, Mirtcheva R, *et al.* CT screening for lung cancer: frequency and significance of part-solid and nonsolid nodules. Am J Roentgenol 2002;178:1053-7.

[23] Varoli F, Vergani C, Caminiti R, *et al.* Management of solitary pulmonary nodule. Eur J Cardiothorac Surg 2008;33:461-5.

[24] De Cicco C, Bellomi M, Bartolomei M, *et al.* Imaging of lung hamartomas by multi detector computed tomography and positron emission tomography. Ann Thorac Surg 2008;86:1769-72.

[25] Roviaro GC, Varoli F, Vergagni C, Maciocco M. State of the art in thoracoscopic surgery: a personal experience of 2000 videothoracoscopic procedures and an overview of the literature. Surg Endosc 2002;16:881-92.

[26] Landreneau RJ, Mack MJ; Hazelrigg SR, *et al.* Video-Assisted Thoacic Surgery: basic technical concepts and intercostals approach strategies. Ann Thorac Surg 1992;54:800-7.

[27] Solaini L, Prusciano F, Bagioni P, *et al.* Video-assisted thoracic surgery (VATS) of the lung: analysis of intraoperative and postoperative complications over 15 years and review of the literature. Surg Endosc 2008;22:298-310.

[28] Shah RM, Spirn PW, Salazar AM, *et al.* Localization of peripheral pulmonary nodules form thoracoscopic excision: value of CT-guided wire placement. Am J Roentgenol 1993;161:279-83.

[29] Kanazawa S, Ando A, Yasui K, *et al.* Localization of pulmonary nodules for thoracoscopic resection: experience with a system using a short hookwire and suture. Am J Roentgenol 1998;170:332-4.

[30]   Mack MJ, Shennib H, Landreneau RJ, Hazelrigg SR. Techniques for localization of pulmonary nodules for thoracoscopic resection. J Thorac Cardiovasc Surg 1993;106:550-3.

[31]   Paci M, Annessi V, Giovanardi F, *et al.* Preoperative localization of indeterminate pulmonary nodules before videothoracoscopic resection. Surg Endosc 2002;16:509-11.

[32]   Ambrogi MC, Dini P, Boni G, *et al.* A strategy for thoracoscopic resection of small pulmonary nodules. Endosc Surg 2005;19:1644-7.

[33]   Hung GU, Hsu HK, Kao CH, Chen KY, Chiu JS. Asymptomatic port-site metastasis following video-assisted thoracoscopic surgery detected by FDG-PET/CT. Clin Nucl Med 2010;35:552-3.

[34]   Molins L, Fibla JJ, Mier JM, Sierra A. Outpatient thoracic surgery. Thorac Surg Clin 2008;18:321-7.

[35]   Rocco G, Romano V, Accardo R, *et al.* Awake single-access (uniportal) video-assisted thoracoscopic surgery for peripheral pulmonary nodules in a complete ambulatory setting. Ann Thorac Surg 2010;89:1625-8.

[36]   Swanson SJ, Jaklitsch MT, Mentzer SJ, *et al.* Management of the solitary pulmonary nodule: role of thoracoscopy in diagnosis and therapy. Chest 1999;116:S523-S4.

[37]   Jimenez MJ. The Spanish Video-Assisted Thoracic Surgery Study Group. Prospective study on video-assisted thoracoscopic surgery in the resection of pulmonary nodules: 209 cases from the Spanish video-assisted thoracic surgery: a five-year experience. Eur J Cardio-thorac Surg 2001;19:562-5.

[38]   Marasugi M, Onuki T, Ikeda T, Kanzaki M, Nitta S. The role of video-assisted thoracoscopic surgery in the diagnosis of the small peripheral pulmonary nodule. Surg Endosc 2001;15:734-6.

[39]   Cardillo G, Regal M, Sera F, *et al.* Videothoracoscopic management of the solitary pulmonary nodule: a single-institution study on 429 cases. Ann Thorac Surg 2003;75:1607-12.

[40]   Ciriaco P, Negri G, Puglisi A, *et al.* Video-assisted thoracoscopic surgery for pulmonary nodules: rationale for preoperative computed tomography-guided hookwire localization. Eur J Cardiothorac Surg 2004;25;429-33.

[41]   Mineo TC, Ambrogi V, Paci M, *et al.* Tranxiphoid bilateral palpation in video-assisted thoracoscopic lung metastasectomy. Arch Surg 2001;136:783-8.

[42]   Pastorino U, Buyse M, Friedel G, *et al.* Long term results of lung metastasectomy: prognostic analyses based on 5206 cases. J Thorac Cardiovasc Surg 1997;113:37-49.

[43]   Pfannschmidt J, Dienemann H, Hoffmann H. Surgical resection of pulmonary metastases from colorectal cancer: a systematic review of published series. Ann Thorac Surg 2007;84:324-38.

[44]   Crow J, Slavin G, Kreel L. Pulmonary metastasis: a pathologic and radiologic study. Cancer 1981;47:2595-602.

[45]   De Giacomo T, Rendina EA, Venuta F, Ciccone AM, Coloni GF. Thoracoscopic resection of solitary lung metastases from colorectal cancer is a viable therapeutic option. Chest 1999;115:1441-3.

[46]   Carballo M, Maish MS, Jaroszewski DE, Holmes CE. Video-assisted thoracic surgery as a safe alternative for the resection of pulmonary metastases: retrospective cohort study. J Cardiovasc Thorac Surg 2009;4:1-13.

[47]   Lin JC, Wiechmann RJ, Szwerc MF, *et al.* Diagnostic and therapeutic video-assisted thoracic surgery resection of pulmonary metastases. Surgery 1999;126: 636-42.

[48]   Landreneau RJ, De Giacomo T, Mack MJ, *et al.* Therapeutic video.assisted thoracoscopic surgical resection of colorectal pulmonary metastases. Eur J Cardiothorac Surg 2000;18:671-7.

[49]   Nakajima J, Murakawa T, Fukami T, Takamoto S. Is thoracoscopic surgery justified to treat pulmonary metastasis from colorectal cancer? Interact Cardiovasc Thorac Surg 2008;7:212-7.

[50]   Gossot D, Radu C, Girard P, *et al.* Resection of pulmonary from sarcoma: can some patients benefit from a less invasive approach? Ann Thorac Surg 2009;87:238-43.

[51]   Guidicelli R, Thomas P, Lonjon T, *et al.* Video-assisted minithoracotomy versus muscle-sparing thoracotomy for performing lobectomy. Ann Thorac Surg 1994;58:712-8.

[52]   Landreneau RJ, Wiechmann RJ, Hazelrigg SR, *et al.* Effect of minimally invasive thoracic surgica approaches on acute and chronic postoperative pain. Chest Surg Clin North Am 1998;8:891-906.

[53]   Hazelrigg SR; Nunchuck SK, Landreneau RJ, *et al.* Cost analysis for thoracoscopy: thoracoscopic wedge rresection. Ann Thorac Surg 1993;56:633-5.

[54]   McCormack PM, Ginsberg KB, Bains MS, *et al.* Accurancy of lung imaging in matstases with implications for the role of thoracoscopy. Ann thorac Surg 1993;56:863-6.

[55]   Mineo TC, Pompeo E, Ambrogi V, Pistolese C. Video-Assisted approach for transxiphoid bilateral lung metastasectomy. Ann Thorac Surg 1999;67:1808-10.

[56]   Pompeo E, Mineo TC. Awake pulmonary metastasectomy. J Thorac Cardiovasc Surg 2007;133:960-6.

[57]   Suzuki K, Kusumoto M, Watanabe S, Tsuchya R, Asamura H. Radiologic classification of small adenocarcinoma of the lung: radiologic-pathologic correlation and its prognostic impact. Ann Thorac surg 2006;81:413-9.

[58]   Shennib HA, Landreneau RJ, Mulder DS, Mack M. Video-assisted thoracoscopic wedge resection of T1 lung cancer in high-risk patients. Ann Surg 1993;218:555-60.

[59]   Shennib H, Bogart J, Herndon JE, *et al.* Video-assisted wedge resection and local radiotherapy for peripheral lung cancer in high-risk patients: The Cancer and Leukemia Group B (CALGB) 9335, a phase II, multi-institutional cooperative group study. J Thorac Cardiovasc Surg 2005;129:813-8.

[60]   Jensik RJ, Faber LP, Kittle CF, Meng RL. Survival following resection for a second primary bronchogenic carcinoma. J Thorac Cardiovasc Surg 1981;82:658-68.

[61]   Stair JM, Womble J, Schaefer RF, Read RC. Segmnetal pulmonary resection for cancer. Am J Surg 1985;150:659-65.

[62]   Lung Cancer Study Group. Randomized trial of lobectomy versus limited resection for T1 N0 non-small cell lung cancer. Ann Thorac Surg 1995;60:615-23.

[63]   Landreneau RJ, Sugarbaker DJ, Mack MJ, *et al.* Wedge resection versus lobectomy for stage I (T1 N0 M0) non-small cell lung cancer. J Thorac Cardiovasc Surg 1997;113:691-700.

[64]   Koike T, Yamato Y, Yoshiya K, Shimoyama T, Suzuki R. Intentional limited pulmonary resection for peripheral T1 N0 M0 small-sized lung cancer. J Thorac Cardiovasc Surg 2003;125: 924-8.

[65]   Okada M, Koike T, Higashiyma M, *et al.* Radical sublobar resection for small-sized non-small cell lung cancer: a multicenter study. J Thorac Cardiovasc Surg 2004;132:769-75.

[66]   El-Sherif A, Gooding WE, Santos R, *et al.* Outcomes of sublobar resection versus lobectomy for stage I non-small cell lung cancer: a 13-year analysis. Ann Thorac Surg 2006;82:408-16.

[67]   Sienel W, Dango S, Kirschbaum A, *et al.* Sublobar resections in stage IA non-small cell lung cancer: segmentectomies result in significantly better cancer-related survival than wedge resections. Eur J Cardiothorac Surg 2008;33:728-34.

[68]   Buckingham WW, Beatty AJ, Brasher CA, Ottosen P. The technique of administering epidural anesthesia in thoracic surgery. Dis Chest 1950;17:561-8.

[69]   Al-Abdullatief M, Wahood A, Al-Shirawi N, *et al.* Awake anaesthesia for major thoracic surgical procedures: an observational study. Eur J Cardiothorac Surg 2007;32:346-50.

[70]   Tacconi F, Pompeo E, Sellitri F, Mineo TC. Surgical stress jormones response is reduced after awake videothoracoscopy. Interact Cardiovasc Thorac Surg 2010;10:666-71.

[71]   Vanni G, Tacconi F, Sellitri F, *et al.* Impact of awake videothoracoscopic surgery on post-operative lymphocyte responses. Ann Thorac Surg 2010;90:973-8.

[72]   Pennathur A, Luketich JD, Abbas G, *et al.* Radiofrequency ablation for the treatment of stage I non-small cell lung cancer in high-risk patients. J Thorac Cardiovasc Surg 2007;134:857-64.

[73]   Timmerman R, Papiez L, McGarry R, *et al.* Extracranial stereotactic radioblation: results of a phase I study in medically inoperable stage I non-small cell lung cancer. Chest 2003;124:1946-55.

[74]   Guckenberger M, Heilman K, Wulf J, *et al.* Pulmonary injury and tumor response after stereotactic body radiotherapy (SBRT): results of a serial follow-up CT study. Radiother Oncol 2007;85:435-42.

[75]   Pennathur A, Luketich JD, Heron DE, *et al.* Stereotactic radiosurgery for the treatment of lung neoplasm: experience in 100 consecutive patients. Ann Thorac Surg 2009;88:1594-600

[76]   Hiraki T, Gobara H, Iishi T, *et al.* Percutaneous radiofrequency ablation for clinical stage I non-small cell lung cancer: results in 20 nonsurgical candidates. J Thorac Cardiovasc Surg 2007;134:1306-12.

[77]   Pennathur A, Abbas G, Gooding WE, *et al.* Image-guided radiofrequency ablation of lung neoplasm in 100 consecutive patients by a thoracic surgical service. Ann Thorac Surg 2009;88:1601-8.

[78]   Grills IS, Mangona VS, Welsh R, *et al.* Outcomes after sterotactic lung radiotherapy or wedge resection for stage I non-small cell lung cancer. J Clin Oncol 2010;28:928-35.

CHAPTER 7

Awake Non-Resectional Lung Volume Reduction Surgery

Eugenio Pompeo[*], Ilaria Onorati and Tommaso Claudio Mineo

Department of Thoracic Surgery, Emphysema Center, Policlinico Tor Vergata University, Rome, Italy

Abstract: Lung Volume Reduction Surgery (LVRS) is now a well established procedure, which can considerably improve dyspnea, pulmonary function, exercise capacity, quality of life and survival in selected patients with severe emphysema, particularly when the upper lung lobes are predominantly involved. The standard operation entails unilateral or bilateral, staple non-anatomical resection of the most emphysematous lung tissue, carried out by median sternotomy or thoracoscopic approaches through general anesthesia and single-lung ventilation (resectional LVRS).

Operative mortality and morbidity of resectional LVRS have been higher than those observed following the majority of other thoracic surgery procedures. It seems reasonable to assume that, in anatomically and physiologically fragile subjects such as candidates to LVRS, determinants of operative mortality and morbidity may include not only the surgical trauma deriving from resection of emphysematous lung tissue, but also general anesthesia.

We have developed a non-resectional LVRS method that can be carried out through sole thoracic epidural anesthesia in fully awake patients. This technique has proved to offer lower morbidity and clinical benefits that paralleled those of resectional LVRS.

Keywords: Emphysema, VATS, LVRS.

INTRODUCTION

Pulmonary emphysema is a chronic disease that is mostly secondary to the effects of cigarette smoking and in advanced stage can lead to severe disability and early death.

Standard medical treatment offers only modest symptom relief and no intervention except smoking cessation or long-term supplemental oxygen therapy has been shown to alter emphysema progression [1].

Lung Volume Reduction Surgery (LVRS) is now a well established procedure, which can considerably improve dyspnea, pulmonary function, exercise capacity, quality of life and survival in selected patients with severe emphysema, particularly when the upper lung lobes are predominantly involved [2-10].

Typically, the operation entails unilateral or bilateral, non-anatomical staple resection of the most emphysematous lung tissue carried out by median sternotomy [11] or thoracoscopic approaches [12, 13] through general anesthesia and single-lung ventilation (resectional LVRS).

Operative mortality and morbidity of resectional LVRS have been higher than those observed following the majority of other thoracic surgery procedures. In particular, the mortality rate ranged widely, from 2.5% up to 19% [14], whereas in the largest multicenter randomized study, the National Emphysema Treatment Trial (NETT)[7], 90-day mortality was 5.5%. In addition, following resectional LVRS, up to 90% of the patients are likely to develop an air leak lasting at least 7 days, whereas major complications, including the need for reintubation, tracheostomy, ventilatory support for more than 2 days or pneumonia within 30 days from surgery, can occur in about 30% of the patients [15]. As a result, the cost-effectiveness of LVRS has been questioned due to frequently prolonged hospitalization times and high costs [16].

*Address correspondence to Eugenio Pompeo: Department of Thoracic Surgery, Policlinico Tor Vergata University, Rome, Italy. E-mail: pompeo@med.uniroma2.it

It seems reasonable to assume that in anatomically and physiologically fragile subjects such as candidates to LVRS, determinants of operative mortality and morbidity may include not only the surgical trauma deriving from resection of emphysematous lung tissue, but also the need for general anesthesia per se, which can be associated with difficulties at weaning and an increased risk of early postoperative respiratory failure.

For these reasons, alternative surgical and non-surgical lung volume reduction methods that might provide similar clinical benefit such as resectional LVRS with fewer risks, are currently being actively investigated [17-20].

In an attempt to minimize both surgical and anesthesiological traumas, we have developed a non-resectional LVRS technique that can be carried through Thoracic Epidural Anesthesia (TEA) alone in fully awake patients and that has proved to offer clinical benefits that seem to parallel those achieved with resectional LVRS [21-23].

The aim of this chapter is to describe this surgical technique and discuss the results.

SURGICAL PATHOPHYSIOLOGY OF EMPHYSEMA

Emphysema is defined as an abnormal, irreversible enlargement of air spaces distal to the terminal bronchioles associated with destruction of their walls and development of blebs and bullae. Destruction of alveolar walls decreases alveolar elastic recoil and traction support of non-cartilaginous small bronchi, leading to early expiratory collapse of the airways and increased airflow resistance. This cascade of detrimental effects induces gas trapping and hyperinflation in overly compliant emphysematous lung regions.

As a result of the lung hyperinflation, which is worsened by exercise (dynamic hyperinflation), remodeling of the thoracic cage with upward-outward repositioning of the ribs and flattening of the diaphragm occur, causing a dysfunctional interaction between the chest wall and the lungs and an impairment in ventilatory mechanics. In fact, the lungs become functionally restricted by the chest wall and dynamic hyperinflation hampers the capacity of the chest wall to lower pleural pressure sufficiently to expand the oversized lungs to supernormal volumes.

Moreover, since capillary-rich alveolar walls are destroyed, emphysematous areas have high ventilation/perfusion ratios, creating physiologic dead space that increases the work of breathing and impairs gas exchange. In addition, regional lung hyperinflation causes compression of more normal lung areas that are better perfused, resulting in low ventilation/perfusion ratios and further impairment in gas exchange eventually leading to hypoxemia [24]. Because of impaired respiratory function and mechanics, oxygen consumption and resting energy expenditure are increased in emphysema further increasing oxygen cost of breathing and substrate oxidation that favors lipid catabolism [25].

Finally, destruction of lung tissue, as seen in emphysema, also adversely affects cardiovascular function. A decreased cross-sectional area of the pulmonary capillary bed leads to increased pulmonary vascular resistance and increased right ventricular afterloads [26] whereas compressive effects of hyperinflated lungs and flattened diaphragm can reduce venous return from the inferior vena cava and hamper diastolic filling of the heart chambers [27] (Fig. **1**).

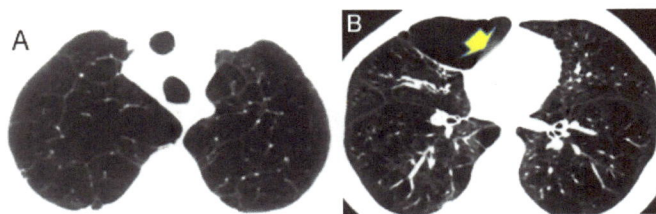

Fig. 1. CT of the chest showing upper-lobe predominant diffuse emphysema (A) with relatively better preserved lower lobes (B). Compression of the right ventricle is exerted by a bulla in the middle lobe (arrow).

Physiologic effects of LVRS. When a portion of a severely hyperinflated emphysematous lung is surgically removed or plicated, the remaining lung tissue stretches within the thorax. An unchanged chest wall operating on a smaller lung restores the elastic recoil [28] and expiratory flow at any given lung volume increases due to increased airway traction and delayed airway closure. Reduced thoracic gas compression and improved expiratory flow translates into improvement of chest wall and diaphragm configuration and mechanics [29] (Fig. **2**), improvement of ventilation perfusion mismatch, and possibly a reduced impediment to venous return with better right ventricular filling [30]. In addition, the improved efficiency of respiratory muscles achieved by LVRS decreases proportional oxygen consumption of respiratory muscles and resting energy expenditure and these improvements correlate with the reduction of Residual Volume (RV)[31]. Clinical benefit of LVRS include long lasting relief from dyspnea and meaningful improvements in forced expiratory volume in one second (FEV$_1$), RV, six minute walking test distance and quality of life measurements [2-10].

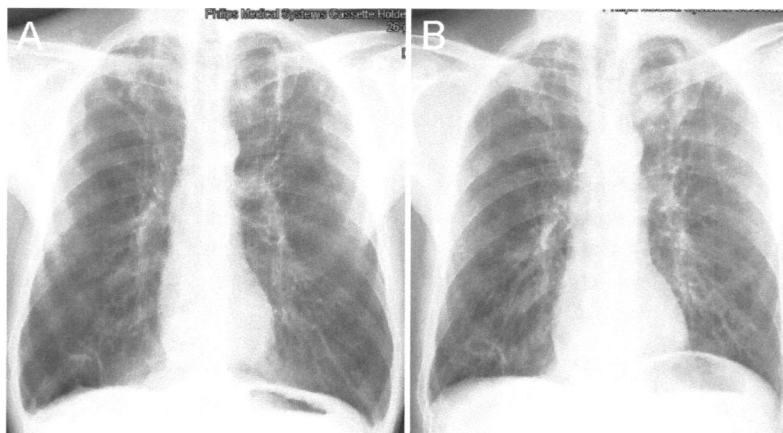

Fig. 2. Chest roentgenogram showing severe lung hyperinflation with flattened diaphragms before unilateral awake left LVRS (A) and postoperative improvement in chest wall and left hemi-diaphragm configuration (B).

HISTORICAL PERSPECTIVE

Anatomic changes caused by pulmonary emphysema were well described by Laennec in 1834 [32], although previous descriptions by Baillie and others already existed [33]. These pathologic descriptions served as the basis for understanding of the emphysematous disease in the early part of the 20th century, although it was not until the latter half of the century that its pathophysiology was fully elucidated.

Since the early 1900s, various operations were proposed to relieve dyspnea or treat the distended chest and flattened diaphragm recognized to be associated with emphysema. Amongst these, costochondrectomy, thoracoplasty, phrenic nerve interruption, and denervation procedures such as glomectomy and lung hilum stripping were initially enthusiastically embraced by their proponents based on anecdotal reports of subjective improvement but were then inexorably discarded, due to improper physiopathologic bases [34].

In 1959, Brantigan and colleagues [35] proposed LVRS as a surgical procedure aimed at removing the most emphysematous lung areas, by non-anatomical resection (resectional LVRS) and through staged thoracotomy, to help restore radial traction on terminal bronchioles, thus improving respiratory airflow obstruction and diaphragmatic excursion. In a first 33-patient series [36], satisfactory symptomatic improvement occurred in most patients although the lack of objective methods to measure clinical benefits and a 16% mortality rate led to severe criticisms [34] and abandonment of the Brantigan operation for decades.

The revival of surgical treatment for emphysema at the beginning of the 90's includes data on results of thoracoscopic contraction of emphysematous bullae by carbon dioxide laser [37] or argon beam coagulator [38] to achieve a sort of volume reduction. In 1994, taking advantage of considerations based on their experience with lung transplantation, Cooper and coworkers [11] were convinced of the correct pathophysiologic basis of Brantigan's operation and proposed a modified resectional LVRS technique entailing simultaneous, bilateral, buttressed staple resection, through median sternotomy. This revised operation resulted in an impressive 82% improvement in FEV_1 associated with significant benefits in dyspnea index, exercise capacity and quality of life measurements that reinvigorated interest for LVRS. Subsequently, thoracoscopic resectional LVRS carried out in either a unilateral or bilateral fashion was also proposed and rapidly adopted by several surgeons in an attempt to minimize surgical trauma [39-42]. Thereafter, laser contraction was essentially abandoned because of inferior results and complications achieved by this technique when compared to resectional LVRS [43].

As far as the development of plication methods is concerned, lung plication was already adopted by Brantigan *et al.* [36] who employed both resections and plications of emphysematous lung regions to achieve an adequate volume reduction.

In 1992 Crosa-Dorado *et al.* [44] proposed an original multiple fold plication method of bullous regions, performed by thoracotomy, whereas in 1997, Swansson *et al.* [45] modified this technique for videothoracoscopic application. A slightly different fold plication LVRS method was proposed by Iwasaki and coworkers [46] in 1999.

In 2006, we published the results of the first series of non-resectional LVRS carried out in fully awake patients using an original introflexive plication method [21].

PATIENT SELECTION

Potential candidates for awake LVRS are all patients with chronic obstructive pulmonary disease who are suffering from severe shortness of breath with low exertion or even at rest despite maximized medical treatment.

Initial screening entails medical history, routine digital chest roentgenograms and standard pulmonary function tests. On this basis, about 70% of potential candidates are turned down mainly due to predominant chronic bronchitis with excessive sputum production, insufficient severity of emphysema or too uniform emphysematous destruction throughout the lungs.

Patients who are found to be potentially eligible must undergo High-Resolution Computed Tomography (HRCT), lung volume measurements with body plethysmography and assessment of diffusing capacity for carbon monoxide with the single-breath technique.

A diagnosis of end-stage emphysema with disabling dyspnea, moderate to severe obstructive defect with a predicted FEV_1 ≤40%, and a predicted RV>180% despite maximal medical therapy are standard inclusion criteria (Table **1**). Smoking cessation for at least 4 months is not only an obligatory prerequisite aimed at reducing operative risks, but can reveal a good indicator of the patient's real motivation to face the burden of a surgical procedure and make every effort to improve his/her rapidly deteriorating clinical condition [4].

Table 1. Indications for awake LVRS.

Appropriately informed consent to undergo an awake procedure.

No contraindication for TEA.

No history of severe anxiety symptoms, panic attacks or psychiatric disturbances.

Diffuse emphysema graded as severe and heterogeneous at the HRCT.

Dyspnea score ≥3 according to the MMRC.

No significant sputum production, clinically significant bronchiectasis or asthma.

Severe obstructive ventilatory defect with FEV_1<50% and RV≥180%.

Age ≤ 80 years.

PaCO$_2$ < 55 mmHg.

D$_L$CO > 20% predicted.

American Society of Anesthesiology score ≤ 3.

No comorbid condition that would significantly increase operative risk including acute pneumonia, unstable angina, severe arrhythmia, acute renal failure or neoplastic disease with life expectancy < 12 months.

No previous pleurodesis or thoracotomy in the hemithorax targeted for LVRS.

Abstinence from cigarette smoking for at least 4 months.

TEA: thoracic epidural anesthesia; HRCT: high resolution computed tomography of the chest; MMRC: Modified Medical Research Council dyspnea score; FEV$_1$: forced expiratory volume in one second; RV: plethysmographic residual volume; PaCO$_2$: arterial carbon dioxide tension; D$_L$CO: diffusion capacity for carbon monoxide.

Inspiratory resistance of the airways had also been proposed as a physiologic marker indicating the most suitable candidates for LVRS with lowest values predicting maximal benefit due to *pure* emphysematous damage without significant bronchitis [47].

However, physiologic factors are not the most useful selection criteria for LVRS due to the poor correlation commonly observed between pulmonary function measures and morphologic pattern of the emphysematous damage.

Severe hypoxemia is rarely observed in patients with heterogeneous emphysema, and patients with room-air PaO$_2$ values of 60-65 mmHg can easily tolerate an awake LVRS procedure. In the same way, hypercapnia with PaCO$_2$>50 mmHg is quite rarely observed in these patients; nonetheless it must be kept in mind that permissive hypercapnia can occur during awake LVRS and, though well tolerated by most of patients, it can rarely induce agitation and neurological disturbances requiring deeper intraoperative sedation or even conversion to general anesthesia.

Radiologically, ideal candidates for awake LVRS have hyperinflated lungs with flattened diaphragms on chest radiography and HRCT findings of emphysema preferably predominant in the upper lobes, intermingled with better preserved and functionally recruitable lung tissue (within-lung heterogeneity). An asymmetric distribution of emphysema with more severe emphysematous destruction in one lung (between-lung heterogeneity) is an elective indication for unilateral treatment (Fig. **3**).

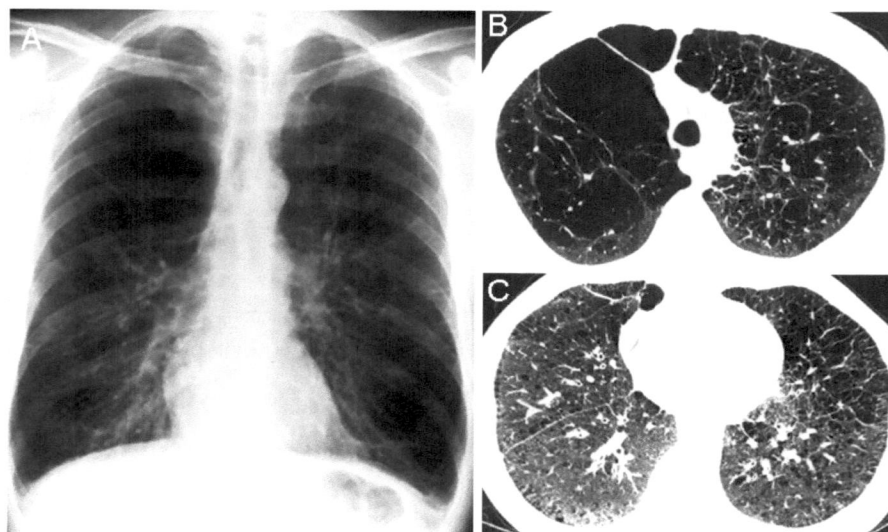

Fig. 3. Radiologic features of an ideal candidate for awake unilateral LVRS. Chest roentgenogram shows signs of lung hyperinflation with flattened diaphragm (A). HRCT of the chest shows severe emphysema with asymmetric distribution predominant in the right upper lobe (B) and relatively better preserved tissue in the middle and lower lung regions (C).

Patients with homogeneous emphysema and no target areas are mostly excluded. In particular, the combination of homogeneous emphysema with FEV_1<20% and D_LCO less than 20% identifies a subgroup at high-risk for death after LVRS and who should be excluded [48].

SURGICAL TECHNIQUE

Anesthesia. The objective of TEA is to achieve somatosensory and motor block between T1-T8 levels. In particular, motor block of the intercostal muscles with preserved diaphragmatic motion is pursued. The thoracic epidural catheter is inserted at T4 level following oral premedication with 7.5 mg midazolam. In the operating room, patients receive a continuous infusion of ropivacaine 0.5% and sufentanil 1.66 μg/mL into the epidural space at a rate of 5mL/h. During the procedure, patients breath O_2 through a Venturi mask/face to keep oxygen saturation above 90%. Whenever coughing reflexes disturb the ongoing surgical maneuvers, additional conscious sedation with an opioid such as remifentanil is highly effective in this regard. During wound closure, the anesthetic regimen is changed to ropivacaine 0.16% and sufentanil 1 μg/mL at 2-5 mL/h. Infusional regimen entails lactated Ringer's solution at 2 mL·Kg^{-1}·h^{-1}.

Surgical approach. One-stage bilateral LVRS has been shown to produce a greater magnitude of improvements in FEV_1, RV, subjective dyspnea, exercise tolerance and prednisone independence when compared to unilateral treatment and has been recommended by some surgeons [49]. Instead, unilateral LVRS has been conventionally relegated to the role of a *by necessity* approach, to be preferred in patients with previous thoracic surgery or pleurodesis on the side targeted for the operation, older patients, or in those most severely debilitated and considered unfit for a simultaneous bilateral procedure [50]. However, initial unilateral LVRS followed by subsequent completion of the bilateral treatment delayed until benefits achieved with the first operation are weaned, is an alternative elective strategy of treatment, which has been shown to have a rationale for the following reasons:

-   The magnitude of improvements following unilateral treatment usually exceeds those of the bilateral operation by more than half. This finding suggests an interdependence effect between the hemithoraxes as a function of the compliance of the lungs and the mobility of the mediastinum [51].

-   An asymmetric distribution of emphysema between the lungs with one lung being more severely destroyed and/or hyperinflated than the contralateral one is quite frequently recognizable at HRCT and in these instances, benefits of unilateral LVRS can compare with those achieved by bilateral treatment [13].

-   Postoperative deterioration in FEV_1 has been shown to be greater after bilateral than after unilateral LVRS [52], thus suggesting a role for a staged bilateral approach with the second reduction delayed until the patient's clinical condition returns to the initial preoperative status. In this respect there is some evidence that improvements in FEV_1, FVC, 6-minute walking test distance and RV were more stable after staged unilateral than after one-stage bilateral LVRS [53].

-   Although previous retrospective studies have shown no advantage for the unilateral approach in terms of mortality and morbidity when compared to the bilateral treatment, no randomized study has been performed in this setting. Thus it seems reasonable to assume that a unilateral operation is associated with less postoperative pain, less risk of prolonged air leaks and an easier perioperative mobilization of the patient.

We consider a simultaneous bilateral awake operation poorly tolerable and prefer an intentional staged unilateral awake LVRS in all instances.

Awake non-resectional LVRS. The patient is placed in the lateral decubitus position as for thoracotomy. Neither axillary roll or table flexion are not used to ensure the patient a comfortable position during the awake procedure and to facilitate ventilation of the dependent lung.

The video monitor is placed at the head of the table and the surgical team consists of two surgeons and one assistant nurse. A complete set for 24Ch chest tube insertion is kept ready on the nurse's table. Four flexible trocars are inserted in the targeted hemithorax. For typical upper-lobe LVRS, the camera port is placed in the sixth intercostal space along the midaxilllary line while operating ports for ring forceps and the endoscopic staplers are placed in the third and fifth intercostal space along the anterior axillary line, and in the fourth intercostal space along the posterior axillary line.

A 30°, 10 mm camera is employed to improve oblique vision during spontaneous ventilation. The pleura is entered bluntly with straight Crile forceps, taking care to avoid tearing the underlying emphysematous lung. As soon as the trocar incisions are carried out and the pleural cavity is explored confirming the possibility to perform the operation by the awake approach, we now prefer to immediately insert one chest tube connected to water seal just below the camera port. This is because we have found that periodical re-expansion of the lung for a few minutes can limit risks of an excessive rise of end-operative $PaCO_2$, particularly if the operating time is expected to be somewhat prolonged or the preoperative functional reserve of the patients is greatly impaired. Whenever pleural adhesions are found they are coagulated and cut thoracoscopically. Limited apical adhesions, which do not hamper lung plication from being carried out, are not divided to facilitate end-operative lung re-expansion.

Following the insertion of the 3rd trocar, the lung is carefully inspected and palpated by 2 ring forceps (Fig. 4) to aid its collapse.

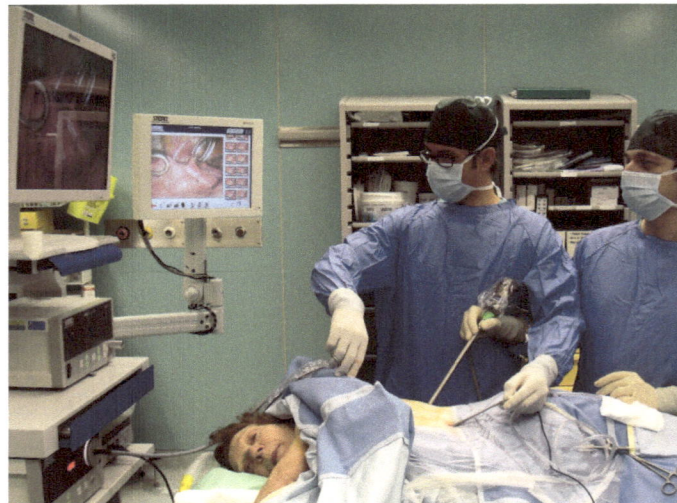

Fig. 4. Position of the patient and operative set-up with camera and two ring forceps inserted for lung palpation.

The goal of LVRS is to reduce as much lung volume while sparing as much functioning tissue as possible. The most destroyed lung regions targeted for plication usually correspond to the lung regions that fail to deflate after creation of the surgical pneumothorax.

During lung inspection and palpation, unnecessary manipulation of the lung is avoided to minimize any trauma to the fragile emphysematous lung tissue, which can increase the development of air leaks postoperatively.

Redundant lung edges of the most emphysematous target areas are gently grasped by two ring forceps and introflexed with cotton swabs. Thereafter, both lung edges are grasped together by a single ring forceps and a 45 mm, 'non-cutting' endostapler is applied on the plicated lung region, starting at the apex of the upper lobe. In a similar manner, 2 other cartridges are fired in the ventral and dorsal side of the targeted area to perform a linear, interrupted suture line (Fig. 5). As a result, the upper lobe volume is reduced by more than 50% with no tissue resection (Fig. 6). The plication line follows a curvilinear shape to allow remodeling of the underlying lung, so that it can easily re-expand and completely fill the pleural cavity at the end of the procedure. In patients with lower lobe emphysema, multiple smaller plications are generally carried out in both the middle and lower lobe to reduce the overall lung volume. The presence of small air leaks does not require any treatment and are expected to stop within a few days whereas large air leaks can require re-stapling of the leaking site. At the end of the procedure, one or two chest tubes are inserted and the patient is asked to cough repeatedly while the camera port is occluded with a gauze to obtain lung re-expansion under thoracoscopic vision (Fig. **7**). Trocar incisions are then sutured in a standard manner (Video 1).

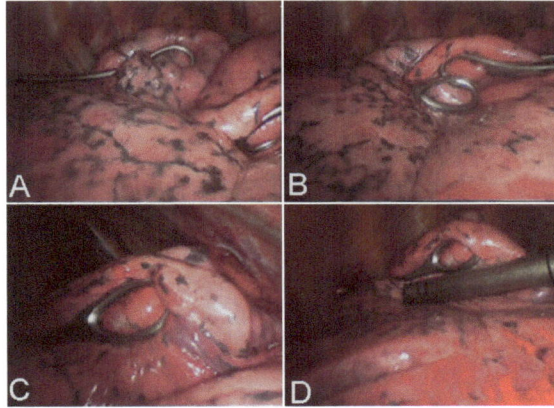

Fig. 5. Distant edges of the lung region to be plicated are grasped ventrally and dorsally by ring forceps starting at the lung apex (A). The grasped edges are then gently approximated (B), grasped together by a single ring forceps (C) and sutured by a non-cutting endoscopic stapler (D).

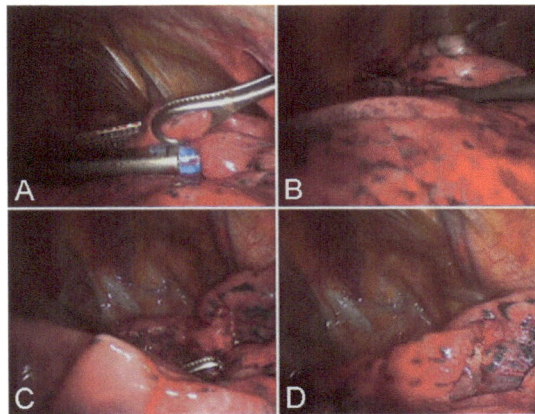

Fig. 6. Another two cartridges are fired; one ventrally (A) and one dorsally (B) along a single ideal line to accomplish a linear but interrupted suture. At end-procedure, the upper lobe is reduced by 60-70% in volume whereas the remaining lung can adequately re-expand (C, D).

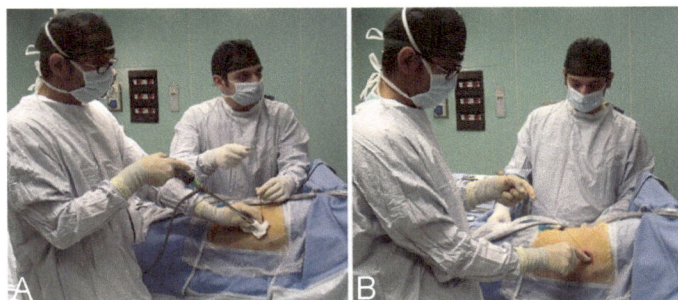

Fig. 7. At end-procedure, after placement of the chest tube(s), one stitch is passed through the camera port and is left untied; the camera is reinserted keeping the port air-tight with a gauze (A). The patient is then asked to cough repeatedly to obtain full lung re-expansion under direct vision. Both the camera and flexible trocar are then extracted rapidly while the underlying stitch is tied (B).

Complications. Intraoperative complications during awake LVRS are rare and include panic attacks and intolerable hypercapnia. Conversion to general anesthesia is seldom required since in most of these instances a simple increase of sedation with sub-hypnotic boluses of propofol is sufficient to allow uneventful completion of the procedure. Bleeding from the suture lines or from the division of improperly coagulated vascularized adhesions can also occur and is usually easily controlled thoracoscopically.

During the surgical maneuvers and adhesiolysis, care must be paid to avoid to injury to nerve structures, such as the phrenic nerve, the sympathetic chain, the vagus and intercostal nerves.

Perioperative morbidity of awake non-resectional LVRS is minimal and is mainly due to prolonged air leaks, which occur in less than 20% of patients [54]. These findings compare favorably with results of resectional LVRS showing prolonged air leaks in nearly 30% of operated patients [55]. Even though air leaks do not seem associated with operative mortality, their importance should not be underestimated since they can promote other complications including gross subcutaneous emphysema, atelectasis, lung infection and even respiratory failure. Moreover, in patients with postoperative air leaks, hospitalization can be prolonged and thus eventual procedure-related costs will be higher than those of patients with an unremarkable postoperative course. Other early complications that can occur following LVRS include pneumonia, bleeding, respiratory failure, arrhythmias, and gastrointestinal complications. Amongst late complications, respiratory failure, pulmonary hypertension [56], secondary pneumothorax [57], metalloptysis [58] (*i.e.* asymptomatic expectoration of steel staples), inflammatory pseudotumor, and development of giant bullous emphysema [59] have been reported with resectional LVRS but have not been reported following the awake operation.

Results. In a comparative analysis [54], the perioperative outcome of 66 patients undergoing awake unilateral LVRS at our University (Fig. **8**) was compared with that of 66 patients undergoing standard LRS through general anesthesia. Prolonged air-leak occurred in 18% of the patients in the awake group vs 40% in the control group and its overall duration was 5.2 days versus 7.9 days, respectively. As a consequence mean hospital stay was significantly shorter in the awake group (6.3 days vs 9.2 days, respectively)..

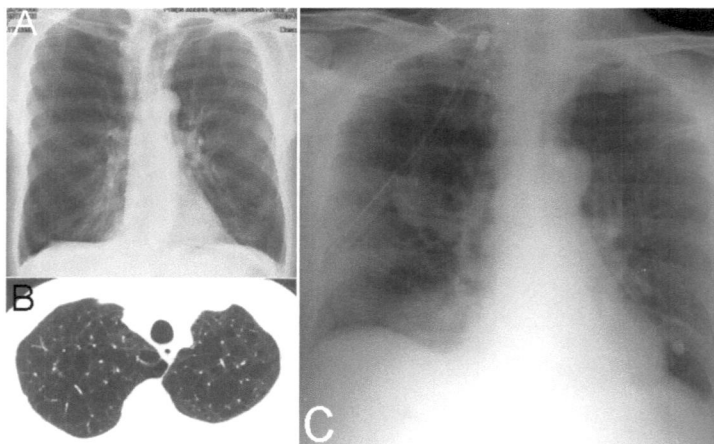

Fig. 8. Radiological images of a patient with severe emphysema before (A, B) and 12h after (C) unilateral, awake right LVRS, showing immediate reconfiguration towards normality of the right hemidiaphragm.

Univariate analysis indicated resectional LVRS, higher severity of emphysema and lower diffusion capacity for carbon monoxide as significant predictors of prolonged air leak whereas at multivariate testing, high severity of emphysema was the most important factor predicting occurrence of prolonged air leaks. Awake non-resectional LVRS is commonly quickly performed and well tolerated by patients although it may prove somewhat more technically demanding than the equivalent operation performed through general anesthesia and one-lung ventilation. The reasons for this are multifactorial and include the partial ventilation of the operated lung, unadvertently triggered coughing reflexes caused by stretching of the lung hilum, and the maintained diaphragmatic motion that can all disturb surgical maneuvering. In another series on awake LVRS, clinical outcome including the multidimensional BODE index was analyzed [22]. Conversion to thoracotomy was not necessary while conversion to general anesthesia was required in 2 patients due to panic attack and severe hypercapnia in one patient each. Partial failure of epidural analgesia occurred in 3 patients who required additional perioperative injection of local anesthetics.

Oxygenation remained satisfactory throughout the procedure. On the other hand, permissive hypercapnia developed at the end of the operation in some patients although, in most of them, it did not require any treatment and resolved within the first postoperative hours (Fig. **9**). All patients were allowed to drink, eat and walk within a few hours after the operation and physiotherapy was commonly started the same day as surgery.

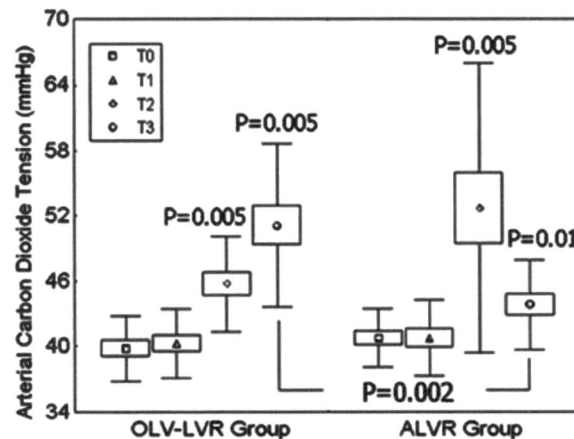

Fig. 9. Perioperative behavior of arterial carbon dioxide tension ($PaCO_2$) in patients undergoing LVRS through general anesthesia and one-lung ventilation (OLV-LVR) or awake anesthesia (ALVR) at 4 time intervals: before the operation (T0); after creation of the surgical pneumothorax (T1); at end-procedure (T2) and 1h postoperatively (T3). Results show that at end-procedure, $PaCO_2$ is higher in the awake group. One hour after the operation it returns towards baseline values in awake patients whereas it continues to increase in the non-awake group.

There was no ninety day mortality whereas median hospital stay was 6 days with 29% of the patients discharged within 4 days and 74% within 6 days. At 12 months, significant clinical improvements were observed in most patients and lasted for more than 2 years. In particular, there was a significant reduction in RV, which was associated with improvements in six minute walking test distance; absolute improvements in FEV, FVC and RV were 0.34L, 0.50L and 1.10L, respectively. The BODE index decreased postoperatively and remained significantly improved for more than 2 years. During follow-up, contralateral LVRS due to FEV_1 decline towards the baseline value or reappearance of incapacitating dyspnea was carried out in 24% of the patients (Fig. **10**). Actuarial survival was 83% at 3 years.

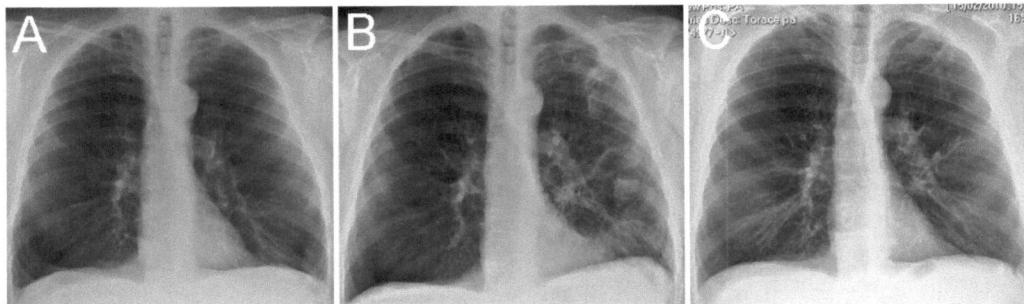

Fig. 10. Chest roentgenograms performed before unilateral, left awake LVRS (A) as well as 12 months (B) and 36 months (C) after the operation, showing relative stability of chest wall and diaphragm reconfiguration over time. Clinically, the patient is still meaningfully improved at 3 years.

Redo awake lung volume reduction. Optimal management of emphysematous patients who have lost benefits achieved after previous, successful LVRS, is a clinical dilemma since most of these subjects are older than 65 years and cannot be inserted in a waiting list for lung transplantation. The desperate clinical conditions of some of these patients have led us to consider lung volume reduction-reoperations in stringently selected instances. In particular, amongst 17 patients with radiological evidence of distinct regional lung hyperinflation undergoing LVRS reoperations (Fig. **11**), 5 patients underwent awake lung plication performed under sole (TEA). Amongst these patients, there was no hospital mortality and clinically meaningful improvements in FEV_1, FVC, RV, six-minute walking test and modified Medical Research Council dyspnea index occurred for up to 12 months. At six-months FEV_1 increases greater than 200mL occurred in 2 patients [60].

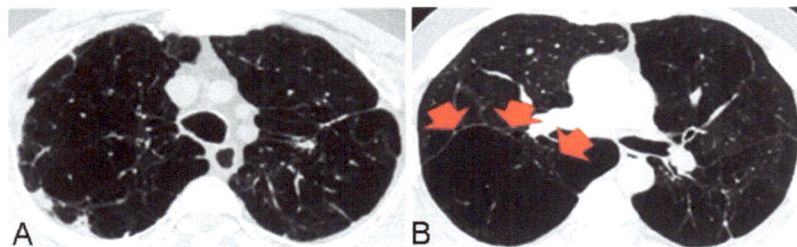

Fig. 11. HRCT of a patient who already underwent bilateral resectional LVRS (A) and developed severe, regional hyperinflation of the right superior segment of the lower lobe (B, red arrows), which represented an ideal target for awake redo LVRS.

Awake bullectomy. Bullectomy is a well established procedure that has been performed for decades, mostly in patients with localized large bullae. It can be assumed to represent the ideal type of LVRS technique, since both removal of non-functioning hyperinflated tissue and respect for underlying better preserved lung are maximized by bullectomy.

Staple excision of emphysematous bullae through general anesthesia is the most commonly employed method for bullectomy [61] whereas, so far, awake bullectomy has been anecdotally reported only in patients with secondary pneumothorax [62].

We recently reported [63] on a novel awake non-resectional LVRS method developed to plicate large, isolated emphysematous bullae (bullaplasty). In this way, even giant bullae of more than 1000 mL in volume have been easily and successfully treated (Fig. **12**) (**Video 2**).

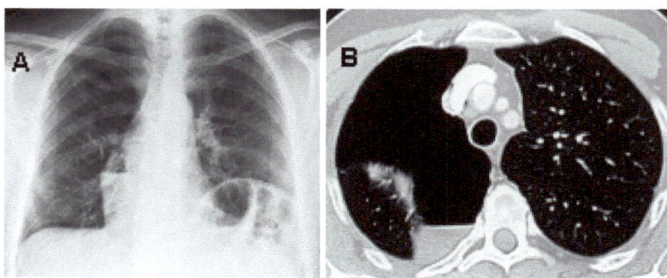

Fig. 12. Chest roentgenogram (A) and HRCT (B) of a huge emphysematous bulla mimicking right hydro-pneumothorax, successfully managed by awake bullaplasty.

In patients with bullous emphysema, preoperative work-up includes spirometry with plethysmography, analysis of blood gases and computed tomography with algorithm for quantitative measurement of the bulla volume. During the operation, oxygenation slightly deteriorated but returned towards baseline values 1 h after surgery. Technical feasibility and patient satisfaction with the awake anesthesia was scored as satisfactory and so far we have had no hospital mortality with this operative method. On average, hospital stay following awake bullaplasty is limited to 2-3 days.

Significant improvements in FEV_1, RV, six minute walking test and subjective dyspnea were observed at 6 months and remained stable during the follow-up at 12 and 24 months.

COMMENT

LVRS has considerably evolved since when Brantigan *et al.* [22] performed manual non-anatomical LVRS through thoracotomy. Several technical refinements and substantial improvements in perioperative management that include multidisciplinary cooperative efforts of surgeons, anesthesiologists, pneumologists, radiologists, and cardiologists have led to satisfactory results, which are reported with different surgical methods and approaches. However, so far, none of these approaches and methods have proved capable of eliminating the meaningful LVRS-related mortality and morbidity, and particularly the occurrence of postoperative air leaks that continues to be the most common complication, resulting in about 30% of the patients still hospitalized or in rehabilitation facilities 1 month after the operation [15, 16]. This procedure-related morbidity is probably independent of the technical measures adopted in an attempt to limit the occurrence of air leaks, including staple line buttress [55, 64, 65], use of biological sealant [55] and additional operating methods [66, 67].

For this reason, alternative non-surgical lung volume reduction methods including bronchoscopic one-way valves [68, 69], use of airway sealants or endobronchial spigots and plugs [70], as well as endobronchial bypass methods allowing for the trapped air to escape by way of an alternative route through bronchial stents and fenestrations [71], have been proposed.

So far, none of these methods has proved capable of achieving clinical results similar to those associated with surgical LVRS.

Awake non-resectional LVRS constitutes a surgical alternative to resectional LVRS and one further step in the attempt to minimize both surgical and anesthesiological trauma. It is likely that the smooth postoperative course observed after awake LVRS reflects the rapid recovery achieved by prompt resumption of main daily-life activity and the relatively low rate of prolonged air leaks, which compares favorably with larger series data [6, 55].

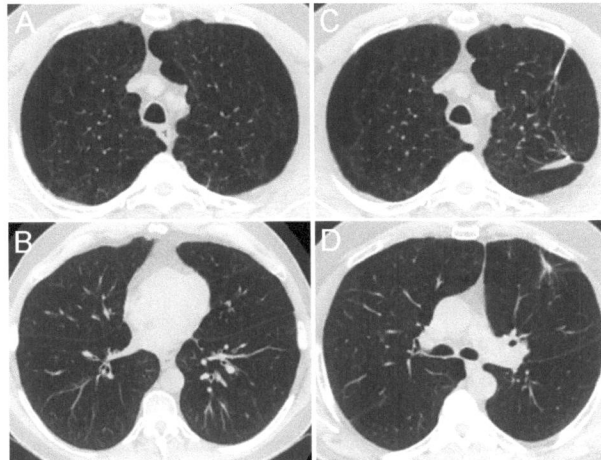

Fig. 13. Preoperative HRCT of the chest shows severe upper-lobe predominant emphysema (A) with better preserved lower lung regions (B). Postoperative CT shows significant reduction in overall lung volume with minimal peripheral scarring resulting from introflexive plication (C, D). The non-resectional nature of the operation as well as peripheral suturing sparing the central part of the lung may both account for the reduced incidence of postoperative air leaks.

The awake non-resectional LVRS technique maintains the basic concepts outlined by Brantigan *et al.* [36] and refined by Cooper *et al.* [11] for resectional LVRS, including a reduction of 20%-30% of the lung volume, suturing along a single ideal line and use of stapling devices (Fig. **13**). However, it also adds some differences that might have contributed to reduce the incidence and duration of air leaks. They include avoidance of discontinuation of visceral pleura, a four-fold buttressed suture line as well as accomplishment of superficial and interrupted sutures in the lung that do not involve central lung areas, are less rigid and thus facilitate filling of the pleural cavity by the remodeled lung. In this way the degree of overall reduction in lung volume can parallel that achieved by resectional LVRS as suggested by the fairly well matched clinical results (Tables **2** and **3**).

Table 2. Results of resectional LVRS performed through general anesthesia.

First author	Year	N	Surgical approach	Mortality (%)	Hospital stay (days)	ΔFEV_1 (%)	ΔRV (%)
Mc Kenna [49]	1996	87	VATS, unilateral	3	11.4	31	-
Naunheim [72]	1996	50	VATS, unilateral	2	13	35	33
Keenan [39]	1996	57	VATS, unilateral	2	17	27	16
Kotloff [40]	1996	80	Sternotomy, bilateral	13.8	22	41	28
		40	VATS, bilateral	2.5	15	41	23
Bingisser [12]	1996	20	VATS, bilateral	0	15	42	24
Mc Kenna [73]	1997	154	VATS, bilateral	4	11	52	-
Pompeo [4]	2000	30	VATS, unilateral/bilateral	3.3	13.6	53	25
Ciccone [6]	2003	250	Sternotomy, bilateral	4.8	9	57	31
NETT [7]	2003	511	Variable*, bilateral	2.2	10	-	-
Mineo [13]	2005	97	VATS, unilateral	1	9	36	20
Meyers [50]	2008	43	Thoracotomy, unilateral	2.3	8	32	23

FEV_1=forced expiratory volume in one second; N=number of patients; RV=residual volume. *Multicenter trial including sternotomy, VATS and thoracotomy approaches.

Table 3. Results of thoracoscopic non-resectional LVRS.

First author	Year	N	Anesthesia	Surgical approach	Mortality (%)	Hospital stay (days)	ΔFEV_1 (%)	ΔRV (%)
Swanson [45]	1997	32	General	Unilateral/bilateral	0	7	29	-
Iwasaki [46]	1999	20	General	Unilateral	0	11.5	34	-
Pompeo [22]	2007	42	Awake, epidural	Unilateral	0	6	39	22

FEV_1=forced expiratory volume in one second; N=number of patients; RV=residual volume.

One-lung ventilation under general anesthesia was deemed necessary for surgical LVRS. However, several adverse effects can derive from this type of anesthesia including an increased risk of pneumonia, impaired cardiac performance, neuromuscular problems and multifactorial mechanical ventilation injury [74]. Furthermore, general anesthesia with instrumentation of the airways can elicit bronchospasm and life threatening complications including tracheal rupture [75, 76]. Most of these adverse effects could be avoided by using (TEA) in awake patients.

On the other hand, it is still commonly believed that an open pneumothorax is poorly tolerated by patients with severe emphysema. Our findings indicates that this concern is likely to be overestimated. In fact, simple administration of oxygen through a Venturi mask prevents hypoxemia in the vast majority of patients while permissive hypercapnia, though commonly observed, does not compromise optimal feasibility of the procedure.

One physiological effect that might contribute to keep respiratory function satisfactory throughout awake procedures is the maintained diaphragmatic motion that contrasts with the compression of the dependent lung by abdominal pressure occurring during general anesthesia through the paralyzed diaphragm.

CONCLUSION

In conclusion, results of novel evolutionary methods [77] of the initial Brantigan operation confirm the idea that reducing the lung volume in severely emphysematous subjects can improve lung function and quality of life. Awake non-resectional LVRS is one of the most promising applications of awake thoracic surgery and the one potentially offering significant clinical advantages when compared to other newly developed non-surgical lung volume reduction methods [78].

REFERENCES

[1]   Barnes PJ. Prospects for new drugs for chronic obstructive pulmonary disease. Lancet 2004;364:985-96.

[2]   Criner GJ, Cordova FC, Furakawa S, *et al.* Prospective randomized trial comparing bilateral lung volume reduction surgery to pulmonary rehabilitation in severe chronic obstructive pulmonary disease. Am J Respir Crit Care Med 1999;160:2018-27.

[3]   Geddes D, Davies M, Koyama H, Hansell D, *et al.* Effect of lung volume reduction surgery in patients with severe emphysema. N Engl J Med 2000;343:239-45.

[4]   Pompeo E, Marino M, Nofroni I, Matteucci G, Mineo TC. Reduction pneumoplasty versus respiratory rehabilitation in severe emphysema: a randomized study. Pulmonary Emphysema Research Group. Ann Thorac Surg 2000;70:948-54.

[5]   Gelb AF, McKenna RJ Jr, Brenner M, Epstein JD, Zamel N. Lung function 5 yr after lung volume reduction surgery for emphysema. Am J Respir Crit Care Med 2001;163:1562-6.

[6]   Ciccone AM, Meyers BF, Guthrie TJ, *et al.* Long-term outcome of bilateral lung volume reduction in 250 consecutive patients with emphysema. J Thorac Cardiovasc Surg 2003;125:513-25.

[7]   National Emphysema Treatment Trial Research Group. A randomized trial comparing lung-volume-reduction surgery with medical therapy for severe emphysema. N Engl J Med 2003;248:2059-73.

[8]   Goldstein RS, Todd TRJ, Guyatt G. Influence of lung volume reduction surgery (LVRS) on health related quality of life in patients with chronic obstructive pulmonary disease. Thorax 2003;58:405-10.

[9]   Miller JD, Malthaner RA, Goldsmith CH, *et al.* Canadian Lung Volume Reduction Surgery Study. A randomized clinical trial of lung volume reduction surgery versus best medical care for patients with advanced emphysema: a two-year study from Canada. Ann Thorac Surg 2006;81:314-20.

[10]   Naunheim KS, Wood DE, Moshenifar Z, *et al.* National Emphysema Treatment Trial Research Group. Long term follow-up of patients receiving lung-volume reduction surgery versus medical therapy for severe emphysema by the National Emphysema Treatment Trial Research Group. Ann Thorac Surg 2006;82:431-4.

[11]   Cooper JD, Trulock EP, Triantafillou AN, *et al.* Bilateral pneumectomy (volume reduction) for chronic obstructive pulmonary disease. J Thorac Cardiovasc Surg 1995;109:106-19.

[12]   Bingisser R, Zollinger A, Hauser M, *et al.* Bilateral volume reduction surgery for diffuse pulmonary emphysema by video-assisted thoracoscopy. J Thorac Cardiovasc Surg 1996;112:875-82.

[13]   Mineo TC, Pompeo E, Mineo D, *et al.* Results of unilateral lung volume reduction surgery in patients with distinct heterogeneity of emphysema between-lungs. J Thorac Cardiovasc Surg 2005;129:73-9.

[14]   DeCamp M, McKenna RJ, Deschamps CC, Krasna MJ. Lung volume reduction surgery. Technique, operative mortality and morbidity. Proc Am Thorac Soc 2008;5:442-6.

[15]   Naunheim KS, Wood DE, Krasna MJ, *et al.* National Emphysema Treatment Trial Research Group. Predictors of operative morbidity and mortality in the National Emphysema Treatment Trial. J Thorac Cardiovasc Surg 2006;131:43-53.

[16]   National Emphysema Treatment Trial Research Group. Cost effectiveness of lung-volume-reduction surgery for patients with severe emphysema. New Eng J Med 2003;348:2092-102.

[17]   Toma TP, Hopkinson NS, Hillier J, *et al*. Bronchoscopic volume reduction with valve implants in patients with severe emphysema. Lancet 2002;361:931-3.

[18]   Rendina EA, De Giacomo T, Venuta F, *et al*. Feasibility and safety of the airway bypass procedure for patients with emphysema. J Thorac Cardiovasc Surg 2003;125:1294-9.

[19]   Yim APC, Hwong TMT, Lee TWL, *et al*. Early results of endoscopic lung volume reduction for emphysema. J Thorac Cardiovasc Surg 2004;127:1564-73.

[20]   Wood DE, McKenna RJ, Yusen RD, *et al*. A multicenter trial of an intrabronchial valve for treatment of severe emphysema. J Thorac Cardiovasc Surg 2007;133:65-73.

[21]   Mineo TC, Pompeo E, Mineo D, *et al*. Awake nonresectional lung volume reduction surgery. Ann Surg 2006;243:131-6.

[22]   Pompeo E, Mineo TC. Two-year improvement in multidimensional body mass index, airflow obstruction, dyspnea and exercise capacity index after nonresectional lung volume reduction surgery in awake patients. Ann Thorac Surg 2007;84:1862-9.

[23]   Tacconi F, Pompeo E, Mineo TC. Duration of air leak is reduced after awake nonresectional lung volume reduction surgery. Eur J Cardiothorac Surg 2009;35:822-8.

[24]   Mora JI, Hadjiliadis D. Lung volume reduction surgery and lung transplantation in chronic obstructive pulmonary disease. Int J Chron Obstruct Pulmon Dis. 2008;3:629-35.

[25]   Donahoe M, Rogers RM, Wilson DO, Pennock BE. Oxygen consumption of the respiratory muscles in normal and in malnourished patients with chronic obstructive pulmonary disease. Am Rev Respir Dis 1989;140:385-91.

[26]   Fira-Mladinescu O, Tudorache V, Mihaicuta S, *et al*. New concepts in the pathogenesis and pathophysiology of COPD. Pneumologia 2007;56:23-31.

[27]   Even P, Sors H, Safran D, *et al*. Hémodynamique des bulles d'emphysème un noveau syndrome: la tamponade cardiaque emphysématouse. Rev Fr Mal Respir 1980;8:117-20.

[28]   Loring SH, Leith DE, Connotti MJ, *et al*. Model of functional restriction in chronic obstructive pulmonary disease, transplantation and lung reduction surgery. Am J Respir Crit Care Med 1999;160:821-8.

[29]   Gorman RB, McKenzie DK, Butler JE, *et al*. Diaphragm length and neural drive after lung volume reduction surgery. Am J Respir Crit Care Med 2005;172:1259-66.

[30]   Mineo TC, Pompeo E, Rogliani P, *et al*. Effect of lung volume reduction surgery for severe emphysema on right ventricular function Am J Respir Crit Care Med 2002;165:489-94.

[31]   Mineo TC, Pompeo E, Mineo D, *et al*. Resting energy expenditure and metabolic changes after lung volume reduction surgery for emphysema. Ann Thorac Surg 2006;82:1205-11.

[32]   Laennec RTH. A treatise on the disease of the chest and of mediate auscultation. Translated by John Forbes. London, UK 1834.

[33]   Baillie M. The morbid anatomy of some of the most important parts of the human body. London: Pronted for J. Johns and G. Nicol 1793; p. 314.

[34]   Naef AP. History of emphysema surgery. Ann Thorac Surg 1997;64:1506-8.

[35]   Brantigan OC, Mueller E. Surgical treatment of pulmonary emphysema. Am Surg 1957;23:789-804.

[36]   Brantigan OC, Mueller E, Kress MB. A surgical approach to pulmonary emphysema. Am Rev Respir Dis 1959;80:194-206.

[37]   Lewis R, Caccavale RJ, Sisler GE. VATS-argon beam coagulator treatment of diffuse end-stage bilateral bullous disease of the lung. Ann Thorac Surg 1993;55:1394-9.

[38]   Wakabayashi A, Brenner M, Kayaleh RA, *et al*. Thoracoscopic carbon dioxide laser treatment of bullous emphysema. Lancet 1991;337:881-3.

[39]   Keenan RJ, Landreneau RJ, Sciurba FC, *et al*. Unilateral thoracoscopic surgical approach for diffuse emphysema. J Thorac Cardiovasc Surg 1996;111:308-16.

[40]   Kotloff RM, Tino G, Bavaria JE, *et al*. Bilateral lung volume reduction surgery for advanced emphysema. A comparison of median sternotomy and thoracoscopic approaches. Chest 1996; 110:1399-406.

[41]   Hazelrigg SR, Boley TM, Magee MJ, Lawyer CH, Henkle JQ. Comparison of staged thoracoscopy and median sternotomy for lung volume reduction. Ann Thorac Surg 1998;66:1134-9.

[42]   Mineo TC, Pompeo E, Simonetti G, *et al*. Unilateral thoracoscopic reduction pneumoplasty for asymmetric emphysema. Eur J Cardiothorac Surg 1998;14:33-9.

[43]   McKenna RJ Jr, Brenner M, Gelb AF, *et al*. A randomized, prospective trial of stapled lung reduction versus laser bullectomy for diffuse emphysema. J Thorac Cardiovasc Surg. 1996;111:317-21.

[44] Crosa-Dorado VL, Pomi J, Perez-Penco EJ. Treatment of dyspnea in emphysema pulmonary remodeling: hemo- and pneumostatic suturing of the emphysematous lung. Res Surg 1992;4:1-4.

[45] Swanson SJ, Mentzer SJ, DeCamp MM, *et al.* No-cut thoracoscopic lung plication: a new technique for lung volume reduction surgery. J Am Coll Surg 1997;185:25-32.

[46] Iwasaki M, Nishiumi N, Kaga K, *et al.* Application of the fold plication method for unilateral lung volume reduction in pulmonary emphysema. Ann Thorac Surg 1999;67:815-7.

[47] Ingenito EP, Evans RB, Loring SH, *et al.* Relation between preoperative inspiratory lung resistance and outcome of lung volume reduction surgery for emphysema. N Engl J Med 1998;338:1181-5.

[48] National Emphysema Treatment Trial Research Group. Patients at high risk of death after lung-volume-reduction surgery. N Engl J Med 2001;345:1075-83.

[49] Mc Kenna, Brenner M, Fischel RJ, Gelb AF. Should lung volume reduction for emphysema be unilateral or bilateral? J Thorac Cardiovasc Surg 1996;112:1331-9.

[50] Meyers BF, Sultan PK, Guthrie TJ, *et al.* Outcomes after unilateral lung volume reduction. Ann Thorac Surg 2008;86:204-12.

[51] Becker MD, Berkmen YM, Austin JHM *et al.* Lung volumes before and after lung volume reduction surgery. Am J Respir Crit Care Med 1998;157:1593-9.

[52] Brenner M, McKenna RJ, Jr, Gelb AF, Fischel RJ, Wilson A. Rate of FEV_1 change following lung volume reduction surgery. Chest 1998;113:652-9.

[53] Pompeo E, Mineo TC. Long-term staged versus one-stage bilateral thoracoscopic reduction pneumoplasty. Eur Cardiothorac Surg 2002;21:627-33.

[54] Tacconi F, Pompeo E, Mineo TC. Duration of air leak is reduced after awake nonresectional lung volume reduction surgery. Eur J Cardiothorac Surg 2009;35:822-8.

[55] DeCamp MM, Blackstone EH, Naunheim KS, *et al.* Patient and surgical factors influencing air-leaks after lung volume reduction surgery: lessons learned from the National Emphysema Treatment Trial. Ann Thorac Surg 2006;82:197-207.

[56] Weg IL, Rossoff L, McKeon K, Graver LM, Scharf SM. Development of pulmonary hypertension after lung volume reduction surgery. Am J Respir Crit Care Med 1999;159:552-6.

[57] Tacconi F, Pompeo E, Mineo TC. Late-onset occult pneumothorax after lung volume-reduction surgery. Ann Thorac Surg 2005;80:2008-12.

[58] Oey I, Waller D. Metalloptysis: a late complication of lung volume reduction surgery. Ann Thorac Surg 2001;71:1694-5.

[59] Iqbal M, Rossof L, McKeon K, Graver M, Scharf SM. Development of giant bulla after lung volume reduction surgery. Chest 1999;116:1809-11.

[60] Tacconi F, Pompeo E, Mineo TC. Late-onset occult pneumothorax after lung volume-reduction surgery. Ann Thorac Surg 2005;80:2008-12.

[61] Benditt JO. Surgical options for patients with COPD: sorting the choice. Respir Care 2006;51:173-82.

[62] Mukaida T, Andou A, Date H, Aoe M, Shimizu N. Thoracoscopic operation for secondary pneumothorax under local and epidural anesthesia in high-risk patients. Ann Thorac Surg 1998;65:924-6.

[63] Pompeo E, Tacconi F, Frasca L, Mineo TC. Awake thoracoscopic bullaplasty. Eur J Cardiothorac Surg 2011;39:1012-17.

[64] Cooper JD. Technique to reduce air leaks after resection of emphysematous lung. Ann Thorac Surg 1994;57:1038-9.

[65] Stammberger U, Klepetko W, Stamatis G, *et al.* Buttressing the staple line in lung volume reduction surgery: a randomized three-center study. Ann Thorac Surg 2000;70:1820-5.

[66] Fischel RJ, McKenna RJ. Bovine pericardium versus bovine collagen to buttress staples for lung reduction operations. Ann Thorac Surg 1998;65:217-9.

[67] Hazelrigg SR, Boley TM, Naunheim KS, *et al.* Effect of bovine pericardial strips on air leak after stapled pulmonary resection. Ann Thorac Surg 1997;63:1573-5.

[68] Yim AP, Hwong TM, Lee TW, *et al.* Early results of endoscopic lung volume reduction for emphysema. J Thorac Cardiovasc Surg 2004;127:1564-73.

[69] Strange C, Herth FJ, Kovitz KL, *et al.* VENT Study Group. Design of the Endobronchial Valve for Emphysema Palliation Trial (VENT): a non-surgical method of lung volume reduction. BMC Pulm Med 2007;7:10.

[70] Brenner M, Hanna NM, Mina-Araghi R, *et al.* Innovative approaches to lung volume reduction for emphysema. Chest 2004;126:238-48.

[71] Cardoso PF, Snell GI, Hopkins P, *et al.* Clinical application of airway bypass with paclitaxel-eluting stents: early results. J Thorac Cardiovasc Surg 2007;134:974-81.

[72] McKenna RJ, Brenner M, Fishel RJ, *et al.* Patient selection criteria for lung volume reduction surgery. J Thorac Cardiovasc Surg 1997;114:957-67.

[73] Naunheim KS, Keller C, Krucylak PE, *et al.* Unilateral video-assisted thoracic surgical lung reduction. Ann Thorac Surg 1996;61:1092-8.

[74] Whitehead T, Slutsky AS. The pulmonary physician in critical care. 7: Ventilator induced lung injury. Thorax 2002;57:635-42

[75] Gómez-Caro Andrés A, Moradiellos Díez FJ, Ausín Herrero P, *et al.* Successful conservative management in iatrogenic tracheobronchial injury. Ann Thorac Surg 2005;79:1872-8.

[76] Conti M, Pougeoise M, Wurtz A, *et al.* Management of postintubation tracheobronchial ruptures. Chest 2006;130:412-8.

[77] Sanchez PG, Kucharczuk JC, Su S, Kaiser LR, Cooper JD. National Emphysema Treatment Trial redux: accentuating the positive. J Thorac Cardiovasc Surg 2010;140:564-72.

[78] Sciurba FC, Ernst A, Herth FJ, *et al.* A randomized study of endobronchial valves for advanced emphysema. N Engl J Med 2010;363:1233-44.

Awake Thoracic Surgery, 2012, 105-118

CHAPTER 8

Awake Lung Biopsy for Interstitial Lung Disease

Luca Frasca, Vincenzo Ambrogi, Paola Rogliani[†], Cesare Saltini[†] and Eugenio Pompeo[*]

Departments of Thoracic Surgery and [†]Pneumology, Policlinico Tor Vergata University, Rome, Italy

Abstract: Lung biopsy has become progressively more important to achieve a definitive diagnosis in patients with Interstitial Lung Disease (ILD) who does not exhibit an easily recognizable clinical-radiological pattern.

Surgical biopsy has been accomplished *via* thoracotomy or Video-Assisted Thoracic Surgery (VATS), which is deemed to offer a lower morbidity, less pain and a shorter hospital stay.

Unfortunately, many ILD patients are considered at high-risk for surgical biopsy due to the need for general anesthesia, which can be poorly tolerated, particularly in patients with compromised respiratory function, pulmonary hypertension and/or immune-suppression.In order to avoid these general-anesthesia-related adverse effects, we have developed a VATS biopsy approach that is performed under thoracic epidural or local anesthesia in awake patients with spontaneous ventilation.

We believe that the introduction of awake VATS biopsy might lead to an easier acceptance of the surgical procedure by both patients and pneumologists and could widen the number of precise pathologic diagnoses, eventually resulting in more targeted therapeutic regimens.

Keywords: Interstitial lung disease, VATS, awake thoracic surgery, lung biopsy, epidural anesthesia.

INTRODUCTION

Interstitial Lung Disease (ILD) is a heterogeneous group of acute and chronic disorders with variable degrees of pulmonary inflammation and fibrosis that involves the pulmonary interstitium, eventually leading to impaired gas exchange through the alveolar septa [1].

Surgical lung biopsy is a necessary step for a confident clinicopathologic diagnosis and more informed decision about therapy, except in cases with a typical clinical-radiological picture. In particular, a definitive diagnosis of *Idiopathic Pulmonary Fibrosis* (IPF) can be established only with the aid of a surgical lung biopsy [2, 3].

Surgical biopsy has been accomplished *via* thoracotomy or Video-Assisted Thoracic Surgery (VATS), which is deemed to offer a lower morbidity, less pain and a shorter hospital stay [4-11]. VATS is usually performed through general anesthesia with a double lumen endotracheal tube to allow collapse of the operated lung [6-8, 10]. The American Society of Anesthesiologists found that the risk of morbidity and mortality using general anesthesia is always present [5, 6]. These risks, which can be considered acceptable when planning major thoracic operations, should be minimized when dealing with minor procedures, such as lung biopsy [6-12].

In order to avoid general-anesthesia-related complications, we have recently started performing VATS biopsy under Thoracic Epidural Anesthesia (TEA) or local anesthesia in awake, spontaneously ventilating patients. TEA can in fact provide optimal pain relief during surgery, avoiding paralysis of respiratory muscles and deep sedation that seem valuable advantages especially in patients with poor pulmonary function. Hereby, we present technical details and discuss the pros and cons of awake VATS lung biopsies in patients with ILD.

*Address correspondence to Eugenio Pompeo: Department of Thoracic Surgery, Policlinico Tor Vergata University, Rome, Italy. E-mail: pompeo@med.uniroma2.it

INTERSTITIAL LUNG DISEASE (ILD)

ILD is defined as a pathologic process characterized by scar tissue proliferation within the lung interstitium, in the absence of known provocation, that progressively involves the entire lung up to clinical evidence of respiratory insufficiency [13]. Exercise-induced breathlessness and chronic dry cough are the prominent symptoms. As the disease progresses, patients invariably become severely limited in their activities and dependent on supplemental oxygen. The estimated incidence of ILD is 30 per 100, 000 per year, whereas the prevalence is almost three times higher, suggesting a mean survival time of approximately 3 years [14, 15].

ILD can be divided into idiopathic, with no known cause [16-18], and secondary, with an identifiable cause or occurring in concomitance with other diseases. Among the former types, IPF is the most common. In 1972, Liebow *et al.* [19] introduced the term of *Usual Interstitial Pneumonia* (UIP) to identify a typical form of IPF characterized by specific histological and radiological features, which differs from other types named *desquamative interstitial pneumonia, bronchiolitis obliterans organizing pneumonia, lymphocytic interstitial pneumonia* and *giant cell interstitial pneumonia*. In 1998, Katzenstein and Fiorelli [20] revised the IPF classification adding another entity termed non-specific interstitial pneumonitis, characterized by absence of heterogeneity or variegated pattern at histology, as well as a better response to therapy and prognosis than that of usual interstitial pneumonia.

Known causes of secondary ILD include the presence of autoimmune diseases [21] such as lupus, rheumatoid arthritis, sarcoidosis and scleroderma; use of drugs such as bleomycin, amiodarone [22], methotrexate, gold, infliximab, etanercept; exposure to radiation therapy for breast cancer, lymphoma, and other cancers; and prolonged contact with polluted environments including asbestos, coal dust, cotton dust, and silica dust.

Current medical regimens have not been shown to improve survival but they are nevertheless routinely employed in an attempt to slow disease progression. Amongst available medications, corticosteroids and immunosuppressives in particular have been associated with significant side effects and morbidity.

As previously mentioned, one major step for ILD treatment is represented by establishing a correct diagnosis. Unfortunately, the diagnosis in these patients is quite difficult for several reasons, and most of the time it is formulated according to exclusion criteria bases on non-histological findings. Finally, ILD is often associated with the presence of undetermined lung nodules whose nature must also be elucidated, thus contributing to mandate surgical biopsy.

NON-HISTOLOGICAL DIAGNOSIS

Diagnostic accuracy of non-histological criteria can be increased by an active interaction between radiologists, clinicians and pathologists [23, 24]. Using High Resolution Computed Tomography (HRCT), ILD may be diagnosed by expert readers whereas a low diagnostic yield is expected in less experienced hands. There are common criteria established by the American Thoracic Society and European Respiratory Society for the diagnosis of IPF without surgical biopsy (Table 1). Such criteria imply the use of spirometry, blood gas analysis, HRCT, Bronchoalveolar Lavage (BAL) and transbronchial biopsy. However, use of the last two tests is still not widely recommended as they are considered not reliable and possibly dangerous, especially in elderly subjects.

Table 1. American Thoracic Society/European Respiratory Society criteria for diagnosis of IPF in the absence of surgical lung biopsy [16].

Major criteria	Minor criteria
Exclusion of other known causes of ILD such as certain drug toxicities, environmental exposure and connective tissue diseases.	Age >50 years
Abnormal pulmonary function studies that include evidence of restriction (reduced VC, often with an increased FEV_1/FVC ratio) and impaired gas exchange (increased $P(A-a)O_2$, decreased PaO_2 with rest or exercise or decreased D_LCO).	Bibasilar, inspiratory crackles (dry or "Velcro"-type in quality)

Table 1: cont....

Bibasilar reticular abnormalities with minimal ground glass opacities on high-resolution computed tomography.	Insidious onset of otherwise unexplained dyspnea on exertion
Transbronchial lung biopsy or BAL showing no features to support an alternative diagnosis.	Duration of illness >3 months

D_LCO: diffusing capacity for carbon monoxide; FEV_1: forced expiratory volume at 1 second; FVC: forced vital capacity; $P(A-a)O_2$: difference between alveolar and arterial oxygen tension; VC: vital capacity.

On these bases, histological diagnosis is progressively becoming more desirable especially to distinguish usual interstitial pneumonia from other idiopathic interstitial pneumonia patterns that prove useful also for prognostic purposes.

Clinical findings. In some instances, the diagnosis can be formulated based on clinical suspicion [25, 26]. Exercise-induced breathlessness interfering with everyday life and chronic dry cough are the prominent symptoms. In most patients, symptoms have been present for more than 6 months before presentation. The onset of symptoms is usually gradual, but they progressively worsen over time.

Digital clubbing develops in 25-50% of patients [26], and Velcro-type fine end-inspiratory crackles that are initially confined to the basal areas are found on chest auscultation [27]. These findings gradually involve the entire lung.

Accurate patient examination may help identify suggestive signs such as systemic sclerosis or polymyositis that can be associated with secondary pulmonary fibrosis, sclerodactily, scleroderma, proximal muscle weakness and telangiectasias.

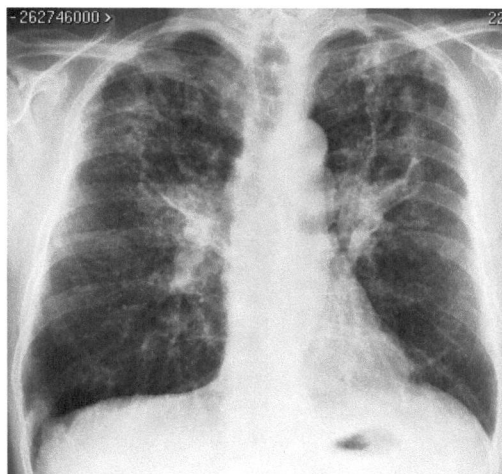

Fig. 1. Standard chest roentgenogram of a patient with ILD predominant in the upper lobes. Histologic diagnosis of silicosis.

Radiologic findings. HRCT is mandatory in every case of suspected ILD since it is more sensitive (>90%) than plain chest radiography (Fig. **1**) and the image pattern of parenchymal abnormalities can often orient the diagnosis [23]. Characteristic HRCT findings may be variably associated and anatomically distributed (Table **2**). They may include ground glass opacities, reticular patterns, consolidation areas (Figs. **2** and **3**), and the presence of associated pathologies such as mediastinal lymphadenopathy. The distinction between usual and non-specific interstitial pneumonia can be anticipated by HRCT, and classic features of honeycombing and basilar distribution orientate the diagnosis towards an usual interstitial pneumonia. Conversely, the presence of diffuse ground glass areas suggests non-specific interstitial pneumonia. The most common radiological finding with more advanced stages of disease is a reticular pattern, characterized by interlacing linear opacities resembling a network [28, 29]. This pattern is often associated with the presence of subpleural honeycombing [28], defined as a cluster or row of cysts (usually <5 mm in diameter) with shared walls. Cysts in the lung are enlarged airspaces surrounded by a wall of variable thickness and composition. Infections, pulmonary edema and hemorrhage cause alveolar filling and typically result in consolidation as well as ground-glass opacities, which are characterized by a hazy increase in lung attenuation through which pulmonary vessels may still be identified [29, 30].

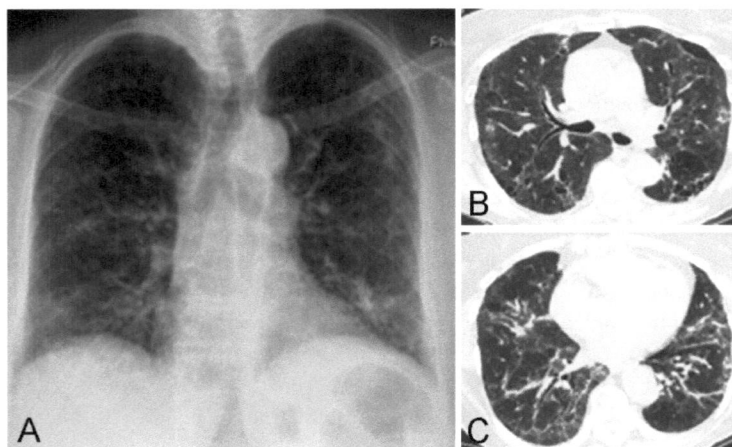

Fig. 2. Typical chest roentgenogram (A) and HRCT (B, C) findings of a patient with nonspecific interstitial pneumonia.

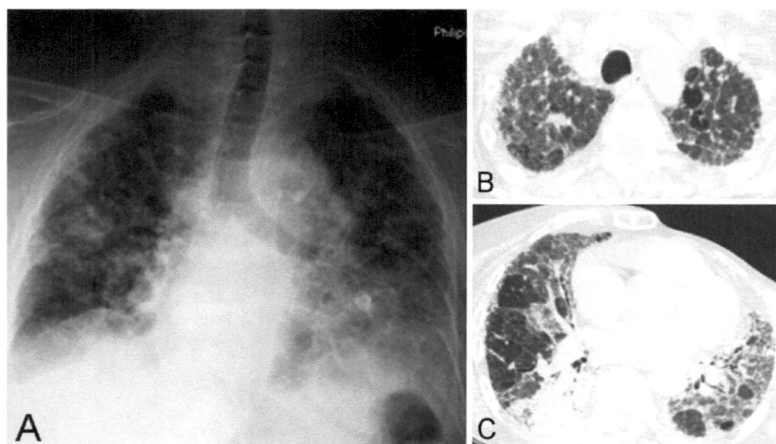

Fig. 3. Typical chest roentgenogram (A) and HRCT (B, C) findings of a patient with usual interstitial pneumonia.

Table 2. Most common anatomic distribution according to the type of ILD.

Prevalent Distribution	ILDs Types
Upper lung predominance	Sarcoidosis, pulmonary Langerhans cell histiocytosis, silicosis, tuberculosis and *Pneumocystis jiroveci* infections.
Central predominance	Sarcoidosis, berylliosis, pulmonary alveolar proteinosis.
Lower lung predominance	IPF, connective tissue disease-associated ILD, asbestosis (also consider chronic aspiration).
Peripheral predominance	IPF, nonspecific interstitial pneumonia, chronic eosinophilic pneumonia, cryptogenic organizing, pneumonia.

Laboratory findings. Laboratory tests in patients with suspected ILD should include a complete blood cell count with differential leukocyte counts, renal and liver function tests, and urinalysis [25]. Patients with a pulmonary hemorrhage syndrome (*e.g.*, microscopic polyangitis), may have iron deficiency anemia. Peripheral eosinophilia may occur in eosinophilic pneumonias, Churg-Strauss syndrome, and some drug reactions. Hypercalcemia is not uncommon in sarcoidosis [31]. Abnormal urine sediment may suggest renal involvement in systemic vasculitis. Certain serologic tests can be diagnostically helpful in the evaluation of patients with suspected ILD. Antineutrophil cytoplasmic antibody and antiglomerular basement membrane antibody assays are helpful in the diagnosis of Wegener granulomatosis and Goodpasture syndrome, respectively. The serum angiotensin-converting enzyme level is frequently elevated in sarcoidosis but it is not specific for this disorder and is not diagnostically useful. Detection of a serum precipitin to an antigen in a patient with suspected hypersensitivity pneumonitis indicates sensitization of the host but this phenomenon does not prove the diagnosis [31, 32]. The brain natriuretic peptide level may be useful in screening for pulmonary hypertension in patients with ILDs and as a prognostic marker [33]. We recommend selective serologic tests depending on the clinical context and considering differential diagnosis.

Pulmonary function test findings. Pulmonary function testing is needed when evaluating patients with suspected ILD and should include assessment of lung volumes, in particular of Vital Capacity (VC) and Total Lung Capacity (TLC) by body plethysmography, diffusing capacity for carbon monoxide (D_LCO), resting arterial blood gases and the 6 minute walk test [25]. Most patients exhibit a restrictive pattern of ventilatory defect with a decrease in D_LCO and low resting PaO_2, which falls on exercise. Nonetheless, pulmonary function may be normal or nearly normal in the early phase of the disease.

Ultrasound evaluation. Echocardiographic evaluation should be considered for patients with ILDs who experience exertional dyspnea or fatigue, particularly if the degree of these symptoms appears disproportionate to the severity of the lung disease [25]. Pulmonary hypertension is common in patients with ILD [34]. Some ILDs may be associated with an intrinsic vasculopathy [35, 36].

Bronchoalveolar lavage. BAL is not always required in the assessment of ILD [37]. It has been performed in the diagnostic work-up of diffuse parenchymal lung disease to rule out infection or tumor. The exclusion of these diseases may orientate the diagnostic strategy toward a surgical biopsy. BAL findings can be helpful in diagnosing ILDs such as pulmonary alveolar proteinosis and pulmonary Langerhans cell histiocytosis [38-40]. In pulmonary alveolar proteinosis, BAL yields a cloudy effluent that contains large amounts of periodic acid-Schiff-positive lipoproteinaceous material, as shown by light microscopy [41]. The presence of 5% or more CD1a-positive cells in the BAL fluid is highly specific for the diagnosis of pulmonary Langerhans cell histiocytosis [42]. BAL findings may sometime be helpful in the diagnosis of pulmonary hemorrhage, eosinophilic pneumonias, berylliosis, hypersensitivity pneumonitis, and some pneumoconioses. BAL cell profiles are not diagnostic in idiopathic interstitial pneumonias [43-46].

LUNG BIOPSY

Although the multidisciplinary integration of clinical and HRCT data is often adequate to yield a confident diagnosis in a significant percentage of patients, these tests are not always deemed sufficient [47] and, in some instances, lung biopsy becomes necessary. Clinical benefit resulting after lung biopsy can be assessed choosing the "change in therapy" as the selected outcome. Indeed, surgical biopsy has made it possible to adjust therapy more appropriately in 18-65% of cases [48-49]. This percentage is even more elevated in immuno-compromised subjects [48]. Surgical biopsy should be ideally performed before initiating immunomodulating therapy, including corticosteroids. A specific issue when performing biopsy in ILD patients is the reliable identification of a usual interstitial pneumonia. According to this aim, the areas of honeycombing as well as normal areas should be avoided whereas areas of intermediate abnormality or those adjacent to honeycomb lung should be preferentially targeted.

Lung biopsy can be achieved by different techniques: transbronchial biopsy with a bronchoscope, percutaneous transthoracic needle biopsy, surgical open or VATS biopsy [46-52]. The first two non-surgical procedures can be conducted by local anesthesia in an outpatient setting. However, they present some major limitations. The specimens retrieved by transbronchial biopsy are unselected, exceedingly small and come from regions adjacent to the bronchial tree, where non-specific fibrosis is frequent but not significant for the diagnosis of ILD. In the case of transthoracic needle biopsy, the most accessible lesions are located in the pleura or in the periphery of the lung parenchyma, which are not optimal for ILD diagnosis. The attempt to reach more central lesions may often be complicated by iatrogenic pneumothorax and hemothorax [50-55]. Furthermore, the specimens provided by transthoracic needle biopsy are small and often prove inconclusive for a specific diagnosis. Nonetheless, these two diagnostic procedures can be helpful to exclude the presence of other pathologic conditions such as infection, malignancy, or sarcoidosis.

Surgical biopsy is performed in the operating room and requires hospitalization. Its main advantages include achievement of a large specimen with less crush artefacts, eventually resulting in an excellent yield rate. However, even surgical lung biopsy can have some limitations. False negatives may occur due to heterogeneity in the histological pattern within the same lung. Thus, a unique biopsy specimen may not be representative of the pathological process and multiple samples retrieved in representative areas of different lobes is advocated. The middle lobe and the lingula, which are the most suitable for biopsy may sometimes reveal a non-specific diagnostic pattern compared to other pulmonary sites. Furthermore, attention must be paid to avoid obtaining small specimens that can prove inadequate to evaluate the overall pathological architecture of the lung. On the other hand, retrieval of larger and multisite biopsies may increase operating time and complications, which can be particularly dangerous in ILD patients, who often suffer from severe cardiopulmonary function impairments with oxygen dependency and pulmonary hypertension [1-3, 47-51].

Open lung biopsy is usually performed through a minithoracotomy, because it is more cosmetic and less painful than posterolateral thoracotomy. Axillary, anterior, or posterior basal minithoracotomy may be alternatively used depending on the best site to biopsy, which should be chosen in advance [4]. However, these approaches reduce the exposure of the lung surface and limit the possibility to reach the biopsy site.

With the evolution of video-assisted technology, VATS procedures can now provide diagnostic results comparable to thoracotomy with less postoperative pain and morbidity [52-57], less operating time and shorter hospital stay [2, 56, 57]. As shown in Table **3**, there are no main differences in the diagnostic yield between open lung biopsy and VATS. It is also evident that thoracotomy resulted in mortality and morbidity rates that were significantly higher than those of VATS [57-63]. However, not all patients can undergo VATS since the presence of adhesions mandates thoracotomy. On the other hand, multilobe lung biopsies are technically easier by VATS than by minithoracotomy, whereas if target areas are sited peripherally in the posterior segment of the lower lobe, they have been preferentially approached by thoracotomy.

Table 3. Surgical biopsy for ILD. Results of major series in the literature.

First Author (Year of Publication)	Method	Patients (N)	Morbidity Rate (%)	Mortality Rate (%)	Diagnostic Yield (%)
Walker (1989)[79]	OLB	61	18	13	34
Bensard (1993)[80]	OLB	21	43	0.05	100
	VATS	22	9	0	95
Ferson (1993)[81]	OLB	28	50	21	100
	VATS	47	19	6	100
Carnochan (1994)[64]	OLB	25	12	0	100
	VATS	25	0	0	100
Bove (1994)[82]	OLB	73	25	25	100
Zegdi (1994)[83]	VATS	64	11	4.7	92
Kramer (1998)[84]	OLB	103	25	20	85
Yamaguki (2004)[58]	VATS	30	10	0	100
Utz (2001) [59]	OLB	44	-	11, 6	100
	VATS	16	-	5	100
Chang (2002)[60]	OLB	61	8	0	100
	VATS	1			98

Table 3: cont....

Tiitto (2005) [61]	OLB	42	2, 4	5, 3	100
	VATS	34	3	0	100
Kreider (2007) [62]	VATS	68	19	4, 4	76, 5
Katlic (2010) [63]	VATS (local anesthesia)	18	5, 5	NR	100

NR=not reported; OLB= open lung biopsy; VATS= video-assisted thoracoscopic surgery.

Regardless of the operative approach, the most common postoperative complications are pleural effusion, pulmonary infection, transient hypoxemia, respiratory failure, prolonged air leak, pneumothorax and pulmonary embolism. Postoperative bleeding can also occur and is facilitated by pulmonary hypertension. Finally, the operation may very occasionally trigger an acute exacerbation of interstitial pneumonitis, which can prove life-threatening, particularly in patients with pulmonary hypertension [53].

So far, no study has clearly determined which patients with ILD are at particularly high risk for surgical lung biopsy.In two randomised controlled trials comparing open lung biopsy versus VATS biopsy [55, 57], there were no differences in operating time, complications or diagnostic yield. Ayed and Raghunathan [57] reported only a significant reduction in hospital stay and analgesic requirement in VATS patients, whereas Miller *et al.* [55] showed no difference in postoperative pain and hospital stay. Cost analysis of VATS versus open lung biopsy showed conflicting results, which are difficult to interpret due to differences in type of analysis and health care delivery [64-67].

AWAKE LUNG BIOPSY

VATS and open lung biopsy are usually conducted under general anesthesia [51, 57-63]. Despite being widely employed, this type of anesthesia is associated with several adverse effects including an increased risk of pneumonia and an impairment in cardiac and neuromuscular performances. In addition, mechanical ventilation can produce injuries through increased airway pressure (barotrauma), lack of re-ventilation (atelectrauma), acute hyperinflation (volutrauma) or release of proinflammatory mediators (biotrauma) [6]. In patients without respiratory insufficiency, these adverse effects may can be usually well tolerated, but in ILD patients with impaired respiratory function, pulmonary hypertension and immune-suppression, they may significantly increase operative risks [16, 54-57].

In order to reduce the adverse effects of general anesthesia, we have recently employed TEA to perform awake VATS biopsies in ILD. All candidates suitable for VATS lung biopsy, who have no contraindications for TEA, are theoretically eligible for an awake approach [11]. However, in the presence of a coagulopathy or a prolonged anticoagulant therapy or vertebral abnormalities, placement of a thoracic epidural catheter may be difficult or even dangerous because of the potential increased risk of spinal hematoma. In all these conditions we prefer local anesthesia only.

An absolute contraindication to the awake approach is represented by severe anxiety or depression. All these aspects should be carefully assessed before proposing an awake procedure and written informed consent should be signed by each patient. The patient should also be warned about the possibility of conversion to general anesthesia or thoracotomy that may be required for technical reasons.

Preoperative work-up. Preoperative work-up is not different from that of patients scheduled for VATS under general anesthesia. Pulmonary function tests including $D_L CO$ are pivotal data in assessing the degree of functional impairments, which defines all ILDs. Blood gas analysis is also very important to evaluate diffusion alterations of the alveolar-capillary membrane [5, 6, 65]. To this regard, high-risk patients are defined as those having a PaO_2 of less than 55 mmHg.

Echocardiography is useful to assess the contractile function of the heart and to have a rough estimation of pulmonary hypertension. Pulmonary hypertension is difficult to predict [34-36]. It occurs with greater frequency in patients who have a FVC of less than 50% and a $D_L CO$ of less than 45% [68].

Radiological work-up includes chest radiography in two projections and HRCT, which is fundamental in targeting the areas most suitable for biopsy [69-71]. In addition, Positron Emission Tomography (PET) has recently been hypothesized to play a role in discriminating areas of reticulation/honeycombing from those with ground glass pattern in ILD patients, possibly facilitating identification of target areas for biopsy (Fig. **4**) [72].

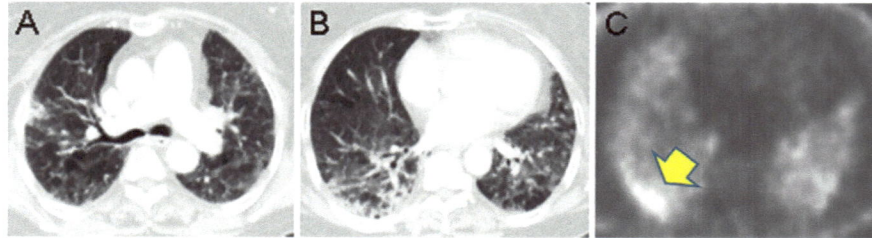

Fig. 4. HRCT showing predominant reticular pattern with scarce consolidation (A, B) associated with elevated 18-fluorodeoxyglucose uptake at PET scan (C, arrow).

Anesthesia. Awake procedures require a calm and cooperative environment. To this purpose, we found low-volume classical or melodic music to be useful in reducing anxiety. The patient should be step-by-step informed about the ongoing surgical procedure. Some patients feel more relaxed if they can follow their vital parameters in the monitor. After insertion of venous and radial artery catheters, TEA is performed with an epidural catheter positioned at T4-T5 level *via* a loss-of-resistance technique and a bolus of 5mg ropivacaine plus 5 µg sufentanyl. Continuous infusion of ropivacaine 2 mg/mL (5 mL/hour) is then started 20 min prior to the operation with the patient lying on the side targeted for biopsy. Pin-prick and warm-cold discrimination tests are usually performed to evaluate the degree of analgesia [5, 6, 65].

Thereafter, the patient's position is changed to contralateral decubitus to start the operation. During the procedure, a Venturi mask is used to keep oxygen saturation above 90%. Whenever a patient declares an unsatisfactory somatosensory block, additional analgesia can be administered through local injection of a 5 mL 50% mixture of ropivacaine (7.5 mg/mL) and bupivacaine (2.5 mg/mL).

In some instances, such as the need for chronic anticoagulant therapy or the presence of vertebral abnormalities, the insertion of the epidural catheter may not be indicated and intercostal blocks should be preferred. These can be performed by local injection of at least 5mL of a 50% mixture of bupivacaine (2.5 mg/mL) and ropivacaine (7.5 mg/mL) at each site chosen for trocar insertion. Supplementary local anesthetic can be delivered locally in the case of pleuric pain or cough.The surgeon should preoperatively explain to the patient that during the operation some discomfort can be induced by the iatrogenic pneumothorax. Although oxygen saturation is commonly maintained at a satisfactory level, a subjective difficulty in ventilation may occur leading to fatigue and tachypnea. For this reason, a chest drain may be previously placed within the pleural cavity at the beginning of the operation, to allow periodic re-expansion of the collapsed lung throughout the procedure.

In extreme cases, a true panic attack can be triggered by dyspena or thoracic pain [5-7, 73]. In these instances, the surgeon reassures the patient about the causes of the increased ventilatory effort and can show in the anesthesiologist's monitor that the main vital parameters remain within satisfactory levels. Mild sedation with midazolam or even intravenous infusion of propofol at subhypnotic dosage may be alternatively useful. Hypercarbia can also occasionally reach intolerable levels resulting in agitation and confusion, thus requiring conversion to general anesthesia. As a rule, a pH of 7.25 is chosen as the low threshold requiring correction. Whenever deemed necessary, conversion to general anesthesia and tracheal intubation is rapidly performed without changing the patient's position but just rotating the table in a semisupine decubitus and taking care to insert the double-lumen tube with the aid of a fiberoptic bronchoscope.

Surgical technique. The patient lies in lateral decubitus with mild trunk elevation and arm freely falling forward, assuming a comfortable position with the face free to facilitate spontaneous breathing and cooperation with the surgical team.

The chest side and the lung area more suitable for biopsy is usually chosen based on radiologic findings. For these reasons trocar accesses should be preliminary foreseen.

The procedure is performed through three flexible, 15 mm, thoracoscopic trocars. The camera port is placed in the eight intercostal space along the midaxillary line. A 30°, 10-mm camera is used to facilitate oblique vision of the lung during spontaneous ventilation. The operating ports are usually placed in the fifth intercostal space along the anterior and posterior axillary lines.

Although the surgical pneumothorax is followed by a nearly complete collapse of the non-dependent lung (Fig. **5**), in awake VATS the surgeon should be trained to harmonize surgical maneuvers with diaphragmatic contractions that inevitably lead to some lung movement. Mechanical stimulation of cartilagineous bronchi during lung manipulation can result in coughing reflexes that must also be taken into account.

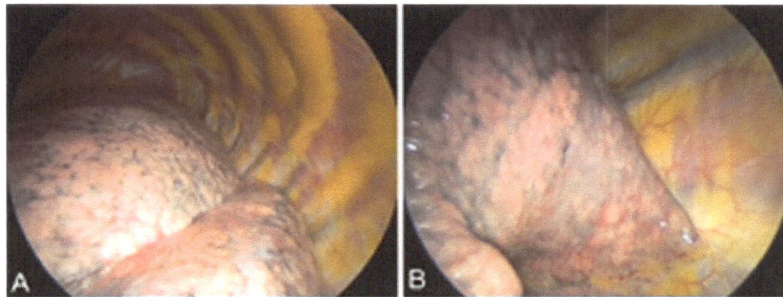

Fig. 5. Intraoperative view showing complete left lung collapse that follows the creation of surgical pneumothorax (A) and typical macroscopic aspect of ILD (B).

The unexpected presence of pleural adhesions may not necessarily imply a conversion to thoracotomy since they can be divided by both blunt and sharp dissection. Otherwise, the decision to convert the operation to an open approach should be rapidly taken at this point to avoid excessively prolonging the overall operative time.

Once the camera has been introduced, the lung is carefully explored visually to identify the most representative areas to be sampled. In this respect we have found not only the HRCT but also the PET findings useful to indicate the areas of active disease [5-9].

Target areas have common morphological features, which the surgeon should familiarize him/herself with. These can appear as subpleural nodularity, honey-combing structures, thickness of visceral pleura, evidence of neoangiogenesis, anelastic parenchyma with increased resistance to palpation, and grayish-colour change. The distribution of the most reliable target areas is related to the various type of ILD, although in most instances the free edges of the lower lobes are frequently involved to a significant extent.

In the case of uniformly distributed disease, the sites most frequently chosen for biopsy are those technically easier to resect. Apical segments of upper and lower lobes in addition to middle and lingular lobes are those most accessible for resection, presenting a narrow, easily suturable pedicle and providing a large quantity of lung tissue. Some authors [74, 75] suggest that lingular and middle lobe sites should be avoided because they are commonly affected by non-specific infectious processes. However, other studies have demonstrated that biopsy samples obtained from the lingula have the same diagnostic yield as those obtained from other lung segments [76].

The lung is grasped with ring forceps and a V-shaped wedge resection is performed by endostapler. Two 45 mm cartridges are usually necessary for each biopsy site. We prefer to employ 4.5 mm staples to resect fibrotic lung tissue due to its increased thickness and lack of elasticity that may result in rupture of the suture line and some bleeding, which is facilitated by pulmonary hypertension. There is considerable variation of biopsy sizes but we agree with Vidone and Libertin [77] that a good general rule regarding the number of biopsies is to select two or three samples of approximately 3x2x1 cm taken from different sites (Fig. **6**).After completion of the wedge resection, the specimens are extracted from the chest through the most anterior port with or without placing them in an endobag. In any case, it is important not to crush or damage the specimens during extraction, to facilitate the subsequent histologic analysis.

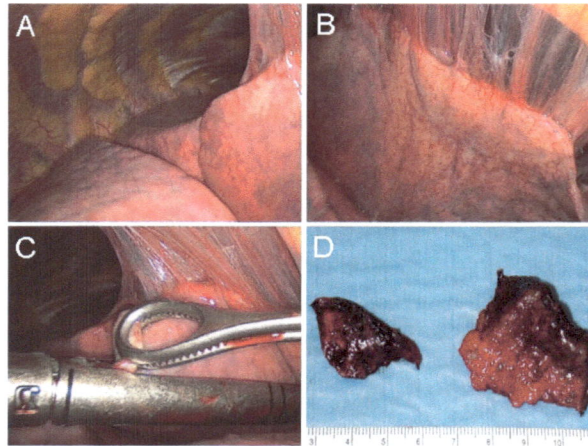

Fig. 6. Intraoperative view showing a collapsed right lung (A); filmy pleural adhesions in the middle lobe (B) do not require to be cut and may facilitate the biopsy (C); multiple surgical specimens after awake lung biopsy (D).

Thereafter, hemostasis and aerostasis are carefully checked. Unless previously positioned, a 28 F chest tube is finally inserted through the most inferior incision and connected to an underwater seal suction with a negative pressure of 20 cm water. A double lumen chest tube associated to a subpleural catheterization can also be employed to optimize postoperative analgesia (Fig. **7**). Finally, the patient is asked to cough repeatedly while the trocar ports are temporarily occluded to restore negative intrapleural pressure and obtain lung re-expansion. Trocar incisions are then sutured in a standard manner.

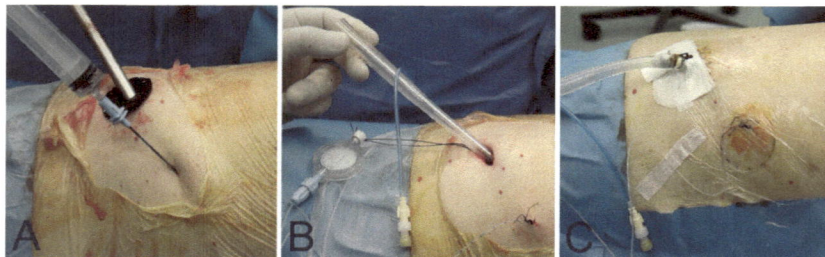

Fig. 7. Subpleural catheterization is performed under thoracoscopic vision in the intercostal space through which the chest tube will be placed (A); A double lumen chest tube is inserted (B); both catheters are connected to an elastomeric device for continuous subpleural-intrapleural analgesia (C).

Care of the specimens. The biopsy sample is sent fresh to the pathologist, who gently injects the lung tissue with formalin using a small gauge needle. Frozen sections are recommended only if coexistence of lung cancer is suspected. A section of the specimen is usually sent to the microbiology department for bacterial, viral, and fungal cultures. Immunohistochemical techniques, in situ hybridisation and polymerase chain reaction can all be performed to increase the diagnostic yields [70, 78].

Postoperative treatment. The epidural catheter is usually removed 24 hours after surgery and continuous intravenous infusion of tramadole (300 mg) [7-9] and ketorolac (90 mg) through a 24-hour elastomeric device is started. Liquid infusion is stopped immediately after the procedure and drinking, eating and ambulation is shortly allowed. The morning after the operation, blood gas analysis and chest radiography are carried out to test the efficacy of ventilation and completeness of lung expansion. If the postoperative course is uneventful and there is no air leak, the patient is discharged 24-48 hours after the procedure.

CONCLUSION

One of the most stimulating phenomena that has followed the introduction of awake operations is the possibility to enroll patients who were considered unfit for an invasive procedure [74]. Patients with ILD clearly fall into this category [62-63] since surgical biopsy performed under general anesthesia has, up to now, resulted in a significant risk of mortality and morbidity.

Awake lung biopsy in ILD represents a new, fully explorable field and so far there are no published series on this particular topic. Katlic *et al.* [63] recently reported excellent results in a series of patients undergoing VATS lung biopsy under sedation with spontaneous ventilation.

We previously investigated the possibilities of awake thoracic surgery in different surgical fields including surgical treatment of patients with severe emphysema [9], lung nodules [10], isolated lung metastases [11] and empyema thoracis [7].

We recently found that lung biopsy in fully awake, spontaneously ventilating patients is feasible and well accepted. In our initial experience, we had no mortality and minimal morbidity, and diagnostic yield was 100%. If these preliminary findings are confirmed this novel option might potentially lead to advocate surgical biopsy at an early stage of ILDs when the possibilities of halting disease progression and maximizing the efficacy of targeted therapy are likely to be the greatest.

REFERENCES

[1]   Fulmer JD. An introduction to the interstitial lung diseases. Clin Chest Med 1982;3:457-73.
[2]   Rena O, Casadio C, Leo F, *et al.* Videothoracoscopic lung biopsy in the diagnosis of interstitial lung disease. Eur J Cardiothorac Surg 1999;16:624-7.
[3]   Riley DJ, Costanzo EJ. Surgical biopsy: its appropriateness in diagnosing interstitial lung disease. Curr Opin Pulm Med 2006;12:331-6.
[4]   Bensard DD, McIntyre RC Jr, Waring BJ, Simon JS. Comparison of video thoracoscopic lung biopsy to open lung biopsy in the diagnosis of interstitial lung disease. Chest 1993;103:765-70.
[5]   Migliore M, Giuliano R, Aziz T, Saad RA, Sgalambro F. Four-step local anesthesia and sedation for thoracoscopic diagnosis and management of pleural diseases. Chest 2002;121:2032-5.
[6]   Mineo TC. Epidural anesthesia in awake thoracic surgery. Eur J Cardiothorac Surg 2007;32:13-9.
[7]   Tacconi F, Pompeo E, Fabbi E, Mineo TC. Awake video-assisted pleural decortication for empyema thoracis. Eur J Cardiothorac Surg 2010;37:594-601.
[8]   Pompeo E, Tacconi F, Mineo D, Mineo TC. The role of awake video-assisted thoracoscopic surgery in spontaneous pneumothorax. J Thorac Cardiovasc Surg 2007;133:786-90.
[9]   Mineo TC, Pompeo E, Mineo D, *et al.* Awake nonresectional lung volume reduction surgery. Ann Surg 2006;243:131-6.
[10]   Pompeo E, Mineo TC. Awake operative videothoracoscopic pulmonary resections. Thorac Surg Clin 2008;18:311-20.
[11]   Mineo TC. Thoracoscopic approach to lung metastases. Minerva Chir 2008;63:511-6.
[12]   Sundarathiti P, Pasutharnchat K, Kongdan Y, Suranutkarin PE. Thoracic epidural anesthesia (TEA) with 0.2% ropivacaine in combination with ipsilateral brachial plexus block (BPB) for modified radical mastectomy (MRM). J Med Assoc Thai 2005;88:513-20.
[13]   Dempsey OJ, Kerr KM, Gomersall L, *et al.* Idiopathic pulmonary fibrosis: an update: QJM 2006;99:643-54.
[14]   Jones, PW, Quirk, FH, Baveystock, CM, *et al.* A self-complete measure of health status for chronic airflow limitation. Am Rev Respir Dis 1992;14:1321-7.
[15]   Raghu, G, Depaso, WJ, Cain, K, *et al.* Azathioprine combined with prednisone in the treatment of idiopathic pulmonary fibrosis: a prospective double-blind, randomized, placebo-controlled clinical trial. Am Rev Respir Dis 1991;144,291-6.
[16]   American Thoracic Society, European Respiratory Society. American Thoracic Society/European Respiratory Society International Multidisciplinary Consensus Classification of the Idiopathic Interstitial Pneumonias. Am J Respir Crit Care Med 2002;165:277-304.

[17]   Meltzer EB, Noble W. Idiopathic pulmonary fibrosis. Orphanet J Rare Dis 2008;26;3-8.

[18]   Fernandez-Perez ER, Daniels CE, Schroeder DR, *et al.* Incidence, prevalence, and clinical course of Idiopathic Pulmonary Fibrosis: a Population-Based Study. Chest 2010 Jan;137:129-37.

[19]   Liebow AA, Carrington CR, Friedman PJ. Lymphomatoid granulomatosis. Hum Pathol 1972;3:457-8.

[20]   Katzenstein AL, Fiorelli RF. Nonspecific interstitial pneumonia/fibrosis. Histologic features and clinical significance. Am J Surg Pathol 1994;18:136-47.

[21]   Fathi M, Lundberg IE. Interstitial lung disease in polymyositis and dermatomyositis. Curr Opin Rheumatol 2005;17:701-6.

[22]   Papiris SA, Triantafillou C, Kolilekas L, *et al.* Amiodarone: review of pulmonary effects and toxicity. Drug Saf 2010;33:539-58.

[23]   Swensen SJ, Aughenbaugh G, Myers JL. Diffuse lung disease: diagnostic accuracy of CT in patients undergoing surgical biopsy of the lung. Radiology 1997;205:229-34.

[24]   Raghu G, Mageto YN, Lockhart D, *et al.* The accuracy of the clinical diagnosis of new-onset idiopathic pulmonary fibrosis and other interstitial lung diseases: a prospective study. Chest 1999;116:1168-74.

[25]   Ryu JH, Daniels CE, Hartman TE, Yi ES. Diagnosis of interstitial lung diseases. Mayo Clin Proc 2007;82:976-86.

[26]   Turner-Warwick M, Burrows B, Johnson A. Cryptogenic fibrosing alveolitis: clinical features and their influence on survival. Thorax 1980;35:171-80.

[27]   King TE Jr, Costabel U, Cordier JF, *et al.* Idiopathic pulmonary fibrosis: diagnosis and treatment. Am J Respir Crit Care Med 2000;161:646-64.

[28]   Lynch D, David Goodwin J, Safrin S, *et al.* Idiopathic Pulmonary Fibrosis Study Group. High-resolution computed tomography in idiopathic pulmonary fibrosis: diagnosis and prognosis. Am J Respir Crit Care Med 2005;172:488-93.

[29]   Ryu JH, Olson EJ, Midthun DE, Swensen SJ. Diagnostic approach to the patient with diffuse lung disease. Mayo Clin Proc 2002;77:1221-7.

[30]   Hansell DM. High-resolution CT of diffuse lung disease: value and limitations. Radiol Clin North Am 2001;39:1091-113.

[31]   American Thoracic Society, European Respiratory Society, World Association of Sarcoidosis and Other Granulomatous Disorders. Statement on sarcoidosis. Am J Respir Crit Care Med 1999;160:736-55.

[32]   Patel AM, Ryu JH, Reed CE. Hypersensitivity pneumonitis: current concepts and future questions. J Allergy Clin Immunol 2001;108:661-70.

[33]   Leuchte HH, Baumgartner RA, Nounou ME, *et al.* Brain natriuretic peptide is a prognostic parameter in chronic lung disease. Am J Respir Crit Care Med. 2006;173:744-50.

[34]   Nathan SD. Pulmonary hypertension in interstitial lung disease. Int J Clin Pract Suppl. 2008;160:21-8.

[35]   Strange C, Highland KB. Pulmonary hypertension in interstitial lung disease. Curr Opin Pulm Med 2005;11:452-455.

[36]   Chaowalit, N, Pellikka, PA, Decker, PA, *et al.* Echocardiographic and clinical characteristics of pulmonary hypertension complicating pulmonary Langerhans cell histiocytosis. Mayo Clin Proc 2004;79:1269-75.

[37]   Meyer KC. The role of bronchoalveolar lavage in interstitial lung disease. Clin Chest Med 2004;25:637-49.

[38]   Reynolds HY. Diagnostic and management strategies for diffuse interstitial lung disease. Chest. 1998;113:192-202.

[39]   British Thoracic Society Standards of Care Committee. The diagnosis, assessment and treatment of diffuse parenchymal lung disease in adults. Thorax 1999;54:S1-S30.

[40]   Presneill JJ, Nakata K, Inoue Y, Seymour JF. Pulmonary alveolar proteinosis. Clin Chest Med 2004;25:593-613.

[41]   Vassallo R, Ryu JH, Colby TV, Hartman T, Limper AH. Pulmonary Langerhans'-cell histiocytosis. N Engl J Med 2000;342:1969-78.

[42]   No authors listed. Clinical guidelines and indications for bronchoalveolar lavage (BAL): report of the European Society of Pneumology Task Group on BAL. Eur Respir J 1990;3:937-76.

[43]   Cushley MJ, Davison AG, du Bois RM, *et al.* The diagnosis, assessment and treatment of diffuse parenchymal lung disease in adults. Thorax 1999;54:S1-S30.

[44]   Martin RJ, Coalson JJ, Rogers RM, *et al.* Pulmonary alveolar proteinosis: the diagnosis by segmental lavage. Am Rev Respir Dis 1980;121:819-25.

[45]   Johnston ID, Prescott RJ, Chalmers JC, Rudd RM. British Thoracic Society study of cryptogenic fibrosing alveolitis: current presentation and initial management. Fibrosing Alveolitis Subcommittee of the Research Committee of the British Thoracic Society. Thorax 1997;52:38-44.

[46]   McElvein RB. The surgical approach to interstitial lung disease. Clin Chest Med 1982; 3:485-90.

[47]   Verschakelen JA. The role of high-resolution computed tomography in the workup of interstitial lung disease. Curr Opin Pulm Med 2010;16:503-10.

[48]   Kramer MR, Berkman N, Mintz B, *et al.* The role of open lung biopsy in the management and outcome of patients with diffuse lung disease. Ann Thorac Surg 1998;65:198-202.

[49]   Qureshi RA, Ahmed TA, Grayson AD, *et al.* Does lung biopsy help patients with interstitial lung disease? Eur J Cardiothorac Surg 2002;21:621-6.

[50]   Berbescu EA, Katzenstein AL, Snow JL, Zisman DA. Transbronchial biopsy in usual interstitial pneumonia. Chest 2006;129:1126-31.

[51]   Marzo C, Guarino C, Cautiero V, *et al.* Transparietal needle biopsy in the diagnosis of isolated lesions of the lung. Arch Monaldi Mal Torace 1988;43:391-407.

[52]   Wall CP, Gaensler EA, Carrington CB, Hayes JA. Comparison of transbronchial and open biopsies in chronic infiltrative lung diseases. Am Rev Respir Dis 1981;123:280-5.

[53]   Moore DJ, McParland CP, Bullock MJ, Cartier Y, Hernandez P. Video-assisted thoracoscopic lung biopsy as a possible cause of acute interstitial pneumonia in a patient with nonspecific interstitial pneumonia. Can Respir J 2004;11:437-40.

[54]   Carrillo G, Estrada A, Pedroza J, *et al.* Preoperative risk factors associated with mortality in lung biopsy patients with interstitial lung disease. J Invest Surg 2005;18:39-45.

[55]   Miller JD, Urschel JD, Cox G, *et al.* A randomized, controlled trial comparing thoracoscopy and limited thoracotomy for lung biopsy in interstitial lung disease. Ann Thorac Surg 2000;70:1647-50.

[56]   Lettieri CJ, Veerappan GR, Helman DL, *et al.* Outcomes and safety of surgical lung biopsy for interstitial lung disease. Chest 2005;127:1600-5.

[57]   Ayed AK, Raghunathan R. Thoracoscopy versus open lung biopsy in the diagnosis of interstitial lung disease: a randomised controlled trial. J R Coll Surg Edinb 2000;45:159-63.

[58]   Yamaguchi M, Yoshino I, Suemitsu R, *et al.* Elective video-assisted thoracoscopic lung biopsy for interstitial lung disease. Asian Cardiovasc Thorac Ann 2004;12:65-8.

[59]   Utz JP, Ryu JH, Douglas WW, *et al.* High short-term mortality following lung biopsy for usual interstitial pneumonia. Eur Respir J. 2001;17:175-9.

[60]   Chang AC, Yee J, Orringer MB, Iannettoni MD. Diagnostic thoracoscopic lung biopsy: an outpatient experience. Ann Thorac Surg 2002;74:1942-6.

[61]   Tiitto L, Heiskanen U, Bloigu R, *et al.* Thoracoscopic lung biopsy is a safe procedure in diagnosing usual interstitial pneumonia. Chest 2005;128:2375-80.

[62]   Kreider ME, Hansen-Flaschen J, Ahmad NN, *et al.* Complications of video-assisted thoracoscopic lung biopsy in patients with interstitial lung disease. Ann Thorac Surg 2007;83:1140-4.

[63]   Katlic MR, Facktor A. Video-assisted thoracic surgery utilizing local anesthesia and sedation: 384 consecutive cases. Ann Thorac Surg 2010;90:240-5.

[64]   Carnochan FM, Walker WS, Cameron EW. Efficacy of video assisted thoracoscopic lung biopsy: an historical comparison with open lung biopsy. Thorax 1994;49:361-3.

[65]   Hazelrigg,SR, Nunchuck SK, Landreneau RJ, *et al.* Cost analysis for thoracoscopy: thoracoscopic wedge resection. Ann Thorac Surg 1993;56:633-5.

[66]   Molin LJ, Steinberg JB, Lanza LA. VATS increases costs in patients undergoing lung biopsy for interstitial lung disease. Ann Thorac Surg 1994;58:1595-8.

[67]   Sugi K, Kaneda Y, Nawata K, *et al.* Cost analysis for thoracoscopy: thoracoscopic wedge resection and lobectomy. Surg Today 1998;28:41-5.

[68]   Ambrosini V, Cancellieri A, Chilosi M, *et al.* Acute exacerbation of idiopathic pulmonary fibrosis: report of a series. Eur Respir J 2003;22:821-6.

[69]   Ayed AK. Video-assisted thoracoscopic lung biopsy in the diagnosis of diffuse interstitial lung disease. A prospective study. J Cardiovasc Surg 2003;44:115-8.

[70]   Ishie RT, Cardoso JJ, Silveira RJ, Stocco L. Video-assisted thoracoscopy for the diagnosis of diffuse parenchymal lung disease. J Bras Pneumol 2009;35:234-41.

[71]   Zhang D, Liu Y. Surgical lung biopsies in 418 patients with suspected interstitial lung disease in China. Intern Med 2010;49:1097-102.

[72]   Groves AM, Win T, Screaton NJ, *et al.* Idiopathic pulmonary fibrosis and diffuse parenchymal lung disease: implications from initial experience with 18F-FDG PET/CT. J Nucl Med 2009;50:538-45.

[73] Pompeo E, Tacconi F, Mineo TC. Comparative results of non-resectional lung volume reduction surgery performed by awake or non-awake anesthesia. Eur J Cardiothorac Surg 2011;39:e51-8.

[74] Miller RR, Nelems B, Müller NL, *et al.* Lingular and right middle lobe biopsy in the assessment of diffuse lung disease. Ann Thorac Surg 1987;44:269-73.

[75] Newman SL, Michel RP, Wang NS. Lingular lung biopsy: is it representative? Am Rev Respir Dis 1985;132:1084-6.

[76] Qureshi RA, Ahmed TA, Grayson AD, *et al.* Does lung biopsy help patients with interstitial lung disease? Eur J Cardiothorac Surg 2002;21:621-6.

[77] Vidone RA, Libertin CR. Laboratory investigation in the diagnosis of pulmonary disease. In: Shields TW, LoCicero J, Reed CE, Feins RH, Eds. General Thoracic Surgery-5th edition. Philadelphia, Lippincott Williams & Wilkins, 2000; pp. 225-44.

[78] Blewett CJ, Bennett WF, Miller JD, Urschel JD. Open lung biopsy as an outpatient procedure. Ann Thorac Surg. 2001;71:1113-5.

[79] Walker WA, Cole FH Jr, Khandekar A, *et al.* Does open lung biopsy affect treatment in patients with diffuse pulmonary infiltrates? J Thorac Cardiovasc Surg 1989;97:534-40.

[80] Bensard DD, McIntyre RC Jr, Waring BJ, Simon JS. Comparison of video thoracoscopic lung biopsy to open lung biopsy in the diagnosis of interstitial lung disease. Chest 1993;103:765-70.

[81] Ferson PF, Landreneau RJ, Dowling RD, *et al.* Comparison of open versus thoracoscopic lung biopsy for diffuse infiltrative pulmonary disease. J Thorac Cardiovasc Surg 1993;106:194-9.

[82] Bove P, Ranger W, Pursel S, *et al.* Evaluation of outcome following open lung biopsy. Am Surg 1994;60:564-70.

[83] Zegdi R, Azorin J, Tremblay B, *et al.* Videothoracoscopic lung biopsy in diffuse infiltrative lung diseases: a 5-year surgical experience. Ann Thorac Surg 1998;66:1170-3.

[84] Kramer MR, Berkman N, Mintz B, *et al.* The role of open lung biopsy in the management and outcome of patients with diffuse lung disease. Ann Thorac Surg 1998;65:198-202.

Awake Thoracic Surgery, 2012, 119-129

CHAPTER 9

Awake Videothoracoscopic Treatment of Pleural Effusion

Francesco Sellitri, Federico Tacconi, Benedetto Cristino and Eugenio Pompeo[*]

Department of Thoracic Surgery, Policlinico Tor Vergata University, Rome, Italy

Abstract: Pleural Effusion (PE) is a common clinical condition, which can greatly affect patients' quality of life. Etiology of PEs can be variable, although in over 70% of cases they prove to be malignant in nature. Video-Assisted Thoracoscopic Surgery (VATS) is now routinely employed for management of recurrent PE and allows a thorough exploration of the pleural cavity, accomplishment of gross multiple biopsies and, whenever required, pleurodesis to prevent recurrences. VATS is usually performed under general anesthesia although this type of anesthesia can be associated with several adverse effects, particularly in the presence of comorbidities such as advanced malignancy, cardiopathy and severe systemic diseases. For this reason, use of local anesthesia in spontaneously ventilating patients has been advocated and we also started a clinical program of VATS carried out through local or Thoracic Epidural Anesthesia (TEA) in fully awake, spontaneously ventilating patients. Awake VATS management of PE requires a single trocar access; it is easily performed and results in optimal patients tolerability, minimal hospitalization and satisfactory outcome.

Keywords: VATS, pleural effusion, talc pleurodesis, thoracic epidural anesthesia, local anesthesia.

INTRODUCTION

Pleural Effusion (PE) is a common clinical condition, which can greatly affect patients' quality of life particularly when symptoms such as dyspnea, cough or chest pain do occur. The etiology of PEs can vary, although in over 70% of cases they prove to be malignant in nature. First line treatments options include simple thoracentesis and chest drainage that deal mainly with evacuation of the effusion, symptom relief and, possibly, establishing a diagnosis.

Surgical management is commonly reserved for recurrent PE, as well as in instances of uncertain diagnosis despite previous non-surgical attempts.

Video-Assisted Thoracic Surgery (VATS) is now routinely preferred for management of recurrent PE since it allows a thorough exploration of the pleural cavity, accomplishment of gross multiple biopsies and, whenever required, pleurodesis to prevent recurrences.

General anesthesia is commonly employed for VATS in this setting although it can be associated with several adverse effects, particularly in the presence of comorbidities such as advanced malignancy, cardiopathy and severe systemic diseases that frequently underlie the development of PE [1].

For this reason, use of local anesthesia in spontaneously ventilating patients has been advocated by some surgeons in this setting [2, 3]. We also started a clinical program of VATS carried out through local or Thoracic Epidural Anesthesia (TEA) in fully awake, spontaneously ventilating patients. The aim of this chapter is to describe indications, technical details and results of this surgical method for management of PE.

ETIOLOGY

According to protein content, PE can be categorized as "transudative" or "exudative". Different etiologies can

---

*Address correspondence to Eugenio Pompeo: Department of Thoracic Surgery, Policlinico Tor Vergata University, Rome, Italy;
E-mail: pompeo@med.uniroma2.it

underline the collection of fluid in the pleural cavity thus explaining its different physical-chemical properties. Transudative PE occurs as a consequence of an increased perfusion pressure at the level of the parietal pleural microcirculation. The most frequent causes are represented by congestive heart failure (Fig. 1), liver cirrhosis and nephrotic syndrome. A reduced level of plasma albumin, which is frequently associated with these conditions, may contribute to fluid transudation, due to the loss of plasma oncotic pressure.

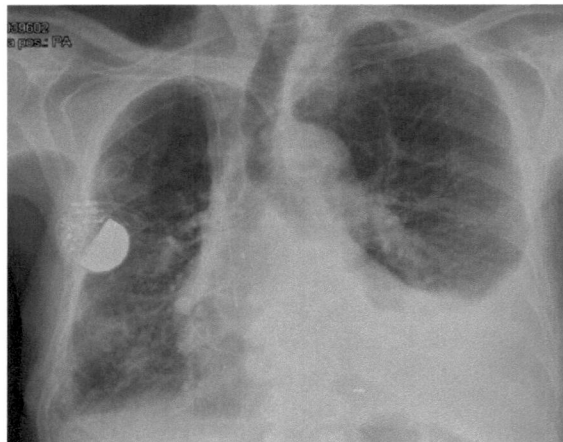

Fig. 1. Radiographic appearance of left pleural effusion related to congestive heart failure in a 76 years-old patient.

Inflammation of the pleural layers is frequently related to underlying pneumonia and can results in vasodilatation and increased vascular permeability. As a consequence, a certain amount of proteins and even blood cells may migrate into the pleural cavity, depending on the extent and severity of the disease process.

Lung cancer, together with breast, ovary and gastric cancer account for the majority of large malignant PEs (Table 1) [9, 10]. In addition, approximately 10% of patients with Hodgkin's lymphoma and 25% of patients with non-Hodgkin's lymphoma have pleural effusions at onset [11]. Malignant PE portends a poor prognosis, with a mean survival of less than 6 months [12]. In these instances, surgical management is merely palliative and aimed at improving quality of life somewhat. Other than metastatic malignancy, a primary pleural mesothelioma should be suspected in patients with recurrent PE, especially if they have a history of long lasting asbestos exposure.

Table 1. Most frequent cancer-related causes of recurrent malignant pleural effusions.

Histology	Arapis [4]	De Campos [5]	Laisaar [6]	Cardillo [7]	Schulze [8]
Metastatic lung cancer	41	132	30	385	15
Metastatic breast cancer	115	137	25	101	44
Metastatic lymphoma	5	34	2	21	1
Metastatic renal cancer	-	11	4	-	2
Other metastatic tumors	104	64	30	50	38
Pleural mesothelioma	8	15	7	54	10

Reported values refer to the total number of patients.

PREOPERATIVE WORK-UP

Laboratory. In a patient with undiagnosed PE, a thoracentesis should be performed as the first diagnostic step. Macroscopic characteristics of pleural fluid can orient diagnosis at simple visual examination. A cloudy or frankly purulent fluid can be suggestive of infection and ongoing transformation into pleural empyema, especially in febrile patients. Bloody fluid is mostly present in patients with recent trauma, malignancy, or pulmonary emboli, whereas milky fluid is suggestive of a chylothorax.

Measurement of biochemical properties such as pH, and the content in protein, glucose and lactated-dehydrogenase (LDH), can vary considerably depending on causative mechanisms. As a rule, exudative PE is characterized by elevated protein and LDH levels, low glucose, and acid pH, which also suggest metabolic activity due to the presence of bacteria and activated leukocytes. The presence of triglycerides and cholesterol is characteristic in chylothorax [13]. Elevated amylase concentration in pleural fluid is common in pancreatitis and esophageal perforation.

Though cultures and strains of the extracted fluid should be routinely obtained to identify infections, these can prove inconclusive in up to 20 % of cases. In a similar manner, cytological examination of the pleural fluid can be quite commonly unrewarding, leading to false negatives in detecting malignancy. In addition, though less frequently, false positives may occur.

Imaging. Clinical diagnosis of PE is usually confirmed by chest radiography. Radiologic appearance is related to both the extent and characteristics of the PE. A scant pleural collection (<400 mL) may become visible as an obliteration of the costophrenic recess on lateral roentgenogram whereas more abundant effusions appear as a lower lobe opacity, with a concave interface towards the lung known as *meniscus* sign. A massive PE can cause a completely opaque hemithorax and is associated with malignancy in up to 90% of instances [14]. Furthermore, these large effusions can cause hemodynamic instability due to a shift or compression of the heart and mediastinal vessels. Loss of diaphragmatic curvature can also occur, more frequently on the left side.

In patients with PE of unknown etiology or suspected malignancy, Computed Tomography (CT) of the chest with or without administration of iodinated contrast [15] makes it possible to accurately evaluate the size and location of the fluid collection(s), to detect underlying parenchymal disease, and to assess thickening of the pleural layers (Figs. **2** and **3**) [13, 16]. Administration of intravenous contrast with a 60-second delay enables an optimal differentiation between pleural thickening and pleural fluid (Fig. **3**), as well as between transudations and exudations, with contrast-enhancement almost always indicating an exudation. Ng and coworkers [17] found that CT scans were able to identify pleural thickening in 94% of patients with PE. Moreover, CT scanning can help distinguish malignant from benign pleural disease with a sensitivity and specificity of 72% and 83%, respectively [18]. Common features of malignant pleural thickening are a nodular pattern, a depth >1 cm, and involvement of the mediastinal pleura (Fig. **4**), whereas the presence of pleural calcifications suggests a benign process. Instead, it may be difficult to differentiate mesothelioma from metastatic pleural malignancies [19]. In this regard, Metinas and coworkers [20] found that, in cases of pleural mesothelioma, the most common CT features were circumferential lung encasement, pleural thickening with irregular pleuropulmonary margins and/or superimposed nodules. Moreover, in up to 70% of cases, there was rind-like extension of the tumor on pleural surfaces. Finally, CT is useful for assessing disease involvement of the chest wall or extension into neighboring structures, such as the superior vena cava and spinal cord [21].

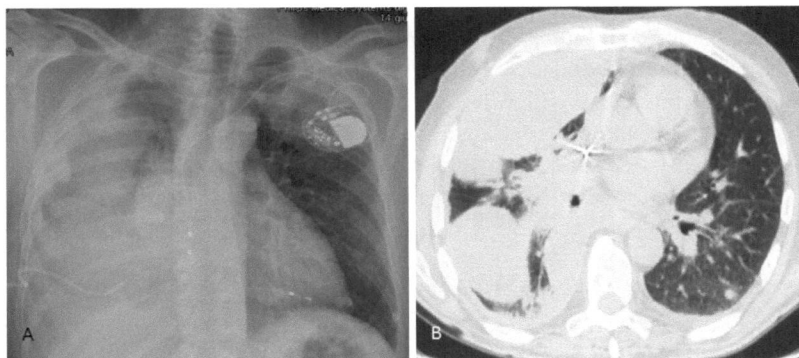

Fig. 2. Roengetenogram (A) and CT-scan (B) appearance of a complex pleural effusion due to metastatic lung cancer. CT-scan helps identify multiple fluid collections, a right lower lobe mass, and a contralateral peripheral nodule.

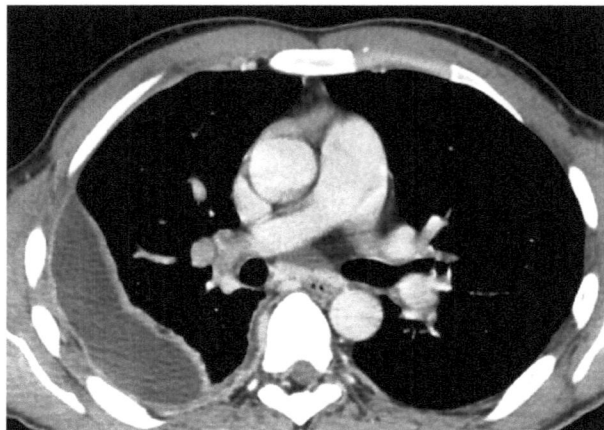

Fig. 3. A 69 years-old patient with pelural effusion of tubercular origin. Note the contrast-enhanced thickening of the visceral pleura.

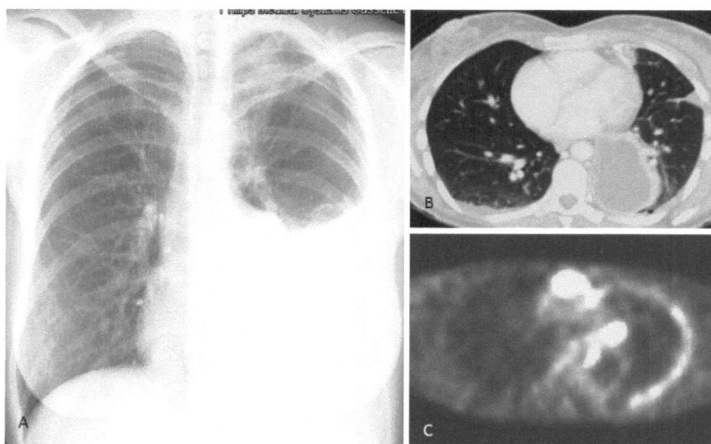

Fig. 4. Roengtenogram (A), CT (B), and PET (C) findings in a patient with malignant pleural effusion arising from breast cancer. Malignant nature is suggested by nodular pleural implants involving the mediastinal pleura and diffuse metabolic activity.

Persistent PE may induce a desmoplastic reaction of the pleural cavity eventually leading to the development of adhesions and septa. Under these circumstances, which are mostly related to either infection or malignancy, the pleural fluid can collect in multiple locations ad is commonly defined as complex PE [14]. Loculations are difficult to identify at simple roentgenogram because they can be misinterpreted as atelectasis or lung consolidation areas. In these instances, ultrasonography may be helpful to visualize the pattern of fibrinous stranding and septations although optimal visualization of complex PEs and their relationship with intrathoracic structures is an elective indication for CT. Positron Emission Tomography (PET) can be integrated with CT, and can improve diagnostic accuracy to differentiate benign from malignant pleural lesions, to detect extrathoracic involvement, and to evaluate the response to therapy [22]. It may also occasionally reveal occult malignancies [23]. To this regard, Duysinx and coworkers [24] found a sensitivity in detecting malignancy of 96.8% and a specificity of 88.5% in patients undergoing a previous non-conclusive CT-scan.

AWAKE VATS MANAGEMENT OF PLEURAL EFFUSIONS

Historical perspective. The term *thoracoscopy* was introduced in clinical practice in the second-half of the XIX century, when the Irish physician Francis Cruise first used a rigid cystoscope to explore the pleural cavity in a young girl with PE of tubercular origin. Nonetheless, Jacobaeus is universally credited as the pioneer of thoracoscopy since he developed a technique for dividing pleural adhesions under thoracoscopic vision to improve the efficacy of Forlanini's artificial pneumothorax in patients with pulmonary tuberculosis [25]. However, with the advent of antimicrobial therapy, alongside the introduction of thoracoplasty as the primary surgical approach in the treatment of pulmonary tuberculosis, the Jacobaues' operation fell into disuse. Nonetheless, thoracoscopy continued to be used mostly for simple procedures, including management of PE.

Fleishmann and coworkers [26] first described their experience with thoracoscopic pleural biopsy in patients' with apparent idiopathic PE, reporting a change in diagnosis in 28% of instances. Bergqvist and Nordestein [27] reported a diagnostic yield over 90% in patients undergoing thoracoscopy for PE of either tubercular or malignant etiology.

Maasen and coworkers [28] used a mediastinoscope instead of the thoracoscope, which also made it possible to grasp small portions of the lung to obtain biopsy samples. A similar technique was also employed by Beaulieu and Deslauriers [29, 30] who inserted the mediastinoscope into the pleural cavity through a cervical incision, and more recently by Rush and Mountain [31] who used multiple intercostals blocks and a standard mediastinoscope introduced *via* a chest uniportal approach to manage different pleural diseases in 46 patients. Other important technical advances in this setting came from the introduction of talc pleurodesis, which was first presented by Swieringa and coworkers [32] in patients with recurrent pneumuothorax, and the use of a two-trocar thoracoscopic approach, which was first described by Rodgers and Talbert [33] in children with mediastinal masses or diffuse lung diseases. Other authors explored the pleural cavity by means of a flexible bronchoscope, an approach which was mainly adopted by interventional pneumologists.

In the early 90's, the advent of video-assistance and dedicated endoscopic instrumentation, made it possible to perform more complex thoracoscopic operations, that were comprehensively included under the denomination of Video-Assisted Thoracic Surgery (VATS) for which general-anesthesia with one-lung ventilation became the standard type anesthesia.

Anesthesia. Premedication is routinely avoided although intravenous midazolam can be administered at a minimum dosage necessary to control emotional stress while maintaining full awareness in patients with anxiety symptoms. Other authors favour preoperative administration of intravenous atropine or aerosolized lidocaine to better control coughing reflexes and arrhythmias [3].

Local anesthesia. In general, we prefer local anesthesia for management of undetermined PEs deemed to be of a benign nature and not requiring a pleurodesis. Other indications for this type of anesthesia include patients with general contraindications for TEA such as spinal deformities or coagulopathies. The intercostal block is accomplished by local injection of anesthesia with 2 % lidocaine mixed with 7.5 % ropivacaine. Thirty to forty mL of this mixture are usually prepared although the use of more than 25-30 mL is rarely necessary. This mixture offers the advantages of both a rapid onset and long duration of the analgesic effect. Injection of anesthetic at the incision site should be performed gradually. In obese patients with a thick chest wall, this maneuver can be performed stepwise under direct visualization, starting with infiltration of the skin and subcutaneous tissue and then continuing with the infiltration of the muscles and ribs. Furthermore, if biopsies have to be taken in the parietal pleura additional injection of the perilesional sub-pleural space can be accomplished either transthoracically under thoracoscopic vision or by direct thoracoscopic puncture.

Thoracic epidural anesthesia. This is preferred when pleural decortication or talc pleurodesis is preoperatively planned. The thoracic epidural catheter is inserted at T4 level using the lateral approach and loss-of-resistance technique. The level and extent of blockade is evaluated using the warm-cold discrimination test 10 minutes after the test-dose injection. Anesthesia is obtained with continuous infusion of ropivacaine 0.5% and sufentanil 1.66 ug/mL into the epidural space, *via* an elastomeric device.

Regardless of the type of anesthesia employed, during the procedure, creation of the surgical pneumothorax is usually well tolerated by patients with PE and oxygenation remains satisfactory throughout the procedure. This might be due to a progressive adaptation of the respiratory system to the chronic condition of lung collapse induced by the effusion.

Should hypoventilation cause a drop in peripheral oxygen saturation below 90%, additional oxygen can be delivered by a Venturi mask. In addition, arterial carbon dioxide level is monitored serially on blood samples obtained *via* a previously placed arterial catheter.

Ideally, there is no need for intraoperative sedation in candidates for awake VATS for PE, mainly due to the short duration of the procedure. Nonetheless, in anxious individuals panic attacks triggered by thoracic pain, dyspnea or hypercapnia can rarely occur intraoperatively. In these instances, administration of midazolam or propofol at subhypnotic dosage can satisfactorily control the situation while maintaining spontaneous ventilation. Whenever additional sedation proves necessary, arterial pressure should be monitored and corrected with plasma expanders if required [3].

At the end of the surgical procedure, the anesthetic regimen is changed to ropivacaine 0.16% and sufentanyl 1 ug/mL at a rate of 2 to 5 mL/hour, to provide postoperative analgesia. The epidural catheter is removed 24 hours after surgery.

Surgical technique. The patient is placed in the lateral decubitus position, with slight rib splitting. The operative field is prepped and draped, taking care to leave the patient's face free to maximize her/his perioperative comfort and facilitate active interaction with the surgeon. However, in management of malignant PEs, we do not allow patients to follow their operation on the monitor, to avoid the afflictive perception of severe intrapleural features.

The first trocar is placed at the 7th or 8th intercostals spaces, on the midaxillary line. After injection of local anesthetics, a 2-cm skin incision is made, and the pleural cavity is entered by blunt dissection along the superior border of the lower rib. In patients with abundant effusions, this maneuver can result in sudden spilling of fluid outside the pleural cavity. In this instance, a Nelaton catheter is immediately inserted blindly to drain part of the pleural fluid, thus limiting its outflow under pressure (Fig. **5**).

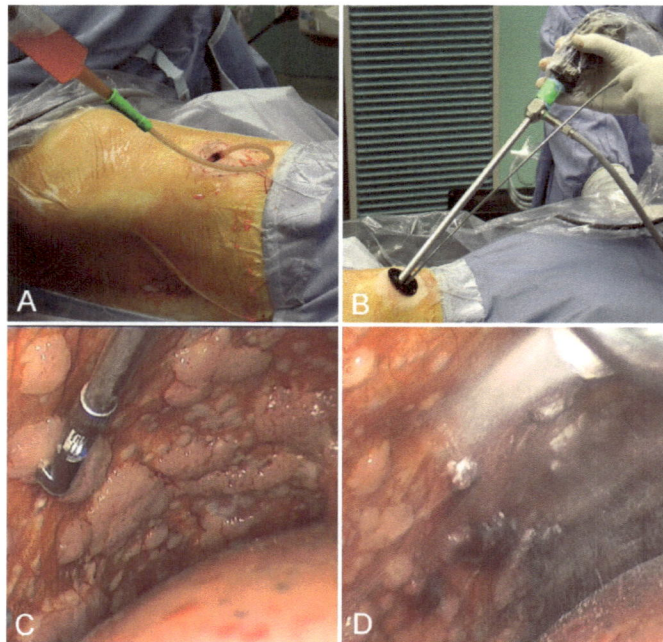

Fig. 5. Single-trocar VATS management for malignant pleural effusion. After initial drainage of the fluid collection (A), a biopsy forceps is inserted coaxially with the 30-degrees camera through a 20-mm trocar port (B). Multiple biopsies are taken (C), and talc is thoroughly insufflated to attain a snow-storm distribution (D) (Video 1).

The index finger is then inserted through the trocar incision to check for the presence of pleural adhesions, and if these are found, to free them circumferentially in a blunt manner. One 20 mm flexible trocar is then inserted and a 30° thoracoscope is introduced for thorough exploration of the pleural surfaces.

Pleural fluid can now be completely removed, irrespective of its amount, since the risk of re-expansion pulmonary edema is counteracted by the establishment of an atmospheric pleural environment due to creation of the surgical pneumothorax [34, 35].

Nonetheless, if there is no contraindication, we routinely administer a 20 mg bolus of intravenous prednison to patients in whom effusion of more than 1, 5 L is drained during awake VATS. Complex PEs are easily drained after debridement of loculations, which can be accomplished with an endoscopic swab introduced coaxially to the camera. If deemed useful, a second trocar access can be made along the same intercostal space, 10-15 cm from the first trocar incision, to facilitate instrumental disruption of pleural adhesions and septa.

Pleural biopsy should be obtained in all instances, since malignancy may occasionally remain occult. As this maneuver can trigger pain and/or cough in patients operated on by local anesthesia, transcutaneous injection of local anesthetics is performed at the level of biopsy site, under thoracoscopic guidance. Multiple biopsies of most representative lesions are accomplished by inserting the biopsy forceps coaxially to the camera (Fig. **5**).

Whenever pleurodesis is deemed necessary, asbestos-free talc powder is insufflated uniformly onto the pleural surface under direct vision to obtain a *snow storm* distribution. To maximize the effectiveness of the procedure, care should be taken not to proceed with talc insufflation unless all fluid collections have been removed. Before starting the pleurodesis it is mandatory to check the capacity of the lung to re-expand satisfactorily, since incomplete lung expansion jeopardizes the usefulness of the maneuver.

After the completion of talc insufflation, a 28 Ch chest tube is inserted and its correct placement along the costovertebral gutter is monitored under thoracoscopic vision. Lung re-expansion is eventually achieved by asking the patients to inhale deeply and cough repeatedly while keeping close airtight the camera port with a gauze. For this purpose, previous placement of a readsorbable, purse string suture at the level of the trocar access makes it possible to rapidly close the skin incision as soon as the scope is retracted, thus avoiding entry of air into the pleural cavity once negative pleural pressure has been re-established by connecting the tube to its water seal chamber. Postoperatively, the tube is removed when chest roentgenogram confirms a satisfactory lung expansion and drained serous fluid is less than 200 mL/24h.

COMMENT

In recent years, VATS procedures in fully awake or spontaneously ventilating patients have regained popularity in the management of a series of thoracic conditions. The rationale for this renewed interest is to avoid the adverse effects of general anesthesia and one-lung ventilation, which include the so-called ventilator-related lung injury as well as the possibility of post-intubation tracheal and esophageal injuries, which can lead to a mortality rate of up to 22 % [36].

Some surgeons advocate VATS operations under local anesthesia with deep sedation. In this regard, Migliore and coworkers [3] employed only propofol administration whereas Katlic and co-workers [2] used a combination of midazolam, fentanyl, and propofol, or ketamine in 244 patients with PEs. The rationale of adding sedation to just local anesthesia is to achieve optimized anesthesia-analgesia, alongside a short-term amnesia. Other alternative analgesia techniques for awake VATS in PE have been occasionally reported. In 2008, Guarracino [37] reported on the use of TEA and non-invasive lung ventilation delivered through bi-level positive airway pressure in a critically-ill patient undergoing VATS for recurrent bilateral PEs, while Piccioni and coworkers [38] published their experience on two cases of malignant PE treatment using thoracic paravertebral anaesthesia.

We prefer to maintain a full consciousness during the operation, since we believe that this proves particularly useful at the end of the procedure when patient cooperation is fundamental in achieving full lung re-expansion. Furthermore, we have reported that most patients undergoing more complex awake VATS procedures [39] are highly satisfied with this approach, thus suggesting a minor role for lack of amnesia in this setting.

Patients with PE represent an ideal target for an awake VATS approach. In fact, on one hand, they usually have a series of relevant medical comorbidities which imply additional anesthesia-related risks; on the other hand, the use of general anesthesia with one-lung ventilation sounds somewhat excessive in the light of the trivial surgical complexity of the procedures most commonly required to manage PEs.

We have found it worth noting that patients with PE tolerate the surgical pneumothorax very satisfactorily and do not develop clinically-relevant hypoxia requiring supportive ventilation. This is likely due to the peculiar status developed by their respiratory system, which is already chronically adapted to the partial ventilatory exclusion of the involved lung.

We have also noticed that, despite the preservation of spontaneous ventilation, the lung remains almost completely deflated, thus making it possible to operate in a surgical field that looks similar to the field obtained with one-lung ventilation.

We hypothesize that a Young-Laplace mechanism, besides the creation of an intrapleural atmospheric environment, might help to explain this finding. Accordingly, it is possible that the alveoli, which have been previously collapsed for a relatively long time, may require higher pressure levels to be re-recruited to ventilation than those acting in physiologic condition, as an effect of their shorter diameter and increased surface tension.

To date, talc and bleomycin are the most frequently employed sclerosants, while tetracyclines have been used in the past [40]. The efficacy of talc pleurodesis in PE has been well documented since Chambers' first experience in 1958 [41] and success rates up to 90% have been reported more recently [42], with a satisfactory safety level (Table 2). In addition, in 2004, a meta-analysis confirmed the superiority of talc poudrage [40], as opposed to bleomycin and tetracycline, with which overall success rates ranged between 60% and 70% [43, 44].

Table 2. Complications in patients with malignant pleural effusion after VATS talc pleurodesis.

Event	First Author					
	Barbetakis [48]	Viallat [42]	Arapis [4]	De Campos [5]	Cardillo [7]	Stefani [49]
Prolonged air leak	9%	-	-	0.5%	0.8%	2.7%
Subcutaneous emphysema	7.5%	0.6%	-	-	1.6%	-
Acute respiratory failure	1.7%	-	-	1.3%	-	-
Persistent pleural space	0.7%	-	-	-	-	-
Bleeding	1%	-	1%	0.4%	0.1%	-
Reexpansion pulmonary edema	0.2%	-	-	2.2%	-	4.1%
Empyema thoracis	0.5%	2.5%	1.5%	2.7%	-	1.4%
Pulmonary embolism	0.5%	-	2%	-	-	-
Fever	-	9.8%	5.3%	2.7%	-	38.8%
Pulmonary infections	-	0.8%	-	0.7%	-	-
Postoperative cardiac disease	0.7%	-	1%	-	0.1%	-

Instillation of pleurodesic agents *via* the tube thoracostomy (slurry) has a low success rate, along with the increased risk of overwhelming infections of the pleural cavity. For this reason, this procedure seems justified exclusively in patients with a life-expectancy of less than 2 months [45, 46]. Moreover, the use of permanent drain systems such as the PleurX drain [47] is not widely available, and their efficacy is still under evaluation.

Talc pleurodesis through awake VATS should be considered as an attractive treatment option in the setting of malignant PE. Indeed, adequate biopsy sampling for tumour characterization, including immunohistochemistry assay and assessment of membrane receptors is feasible by this approach. Thoracoscopic vision also allows optimal distribution of the talc even in relatively inaccessible areas, leading to satisfactory results in most instances (Fig. **6**).

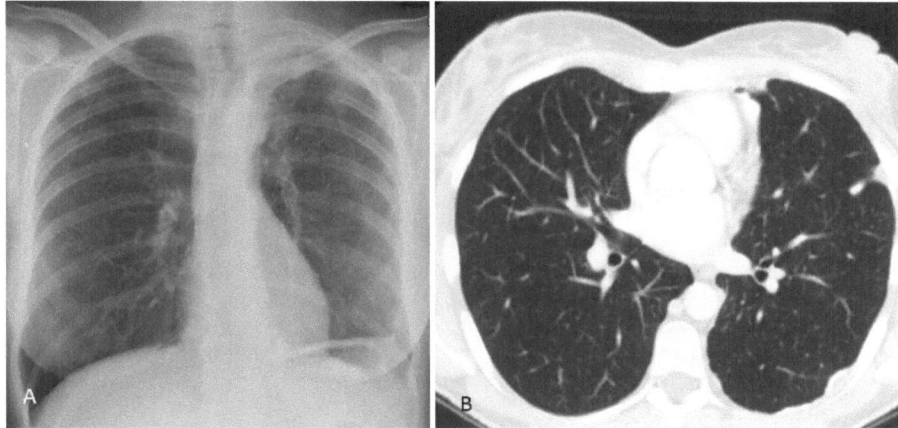

Fig. 6. The same case showed in figure 4. Complete lung re-expansion after awake VATS pleurodesis is showed at roentgenogram (A) and confirmed by CT-scan (B).

In patients with malignant pleural mesothelioma and associated PE, VATS can be employed both for diagnostic purposes, as well as for controlling symptoms by adding talc pleurodesis. In addition, we believe that awake VATS can make it possible to avoid repeated general anesthesia in a short time span when subsequent more aggressive surgical treatment of pleural mesothelioma is planned.

CONCLUSION

Awake VATS management of PE proved safely feasible and could offer some advantages when compared to equivalent procedures performed under general anesthesia.

Although management of PE by medical thoracoscopy through just local anesthesia has been widely reported in the past, awake VATS enhances the versatility of the technique by allowing more complex surgical maneuvers and accurate pleurodesis to be easily performed. In this regard, the possibility to evacuate the effusion and perform both pleural biopsies and talc pleurodesis through a single trocar access under TEA, seems particularly attractive. This simple method can allow reliable management of patients with advanced malignancy in whom optimal palliation may be achieved at the cost of surgical and anesthesiological trauma that is not such greater than with a simple chest drainage.

REFERENCES

[1]   Whitehead T, Slutsky AS. The pulmonary physician in critical care*7: ventilator induced lung injury. Thorax 2002;57:635-42.
[2]   Katlic MR, Facktor MA. Video-assisted thoracic surgery utilizing local anesthesia and sedation: 384 consecutive cases. Ann Thorac Surg 2010;90:240-5.
[3]   Migliore M, Giuliano R, Aziz T, Saad AR, Sgalambro F. Four-step local anesthesia and sedation for thoracoscopic diagnosis and management of pleural diseases. Chest 2002; 121:2032-5.
[4]   Arapis K, Caliandro R, Stern JB, *et al.* Thoracoscopic palliative treatment of malignant pleural effusions. Results in 273 patients. Surg Endosc 2006;20:919-23.

[5]   De Campos JR, Vargas FS, Werebe EC, *et al.* Thoracoscopy talc poudrage: a 15-year experience. Chest 2001;119:801-6.

[6]   Laisaar T, Palmiste V, Vooder T, Umbleja T. Life expectancy of patients with malignant pleural effusion treated with video-assisted thoracoscopic talc pleurodesis. Interact Cardiovasc Thorac Surg 2006;5:307-10.

[7]   Cardillo G, Facciolo F, Carbone M, *et al.* Long-term follow-up of video-assisted talc pleurodesis in malignant recurrent pleural effusions. Eur J Cardiothorac Surg 2002;21:302-6.

[8]   Schulze M, Boehle AS, Kurdow R, *et al.* Effective treatment of malignant pleural effusion by minimal invasive thoracic surgery: thoracoscopic talc pleurodesis and pleuroperitoneal shunts in 101 patients. Ann Thorac Surg 2001;71:1809-12.

[9]   Light RW. The undiagnosed pleural effusion. Clin Chest Med 2006;27:309-19.

[10]   Lee YC, Light RW. Management of malignant pleural effusion. Respirology 2004;9:148-56.

[11]   Romano M, Libshitz HI. Hodgkin disease and non-Hodgkin lymphoma: plain chest radiographs and chest computed tomography of thoracic involvement in previously untreated patients. Radiol Med 1998;95:49-53.

[12]   Haas AR, Sterman DH, Musani AI. Malignant pleural effusion: management options with consideration of coding, billing, and a decision approach. Chest 2007;132:1036-41.

[13]   Rush VW. Pleural effusion: benign and malignant. In: Pearson FG, Cooper JD, Deslauriers J, *et al.*, Eds. Thoracic Surgery. 2nd edition. New York, Churchill Livingstone, 2002; pp. 1157-69.

[14]   Qureshi NR, Gleeson FV. Imaging of pleural disease. Clin Chest Med 2006;27:193-213.

[15]   Pompeo E, Mineo TC. Awake operative videothoracoscopic pulmonary resections. Thorac Surg Clin 2008;18:311-20.

[16]   Yilmaz UM, Utkaner G, Yalniz E. Computed tomographic findings of environmental asbestos-related malignant pleural mesothelioma. Respirology 1998;3:33-8.

[17]   Ng CS, Munden RF, Libshitz HI. Malignant pleural mesothelioma: the spectrum of manifestations on CT in 70 cases. Clin Radiol 1999;54:415-21.

[18]   Lombardi G, Zustovich F, Nicoletto MO, *et al.* Diagnosis and treatment of malignant pleural effusion: A systematic literature review and new approaches. Am J Clin Oncol 2010;33:420-3.

[19]   Bittner RC, Felix R. Magnetic resonance (MR) imaging of the chest: state of art. Eur Respir J 1998;11:1392-404.

[20]   Metintas M, Ucgun I, Elbek O, *et al.* Computed tomography features in malignant pleural mesothelioma and other commonly seen pleural diseases. Eur J Radiol 2002;41:1-9.

[21]   West SD, Lee YCG. Management of malignant pleural mesothelioma. Clin Chest Med 2006;27:335-54.

[22]   Gill RR, Gerbaudo VH, Sugarbaker DJ, Hatabu H. Current trends in radiologic management of malignant pleural mesothelioma. Semin Thorac Cardiovasc Surg 2009;21: 111-20.

[23]   Truong MT, Marom EM, Erasmus JJ. Preoperative evaluation of patients with malignant pleural mesothelioma: role of integrated CT-PET imaging. J Thorac Imaging 2006;21:146-53.

[24]   Duysinx B, Nguyen D, Louis R, *et al.* Evaluation of pleural disease with 18-fluorodeoxyglucose positron emission tomography imaging. Chest 2004;125:489-93.

[25]   Bloomberg AE. Thoracoscopy in diagnosis of pleural effusions. N Y State J Med 1970; 70:1974-7.

[26]   Fleishman SJ, Lichter AI, Buchanan G, *et al.* Investigation of idiopathic pleural effusions by thoracoscopy. Thorax 1956;11:324.

[27]   Bergqvist S, Nordenstein H. Thoracoscopy and pleural biopsy in the diagnosis of pleurisy. Scand J Respir Dis 1966,47:64.

[28]   Maasen W. Thoracoscopy and surgical lung biopsy without initial pneumothorax. Endoscopy 1972,4:95.

[29]   Beaulieu M, Depres JP, Lemieux M. Mediastinopleuroscopy; a new technique for the diagnosis of thoracic diseases. Chirurgie 1972;98:355.

[30]   Deslauriers J, Beaulieu M, Dufour C, *et al.* A new approach to the diagnosis of intrathoracic disease. Society of Thoracic Surgeons, Washington: USA 1976.

[31]   Rush VW, Mountain C. Thoracoscopy under regional anesthesia for the diagnosis and management of pleural disease. Am J Surg 1987;154:274-8.

[32]   Swieringa J, Wagenaar JPM, Bergstein PGM. The value of thoracoscopy in the diagnosis and treatment of disease affecting the pleura and lung. Pneumologie 1974;151:11.

[33]   Rodgers BM, Talbert JL. Thoracoscopy for diagnosis of intrathoracic lesions in children. J Pediatr Surg 1976;11:703-8.

[34]   Loddenkemper R. Thoracoscopy-state of the art. Eur Respir J 1998;11:213-21.

[35]   Brandt HJ, Loddenkemper R, Mai J. Atlas of diagnostic thoracoscopy. New York, USA 1985.

[36]   Minambres E, Buron J, Ballesteros MA, *et al.* Tracheal rupture after endotracheal intubation: a literature systematic review. Eur J Cardiothorac Surg 2009;35:1056-62.

[37]   Guarracino F, Gemignani R, Pratesi G, *et al.* Awake palliative thoracic surgery in a high-risk patient: one-lung, non-invasive ventilation combined with epidural blockade. Anaesthesia 2008;63:761-3.

[38]   Piccioni F, Langer M, Fumagalli L, *et al.* Thoracic paravertebral anaesthesia for awake video-assisted thoracoscopic surgery daily. Anaesthesia 2010;65:1221-4.

[39]   Pompeo E, Mineo TC. Two-year improvement in multidimensional body mass index, airflow obstruction, dyspnea and exercise capacity index after nonresectional lung volume reduction surgery in awake patients. Ann Thorac Surg 2007;84:1862-9.

[40]   Tan C, Sedrakyan A, Browne J, *et al.* The evidence on the effectiveness of management for malignant pleural effusion: a systematic review. Eur J Cardiothorac Surg 2006;29:829-38.

[41]   Chambers JS. Palliative treatment of neoplastic pleural effusions with intercostals intubation and talc instillation. West J Surg Obstet Gynecol 1958;66:26-8.

[42]   Viallat JR, Rey F, Astoult P, Boutin C. Thoracoscopic talc poudrage pleurodesis for malignant effusion: a review of 360 cases. Chest 1996;110:1387-93.

[43]   Walker-Renard PB, Vaughan LM, Sahn S. Chemical pleurodesis for malignant pleural effusions. Ann Intern Med 1994;120:56-64.

[44]   Kennedy L, Rush VW, Strange C, *et al.* Pleurodesis for the treatment of pneumothorax and pleural effusion. Chest 1994;106:125-32.

[45]   Gasparri R, Leo F, Veronesi G, *et al.* Video-assisted management of malignant pleural effusion in breast carcinoma. Cancer 2006;106:271-6.

[46]   Marrazzo A, Noto A, Casà L, *et al.* Video-thoracoscopic surgical pleurodesis in the management of malignant pleural effusion: the importance of an early intervention. J Pain Symptom Manag 2005;30:75-9.

[47]   Efthymiou CA, Masudi T, Thorpe JA, Papagiannopoulos K. Malignant pleural effusion in the presence of trapped lung. Five-year experience of PleurX tunneled catheters. Interact Cardiovasc Thorac Surg 2009;9:961-4.

[48]   Barbetakis N, Asteriou C, Papadopoulou, *et al.* Early and late morbidity and mortality and life expectancy following thoracoscopic talc insufflations for control of malignant pleural effusions: a review of 400 cases. J Cardiothorac Surg 2010;5:27-34.

[49]   Stefani A, Natali P, Casali C, Morandi U. Talc poudrage versus talc slurry in the treatment of malignant pleural effusion. A prospective comparative study. Eur J Cardiothorac Surg 2006;30:827-32.

CHAPTER 10

Awake Thoracoscopic Treatment of Spontaneous Pneumothorax

Gianluca Vanni, Federico Tacconi, Tommaso Claudio Mineo and Eugenio Pompeo[*]

Department of Thoracic Surgery, Emphysema Center, Policlinico Tor Vergata University, Rome, Italy

Abstract: Spontaneous Pneumothorax (SP) is a relatively common condition defined as the presence of air in the pleural space associated with lung collapse.

On an etiologic basis, pneumothorax is classified as spontaneous, traumatic and iatrogenic. The term "spontaneous" indicates that no mechanical injury is recognized as the causative mechanism whereas secondary SP occurs as an acute complication of an underlying lung disease.

The principal goal of treatment is to evacuate air from the pleural space and achieve lung reexpansion. Simple chest drainage is often employed as first line treatment, whereas bullectomy performed by Video-Assisted Thoracic Surgery (VATS) is widely adopted for treatment of recurrent SP. Pleurodesis by pleurectomy or talc insufflation is also commonly associated to bullectomy to reduce risks of recurrence.

VATS is usually carried out through general anesthesia and one lung ventilation, although use of this type of anesthesia can be associated with several adverse effects. Recently, VATS management of SP has been performed with satisfactory results by local anesthesia in spontaneously ventilating patients. In particular, we have began a clinical investigational program entailing VATS bullectomy and pleurectomy performed through sole Thoracic Epidural Anesthesia (TEA) in fully awake patients. In this chapter we describe technical features and results of this novel surgical approach.

Keywords: Pneumothorax, VATS, thoracic epidural anesthesia.

INTRODUCTION

Spontaneous Pneumothorax (SP) is a relatively common condition, which is defined as the presence of air in the pleural space associated with lung collapse (Fig. **1**). The goals of treatment are to evacuate air from the pleural space, achieve lung re-expansion, and prevent recurrence.

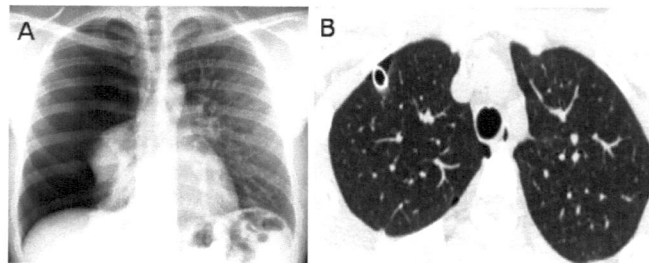

Fig. 1. Right spontaneous pneumothorax with nearly complete lung collapse (A). Complete re-expansion after just drainage placement (B).

Bullectomy through Video-Assisted Thoracic Surgery (VATS) has become a widely accepted therapy for SP [1-21]. The operation is usually carried out through general anesthesia and one-lung ventilation, although in recent years there have been some satisfactory results reported with VATS performed by local or regional anesthesia in spontaneously ventilating patients [2-10].

*Address correspondence to Eugenio Pompeo:** Department of Thoracic Surgery, Emphysema Center, Policlinico Tor Vergata University, Rome, Italy; Email: pompeo@med.uniroma2.it

In 2001, we began a clinical investigational program entailing VATS bullectomy in SP performed through sole Thoracic Epidural Anesthesia (TEA) in awake patients [8, 22-28]. The aim of this chapter is to describe this surgical approach and discuss the results, also taking into account data from the literature.

BASIC CONCEPTS ON PNEUMOTHORAX

Etiology. On an etiologic basis, pneumothorax is classified as spontaneous, traumatic and iatrogenic. The term "spontaneous" indicates that no mechanical injury is recognized as the causative mechanism. In patients with SP, symptoms such as chest pain and dyspnea occur frequently without major physiologic impairments. Occasionally, an uncomplicated pneumothorax may become under tension resulting in respiratory and hemodynamic instability that require an emergency chest tube insertion [29]. SP can be further classified into primary and secondary. Primary SP occurs in subjects without clinically apparent lung disease whereas secondary SP occurs as a complication of a preexisting lung disease, most often pulmonary emphysema.

Primary spontaneous pneumothorax. The annual incidence of primary SP accounts for 12-28 cases per 100.000 men and 1.2-6.0 cases per 100.000 women [12, 30]. Cigarette smoking has been shown to increase the likelihood of developing primary SP in a dose-dependent manner [30]. Overall, the lifetime risk of developing primary SP in smoking males is 12%, compared to 0.1% observed in non-smokers [31-33]. Familiarity may also play a role since over 10% of patients with primary SP have a positive family history for the disease, which has been associated with mutations in a folliculin gene [34-35]. A previous SP increases the likelihood of a new episode that can be expected within 2 years in about 20% of subjects [32].

Primary SP is caused by the rupture of subpleural blebs or small bullae [30, 31-49]. These lesions which are commonly referred as Emphysema-Like Changes (ELC) are predominantly localized at the lung apex and/or in the apical segment of the lower lobes (Fig. **2**) and are mostly observed in young, thin-tall individuals [4, 8, 32, 50-53]. (ELC) are revealed in 76% to 100 % of patients during VATS and in virtually all patients at thoracotomy [32]. In addition, ELC in the controlateral lung have been found in 79% up to 96 % of patients undergoing one-stage bilateral management by median sternotomy [32].

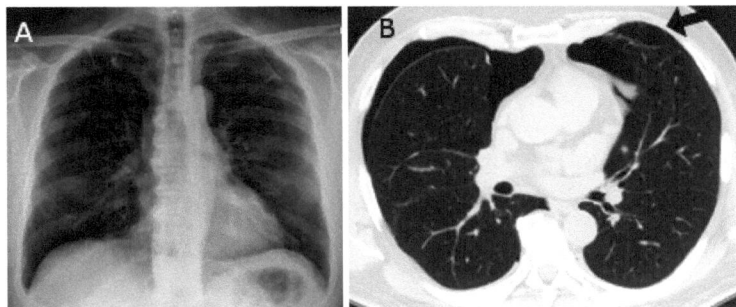

Fig. 2. Bilateral pneumothorax (A, B). Multiple peripheral emphysema-like changes are detected, mostly lying on the lung surface (B, arrow).

The mechanism of ELC formation remains speculative. West [36] hypothesized that ELC preferentially develop at the lung apex due to the higher mechanical stress in this region created by pressure gradients between the lungs' own weight and negative-pleural pressures. Another possible explanation is the degradation of elastic fibers in the lung induced by the smoking-related activation of macrophages and neutrophils, which might induce an imbalance in the protease-antiprotease and oxydant-antioxydant systems [32].

The exact mechanism of ELC rupture is also not fully understood, although it is believed that an abrupt variation in alveolar pressure is the main cause of disruption of the blebs/bullae wall. Changes in atmospheric pressure and exposure to loud music have been also anecdotally reported to facilitate rupture of blebs/bullae [37-39, 50]. Pressure gradients that may develop during scuba diving or flying, are other examples of triggering factors for SP [39].

Secondary spontaneous pneumothorax. Secondary SP occurs as an acute complication of an underlying lung disease (Table **1**) (Figs. **3** and **4**). The incidence of secondary SP in the general population is similar to that of primary SP although in the former, the peak incidence is at 60-65 years of age. In patients with chronic obstructive pulmonary disease, the incidence of secondary SP is about 26 cases per 100.000 individuals/year [33, 40]. However, the probability of developing a secondary SP episode increases as severity of pulmonary emphysema worsens. Indeed, patients with a forced expiratory volume in one second (FEV_1) of less than 1 liter or a ratio of FEV_1 to forced vital capacity of less than 40 % are at greater risk [33]. Cocaine abuse has also been considered a predisposing factor for the development of secondary SP (Fig. **4**), pneumomediastinum, and subcutaneous emphysema [41].

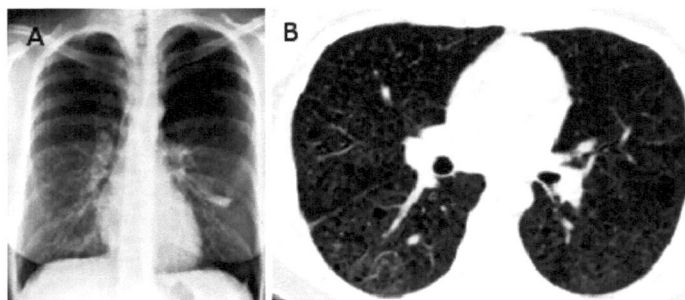

Fig. 3. Left spontaneous pneumothorax (A) in a 27 years-old girl with lymphangio-leiomyomatosis. Diffuse small-sized air cysts are revealed by high-resolution CT-scan (B).

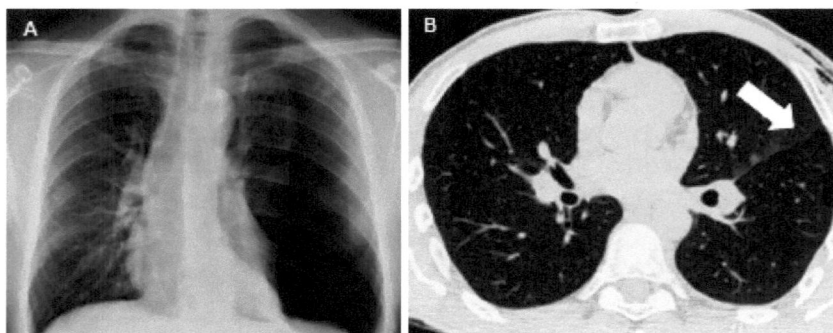

Fig. 4. Left secondary pneumothorax (A) in a young "crack" abuser. CT-scan (B) reveals localized air-filled spaces and inflammatory changes of the major fissure (arrow), consistent with development of an early paraseptal emphysema.

Table 1. Most common causes of secondary pneumothorax.

Chronic airway disease	Bullous emphysema
	Cystic fibrosis
	Severe asthma
Infectious lung disease	Pneumocystis jiroveci pneumonia (AIDS related)
	Active tubercolosis
	Necrotising pneumonia
Interstitial lung disease	Sarcoidosis
	Lymphangio-leiomyomatosis
	Idiopatic pulmonary fibrosis
Connective disease	Rheumatoid arthritis
	Scleroderma
	Marfan's syndrome (Fig. **5**)
Neoplastic disease	Primary lung cancer
	Lung metastases
	Sarcoma
	Lymphoma

Recurrent SP occurring in women in synchrony with the menstrual cycle strongly suggests a diagnosis of catamenial pneumothorax related to the presence of intrathoracic endometriosis [42].

The pathophysiology of secondary SP is mainly addressed to the development of high pressure gradients between alveoli and the interstitium of the lung as it happens with coughing or Valsalva maneuvers that can trigger alveolar disruption. Air from the ruptured alveolus may move into the interstitium of the lung and backward along the bronchovascular bundle to the hilum resulting in pneumothorax. In contrast to the usually indolent clinical course of primary SP, secondary SP can become a life-threatening event, especially in patients with low respiratory reserve in whom hypoxia, hypercapnia and even cardiovascular failure can occur [13, 43, 44, 49]. In patients with a history of previous thoracic surgery, pleurodesis or pleuropulmonary infections, detection of the secondary SP with standard roentgenogram may be hindered and CT-scan should be preferred to allow a precise identification of air collections that can be multiloculated due to pleural adhesions and septa [22, 45, 51] (Figs. **5** and **6**).

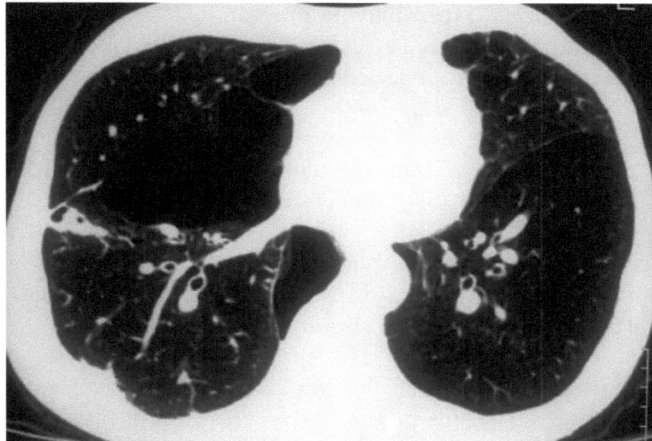

Fig. 5. Loculated right pneumothorax occurring 6 months after lung volume reduction surgery. Note the peculiar location of the air collection, which contraindicated blind chest drainage placement.

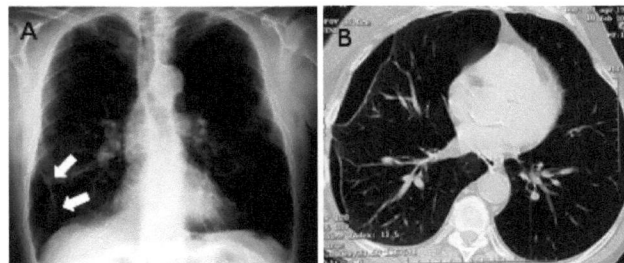

Fig. 6. Loculated pneumothorax occurring after lung volume reduction surgery. Roengtenogram reveals right-sided air-collection of limited size (A, arrows). Precise detection of multiple loculations is allowed by CT-scan (B).

AWAKE VATS MANAGEMENT OF SPONTANEOUS PNEUMOTHORAX

Historical background. The thoracoscope is a lineal descendent of the cystoscope, an instrument conceived in 1806 by Bozzini, to explore the urinary bladder using a candle as a light source [54]. According to Unverricht, Kelling is credited as the first using an endoscope into the pleural cavity of a dog. Interest towards usefulness of the cystoscope in the clinical setting was common in Europe in the early 900s [55]. In 1908 Jacobeus pioneered its use for diagnosis and treatment of a patient with pleural effusion [56] and for 80 years thoracoscopy was performed through hollow tubes under local anesthesia [9].

In 1937, Sattler et al [33] identified areas with little bullae on the visceral pleura using thoracoscopy and they concluded that air leakage leading to SP was due to ruptured bullae. In 1969, Sukhanovsi *et al.* [57]

studied patients with SP, and showed bullous area by means of thoracoscopy; at that time the choice between simple pleural drainage or thoracotomy was decided following thoracoscopic exploration.

In the 1980s, Friedel *et al.* [58] performed thoracoscopy through general anesthesia in 150 patients whereas in 1990, Levi et al [1] introduced VATS for treatment of SP under general anesthesia and one-lung ventilation.

In 1987, Rush *et al.* [59] employed multiple intercostals block to perform simple thoracoscopic procedures in awake patients. In 1997, Nezu *et al.* [2] firstly reported excellent results with awake VATS bullectomy for SP through sole intercostal blocks.

More recently other surgeons have reported on awake VATS management of SP performed by intercostal block or TEA [2-10].

Basic principles of surgical management. The management of SP pivots on evacuation of air from the pleural space, achievement of lung re-expansion and prevention of recurrences. In the published British Thoracic Society guidelines [30], conservative treatment is proposed as the first-line treatment. Conversely, patients who have recurrent pneumothorax or persistent air leaks several days after chest drainage should be regarded as candidates for surgery [30-37, 41, 43-47].

As far as prevention of recurrence is concerned, the estimated risk of recurrent SP is about 0-10% [1, 14, 15, 41, 60] after surgery and 25%-34% [30, 48] after conservative management.

Removal of ELC through staple resection or plication (bullectomy) is the most commonly employed method to eliminate them and prevent recurrences. Bullectomy can be combined with pleurodesis, which can be obtained by partial pleurectomy or pleural abrasion as well as by talc insufflation.

Bullectomy and pleurodesis have been satisfactorily performed by either thoracotomy or VATS. Advocators of VATS believe that it results in less postoperative respiratory impairment, shorter hospital stay and better perioperative quality of life with equivalent outcome. Instead, other surgeons [49-51] continue to prefer thoracotomy in the believe that VATS can be associated with higher rates of complications and recurrence. Since 2001 we have offered awake VATS bullectomy performed by TEA to patients with SP and our indications for this surgical approach are detailed in Table **2**.

Table 2. Main indications to awake VATS management of SP.

Recurrent SP, with or without radiologic evidence of ELC.
First SP episode with radiologic evidence of ELC.
Suboptimal lung re-expansion and/or persistent air-leak after 3 days of chest drainage.
Concomitant controlateral pneumothorax.
Complex, multiloculated pneumothorax occurring after lung surgery in high-risk patients (Figs. **5, 6**).

SP: spontaneous pneumothorax; ELC: emphysema like changes.

Anesthesia. In the operating room, venous and radial artery catheters are inserted. Premedication is usually not necessary although minimal sedation with midazolam and/or remifentanyl is performed in selected instances.

The thoracic epidural catheter is inserted at T4 level *via* a loss-of-resistance technique, and a bolus of ropivacaine 0.5 % plus sufentanyl 5γ is administered immediately after placement. Subsequently, continuous infusion of ropivacaine 0.2% at a rate of 5 mL/h is started, about 20 minutes prior to operation. If necessary, additional injection of local anaesthetics (2-5 mL of ropivacaine 7.5% plus lidocaine 2%) is used to reinforce the analgesia at the incision sites.

During the operation, oxygen addition is usually not necessary although it can be delivered through a Venturi Mask whenever oxygen saturation falls below 90%. The patient must be aware that creation of the surgical pneumothorax can be followed by a certain ventilatory discomfort without significant changes in oxygenation that is attributable to a reduction in vital capacity. In these instances, anxious symptoms may be easily controlled by intravenous administration of low-dose propofol or remifentanyl, the latter being also useful to control excessive intraoperative coughing. Should conversion to general anesthesia become necessary for any technical difficulty, orotracheal intubation is usually carried out without changing the patient's position, with the aid of a fiberoptic bronchoscope.

Perioperatively, fluids are given at a minimum rate to ensure adequate urinary output. At the end of the procedure the patient is immediately transferred to the ward and can start drinking and walking. The epidural catheter is usually left in place for 24 hours. Afterwards thoracic analgesia is assured by continuous intravenous administration of tramadol (200 to 300 mg/24 h) at a rate of 2 ml/h *via* an elastomeric device.

Surgical technique. The patient is placed in full lateral decubitus position with slight trunk elevation and splitting of the intercostal spaces. The operating field is prepped and draped in order to let the patient free to breath comfortably and talk freely with the surgical and anesthesiological staff. The patient is also allowed to follow in the monitor the main vital cardiocirculatory and oxygenation parameters, as well as the ongoing surgical procedure. Immediately before the operation, a chest drainage with water seal system must be kept ready on the operating table to allow immediate tube insertion and lung re-expansion in case of unexpected technical problems requiring rapid conversion to general anesthesia. A 15 mm flexible trocar is inserted in the 7th intercostal space along the midaxillary line for a 30° camera. Two additional ports are placed in the 3rd and 4th intercostals space, in the anterior and posterior axillary lines, respectively. A thorough exploration of the whole lung surface is carried out with the aid of two ring forceps in order to recognize blebs and bullae (Fig. **7**).

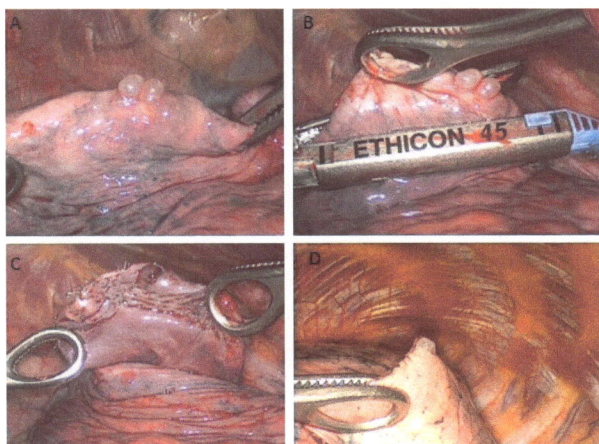

Fig. 7. Awake blebectomy. Spontaneous ventilation helps detecting ELCs, which present as air-filled spaces (A). Plication or resection (B, C) is performed by endostapler. Additional smaller blebs are often found on the apical-posterior segments (D).

Manipulation of the lung is made taking care not to stretch the hilum or compress cartilagineous bronchi, which may trigger cough reflexes. In particular, attention has to be paid to accurately explore the intrafissural lung surface as well as lobar margins, where minimal blebs may easily remain undetected.

Bullectomy is performed with a 45 mm endoscopic stapler. Alternatively, plication of the bullae with a "non cutting" stapler is sometimes preferred whenever the underlying lung tissue is considered at risk for postoperative air leaks. If no ELC are found, "blind" resection of the lung apex is performed (**Video 1**).

Pleural abrasion is our preferred method for pleurodesis. This is commonly performed in the upper third of the pleural cavity by using a mesh abrader although we have more recently used also low-energy argon beam coagulator (Fig. **8**).

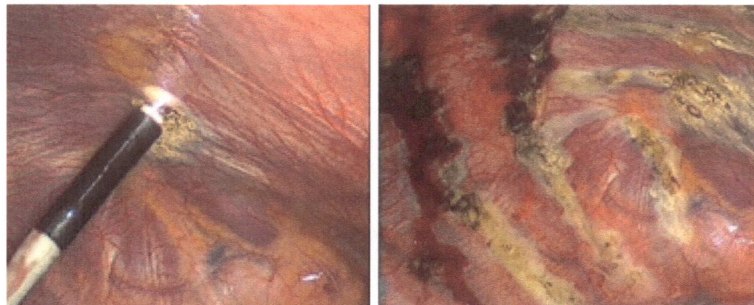

Fig. 8. Awake pleuroablation by Argon-beam coagulator.

While performing abrasion/pleurectomy, care must be taken not to injury the intercostal neuro-vascular bundle and, posteriorly, the sympathetic chain which runs just below the parietal pleura.

In patients with recurrent SP despite previous surgical attempts of treatment, we prefer talc pleurodesis (Fig. **8**).

At the end of the procedure, a 28F chest tube is inserted through the camera port incision and placed on mild suction (-10 cm H_2O). Afterwards, to achieve immediate and complete lung re-expansion we ask the patient to breath deeply and cough repeatedly while temporarily keeping closed the thoracoports with fingers and gauzes.

Pitfalls and complications. Complications of awake VATS in SP are rare. In anxious patients, panic attacks can occur as a consequence of the increased inspiratory load that follows creation of the surgical pneumothorax. Panic attacks can be controlled by administration of intravenous midazolam or propofol at subhypnotic dosage [8]. Minor TEA-related complications such as vomiting, transient urinary retention and mild hypotension can also rarely occur postoperatively although early removal of the epidural catheter minimizes this risk.

Postoperative management. At the end of the procedure, the patient is transferred to the recovery room until when main vital cardiovascular parameters are judged satisfactorily stable by the anesthesiologist. Patients may start drinking water as soon as they are transferred to the ward. On postoperative morning 1, bedside chest roentgenogram is obtained and the epidural catheter is removed. The criteria for chest tube removal and discharge are standardized and include the absence of detectable air-leak on water seal, achievement of complete lung re-expansion, and serum fluid loss not exceeding 200 mL/24 hours. Prior to definitive removal, tube should be clamped for 1-2 hours ans subsequently reopened to help detection of any occult residual air-leak ("provocative clamping" test).

COMMENT

Awake VATS is a particularly attractive surgical approach for treatment of SP because of the simplicity of the surgical procedure and the peculiar features of the patients that are commonly young and healthy [11].

In a small randomized study comparing VATS bullectomy carried out through general anesthesia or TEA, we have shown that the awake operation was easily feasible and well tolerated by the patients [8]. In this study, technical feasibility and satisfaction with the type of anesthesia were comparable between study groups whereas global time spent into the operating room, hospital stay and procedure-related costs were significantly better in the awake group [8]. In addition, awake VATS bullectomy revealed a simple and easy-to-learn operation, particularly if the young surgeons had already matured a certain confidence with equivalent procedures performed through general anesthesia.

The 24-month recurrence rate in our series was 4.5%, a feature that compared favorably with data reported with equivalent procedures performed through general anesthesia (Table **3**).

Table 3. Literature series on VATS management of SP.

First Author	Year	Patients	Anesthesia	Surgical Technique	Hospital Stay (days)	Recurrence (%)
Bertrand [17]	1996	163	General	Bullectomy	6.9	3.6
Nezu [2]	1997	32	Local	Bullectomy	4.3	3.1
		34	General		5.8	5.3
Tschopp [6]	1997	93	Local	Talc pleurodesis	5.6	NA
Passlich [13]	1998	99	General	Bullectomy	8	6.8
Sawada [60]	2005	154	General	Bullectomy/pleural abrasion	8.3	11.7
Cardillo [37]	2006	861	General	Talc pleurodesis/bullectomy	NA	2.4
Pompeo [8]	2007	21	Awake (TEA)	Bullectomy/pleural abrasion	2	4.7
		22	General		3	8
Chen [48]	2008	52	General	Pleural abrasion	4.9	3.3
Ramos Izquierdo [10]	2010	133	Local	Talc pleurodesis	5.6	3
Dubois [64]	2010	72	General	Bullectomy/ talc pleurodesis	4	0

NA: not available; TEA: thoracic epidural anesthesia.

Awake VATS management of SP has been anecdotally reported in recent years, although local analgesia with or without sedation has been most commonly employed [2, 7, 61, 62].

We prefer the use of TEA because of the optimal pain control offered by this type of anesthesia during pleural abrasion or talc insufflation, which may reveal particularly painful in conscious patients. Furthermore, TEA obviates the need for a deep sedation thus allowing an easy intraoperative interaction between the patient and the surgeon that reveal particularly useful at the end-procedure when lung re-expansion must be achieved without the aid of mechanical ventilation.

As far as the elective method for pleurodesis is regarded, pleural abrasion is our preferred option because it combines the advantages of an optimal patient's tolerability with a low risk of recurrence [2, 6, 8, 10]. Recently, pleurectomy by argon-beam pneumodissection, advocated by Song *et al.* [63] has been successfully employed also by our group.

Some surgeons advocate talc pleurodesis even in primary SP because of its effectiveness and low recurrence rate [12, 62, 64]. However, talc pleurodesis resulted poorly effective in presence of bullous areas larger than 2 cm [65, 66] and we have occasionally observed chronic thoracic pain and foreign-body reactions evolving into inflammatory pseudotumors following its use. For these reasons, we now offer talc pleurodesis to patients who previously underwent unsuccessful bullectomy/pleuroabrasion or are deemed at high risk of SP due to occupational reasons.

The prevalence of ELC in patients treated for SP ranges between 76%-100% [8, 12, 67]. Since undetected ELCs are thought to represent an independent predictor of recurrence [63], the question of whether awake VATS can yield optimal recognition of smaller blebs and bullae appears crucial. We believe that accurate exploration of the lung surface is not jeopardized in spontaneously ventilating subjects since we were able to found ELC in up to 90 % of patients. One hypothetical reason is that bullae can remain inflated during awake VATS so facilitating their recognition without the need of mechanical re-ventilation of the lung [8, 68].

Another open question is whether to operate, or not, on patients after their first SP episode. Different factors contribute to the decision-making process in these instances, including the patient's clinical status and preference as well as the surgeon's common practice. Many thoracic surgeons initially favour simple chest drainage while reserving surgical management for recurrences. Nonetheless, the operation can result in lower risk of recurrence with an obvious impact in patients' quality of life [1, 14, 15, 30, 35, 67]. In addition, conservative management can be associated with longer hospital stay and higher costs when compared to immediate surgery [8, 12, 17, 61]. In this respect, the proposal of an awake VATS management might contribute to facilitate the patients' acceptance of immediate surgical treatment leading to an overall reduction of recurrences.

CONCLUSION

In conclusion, we believe that awake VATS under TEA could be now considered a valid and globally minimally invasive option to achieve definitive successful treatment of SP.

REFERENCES

[1]   Levi JF, Kleinmann P, Riquet M, Debesse B. Percutaneous parietal pleurectomy for recurrent spontaneous pneumothorax. Lancet 1990;336:1577-8.

[2]   Nezu K, Kushibe K, Tojo T, *et al.* Thoracoscopic wedge resection of blebs under local anesthesia with sedation for treatment of spontaneous pneumothorax. Chest 1997;111:230-5.

[3]   Mukaida T, Andou A, Date H, *et al.* Thoracoscopic operation for secondary pneumothorax under local and epidural anesthesia in high-risk patients. Ann Thorac Surg 1998;65:924-6.

[4]   Iderbitzi RG, Leiser A, Furrer M, Althaus U. Three years experience in video-assisted thoracic surgery (VATS) for spontaneous pneumothorax. J Thorac Cardiovasc Surg 1994;107:1410-5.

[5]   Mouroux J, Elkaim D, Padovani B, *et al.* Video-assisted thoracoscopic treatment of spontaneous pneumothorax: technique and results of one hundred cases. J Thorac Cardiovasc Surg 1996;112:385-91.

[6]   Tschopp JM, Boutin MC, Astoul P, *et al.* Treatment of complicated spontaneous pneumothorax by simple talc pleurodesis under thoracoscopic and local anesthesia. Thorax 1997;52:329-2.

[7]   Katlic MR. Video-assisted thoracic surgery utilizing local anesthesia and sedation. Eur J Cardiothoraci Surg 2006;30:529-32.

[8]   Pompeo E, Tacconi F, Mineo D, Mineo TC. The role of awake video-assisted thoracoscopic surgery in spontaneous pneumothorax. J Thorac Cardiovasc Surg 2007;133:786-90.

[9]   Katlic MR, Facktor MA. Video-assisted thoracic surgery utilizing local anesthesia and sedation: 384 consecutive cases. Ann Thorac Surg 2010;90:240-5.

[10]   Ramos Izquierdo R, Moya J, Macia I, *et al.* Treatment of primary spontaneous pneumothorax by videothoracoscopic talc pleurodesis under local anesthesia: a review of 133 procedures. Surgical Endosc 2010;24:984-7.

[11]   Janssen JP, Schramel FMNH, Sutedja TG, *et al.* Videothoracoscopic appearance of first and recurrent pneumothorax. Chest 1995;108:330-4.

[12]   Tschopp JM, Rami-Porta R, Noppen M, Astoul P. Management of spontaneous pneumothorax: state of the art. Eur Respir J 2006;28:637-50.

[13]   Passlick B, Born C, Haussinger K, Thetter O. Efficiency of Video-assisted thoracic surgery for primary and secondary spontaneous pneumothorax. Ann Thorac Surg 1998;65:324-7.

[14]   Waller D, Forty J, Morrit G. Video-assisted thoraoscopic surgery versus thoracotomy for spontaneous penumothorax. Ann Thorac Surg 1994;58:372-6.

[15]   Jutley SR, Khalil MW, Rocco G. Uniportal vs standard three port VATS technique for spontaneous pneumothorax: comparison of post operative pain and residual paraesthesia. Eur J Cardiothorac surg 2005;28:43-6.

[16]   Tagaya N, Kasama K, Suziki N, *et al.* Video assisted bullectomy using needlescopic instruments for spontaneous pneumothorax. Surg Endosc 2003;17:1486-7.

[17]   Bertrand PC, Regnard JF, Spaggiari L, *et al.* Immediate and long-term results after surgical treatment of primary spontaneous pneumothorax by VATS. Ann Thorac Surg 1996;61:1641-5.

[18]   Naunheim KS, Mack MJ, Hazelrigg SR, *et al.* Safety and efficacy of video-assisted thoracic surgical techniques for the treatment of spontaneous pneumothorax. J Thorac Cardiovasc Surg 1995;109:1198-203.

[19]   Chan P, Clarke P, Daniel FJ, *et al.* Efficacy of video-assisted thoracoscopic surgery pleurodesis for spontaneous pneumothorax. Ann Thorac Surg 2001;71:452-4.

[20]   Cardillo G, Facciolo F, Giunti R, *et al.* Videothoracoscopic treatment of primary spontaneous pneumothorax: a 6-years experience. Ann Thorac Surg 2000;69:357-62.

[21]   Ignolfsson I, Gyllstedt E, Lillo-Gil R, *et al.* Reoperations are common following VATS for spontaneous pneumothorax: study of risk factors. Interact Cardiovasc Thorac Surg 2006;5:602-7.

[22]   Tacconi F, Pompeo F, Mineo TC. Late-onset occult pneumothorax after lung volume reduction surgery. Ann Thorac Surg 2005;80:2008-12.

[23]   Mineo TC. Epidural anesthesia in awake thoracic surgery. Eur J Cardiothorac Surg 2007;32:13-9.

[24]   Mineo TC, Pompeo E, Mineo D, *et al.* Awake nonresectional lung volume reduction surgery. Ann Surg 2006;243:131-6.

[25]   Pompeo E, Mineo D, Rogliani P, *et al.*Feasibility and results of awake thoracoscopic resection of solitary pulmonary nodules. Ann Thorac Surg 2004;78:1761-8.

[26]   Mineo TC, Pompeo E, Mineo D, *et al.* Results of unilateral lung volume reduction surgery in patients with distinct heterogeneity of emphysema between lungs. J Thorac Cardiovasc Surg 2005;129:73-9.

[27]   Pompeo E, Mineo TC. Awake operative videothoracoscopic pulmonary resections. Thorac Surg Clin 2008;18:311-20.

[28]   Vanni G, Tacconi F, Sellitri F, *et al.* Impact of awake videothoracoscopic surgery on postoperative lymphocyte responses. Ann Thorac Surg. 2010;90:973-8.

[29]   Baumann MH, Sahn SA. Tension pneumothorax: diagnostic and therapeutic pitfall. Crit Care Med 1993;21:177.

[30]   Henry M, Arnold T, Harvey J. BTS guidelines for the management of spontaneous pneumothorax. Thorax 2003;58:S39-S52.

[31]   Jansveld CA, Dijkman JH. Primary spontaneous pneumothorax and smoking. BMJ 1975;4:559-560.

[32]   Shan SA, Heffner J. Spontaneous pneumothorax (review). New Engl J Med 2000;342:868-74.

[33]   Sattler A. Zur Behandlung der Spontanpneumothorax mit besonderer Ber cksichtigung der Torakoskopie. Beitr Klin Tuberk Spezif Tuberkuloseforsch 1937;89:394-408.

[34]   Ohata M, Suzuki H. Pathogenesis of spontaneous pneumothorax: with special reference to the ultrastructure of emphysematous bullae. Chest 1980;77:771-6.

[35]   Chiu HT, Garcia CK. Familial spontaneous pneumothorax. Curr Opin Pulm Med 2006;12:268-72.

[36]   West JB, Matthews FL. Stresses, strains and surface pressures in the lung caused by its weight. I Appl Physiol 1972;32:332-45.

[37]   Cardillo G, Corleo F, Giunti R, *et al.* Videothoracoscopic talc poudrage in primary spontaneous pneumothorax: a single institution experience in 861 cases. J Thorac Cardiovasc Surg 2006;131:322-8.

[38]   Noppen M, Verbanck S, Harvey J, *et al.* Music: a new cause of primary spontaneous pneumothorax. Thorax 2004;59:722-4.

[39]   Smit HJM, Davillè WL, Scramel FM, Schreurs A. Atmospheric pressure changes and outdoor temperature changes in relation to spontaneous pneumothorax. Chest 1999;116:676- 81.

[40]   Luck SR, Raffensperger JG, Sullivan HJ, Gibson LE. Management of pneumothorax in children with chronic pulmonary disease. J Thorac Cardiovasc Surg 1977;74:834-9.

[41]   Maeder M, Ullmer E. Pneumomediastinum and bilateral pneumothorax as a complication of cocaine smoking. Respiration 2003;70:407.

[42]   Korom S, Canyurt H, Missbach A, *et al.* Catamenial pneumothorax revisited: clinical approach and systematic review of the literature. J Thorac Cardiovasc Surg 2004;128:502-8.

[43]   Spector ML, Stern RC. Pneumothorax in cystic fibrosis: a 26-year experience. Ann Thorac Surg 1989;47:204-7.

[44]   Dines DE, Clagett OT, Payne WS. Spontaneous pneumothorax in emphysema. Mayo Clin Proc 1970;45:481-7.

[45]   Bourgoin P, Cousineau G, Lemire P, Hebert G. Computed tomography used to exclude pneumothorax in bullous lung disease. J Can Assoc Radiol 1985;36:341-2.

[46]   Bense L, Eklund G, Wiman LG. Smoking and the increased risk of contracting spontaneous pneumothorax. Chest 1987;92:1009-12.

[47]   Waller D, Forty J, Morrit G. Video-assisted thoracoscopic surgery versus thoracotomy for spontaneous penumothorax. Ann Thorac Surg 1994;58:372-6.

[48]   Chen JS, Hsu HH, Tsai KT, *et al.* Salvage for unsuccessful aspiration of primary pneumothorax: thoracoscopic surgery or chest tube drainage? Ann Thorac Surg 2008;85:1908-13.

[49]   Barker A, Maratos EC, Edmonds L, Lim E. Recurrence rates of video-assisted thoracoscopic versus open surgery in the prevention of recurrent pneumothoraces: a systematic review of randomized and non-randomised trials. Lancet 2007;370:329-35.

[50]   Cole, Kim HK, Han JY, *et al.* Transaxillary minithoracotomy versus video-assisted thoracic surgery for spontaneous pneumothorax. Ann Thorac Surg 1996;61:1510-2.

[51]   Sakurai H. Videothoracoscopic surgical approach for spontaneous pneumothorax: review of the literature. World J Emerg Surg 2008;3:23.

[52]   Czerny M, Salat A, Fleck T, *et al.* Lung wedge resection improves outcome in stage I primary spontaneous pneumothorax. Ann Thorac Surg 2004;77:1802-5.

[53]   Zisis C, Stratakos G. Do we know the ideal surgical treatment for primary spontaneous pneumothorax? Eur J Cardiothorac Surg 2006;29:1067-8.

[54]   Bozzini P. On the illumination of internal cavities. Weimar, Germany 1807.

[55]   Bloomberg AE. Thoracoscopy in perspective. Surg, Gynecol Obst 1978;147:433-43.

[56]   Jacobaeus HC. Possibility of the use of the cystoscope for investigation of serous cavities. Munch Med Wochenschr 1910;57:2090.

[57]   Sukhanovski I. Thoracoscopy in spontaneous pneumothorax. Vest Khir 1969;103:21.

[58]   Friedel H, Wetzger K, Thies WH. New diagnostic thoracoscopy and its possibilities. Z Erk Atmungsorgane 1974;140:313.

[59]   Rush VW. Thoracoscopy under regional anesthesia for the diagnosis and management of pleural diseae. Am J Surg 1987;15:274-8.

[60]   Sawada S, Watanabe Y, Morimoto S. Video assisted thoracoscopic surgery for primary spontaneous pneumothorax. Chest 2005;127:2226-30.

[61]   Sugimoto S, Date H, Sugimoto R, *et al.* Thoracoscopic operation with local and epidural anesthesia in the treatment of pneumothorax after lung transplantation. J Thorac Cardiovasc Surg 2005;130:1219-20.

[62]   Yokoyoma T, Tomoda M, Kanbara T, *et al.* Epidural anesthesia for a patient with catamenial pneumothorax. Masui 2001;50:290-2.

[63]   Song SH, Kim YD, Seok H, Cho JS, Lee JH. Videothoracoscopic parietal pleurectomy with argon pneumodissection. Ann Thorac Surg 2010;90:e64-5.

[64]   Dubois L, Malthaner RA. Video-assisted thoracoscopic bullectomy and talc poudrage for spontaneous pneumothoraces: effect on short-term lung function. J Thorac Cardiovasc Surg 2010;140:1272-5.

[65]   Tschopp JM, Boutin C, Astoul P, *et al.* Talcage by medical thoracoscopy for primary spontaneous pneumothorax is more cost-effective then drainage: a randomized study. Eur Respir J 2002;20:1003-9.

[66]   Tschopp JM, Brutsche M, Frey JG. Treatment of complicated spontaneous pneumothorax by simple talc pleurodesis under local anesthesia. Thorax 1997;52:329-32.

[67]   Scramel FM, Postmus PE, Vanderschueren RG. Current aspect of spontaneous pneumothorax. Eur Respir J 1997;10:1372-9.

[68]   Whitehead T, Slutsky AS. The pulmonary physician in critical care: ventilator induced lung injury. Thorax 2002;57:635-42.

CHAPTER 11

Awake Pleural Decortication for Empyema Thoracis

Federico Tacconi and Eugenio Pompeo[*]

Department of Thoracic Surgery, Policlinico Tor Vergata University Rome, Italy

Abstract: Empyema thoracis is defined as the presence of purulent fluid within the pleural cavity. Despite proper management is still debated, widespread agreement exists amongst thoracic surgeons that an immediate surgery is more likely to result in favorable outcome than conservative treatment.

In recent years, the use of video-assisted thoracic surgery has gained acceptance as a valuable option in this setting, since satisfactory re-expansion of the trapped lung can be achieved in more than 90% of patients with a minimal surgical traumatism.

A further development in the field of minimally-invasive approach for empyema thoracis is represented by the renewed interest in videothoracoscopic operations performed in spontaneous ventilating patients, through local or locoregional anesthesia techniques. In our experience, awake videothoracoscopic decortication performed under thoracic epidural anesthesia proven feasible and well tolerated in most instances. In addition, conversion to thoracotomy was possible in more than 20% of patients without switching to general anesthesia.

In this chapter, we focus on clinical and technical aspect of this novel surgical approach, which could represent a reliable treatment tool especially in high-risk patients with early-stage empyema thoracis.

Keywords: Empyema thoracis, VATS, thoracic epidural anesthesia.

INTRODUCTION

Empyema Thoracis (ET) is defined as the presence of frankly purulent fluid within the pleural cavity [1-6]. In more than 50% of instances, it occurs as the ultimate evolution of a preexisting parapneumonic pleural effusion, mostly because of late or inappropriate treatment, or develops due to superinfection of any pleural collection, irrespective of its origin.

Regardless of the causative mechanism, proper management of ET is still a matter of debate. Adopted protocols can vary widely depending on evolutional stage, clinical presentation, and the surgeon's own habits. However, despite the lack of definitively accepted guidelines, widespread agreement exists amongst thoracic surgeons an immediate surgery is more likely to result in a favorable outcome than repeated attempts of conservative treatment.

The use of Video-Assisted Thoracic Surgery (VATS) has progressively gained acceptance as a valuable option for early treatment of complex pleural effusions and ET, since complete evacuation of the pleural cavity and satisfactory re-expansion of the trapped lung can be achieved in more than 90 % of patients with minimal surgical traumatism [7-29] (Table **1**). A further contribution in reducing the overall invasiveness of the surgical approach in this setting is represented by the growing interest in VATS procedures performed through different types of local/regional anesthesia [29-33], especially in patients with increased risk for general anesthesia and one-lung ventilation.

In this chapter, we focus on the clinical and technical aspects of the surgical management of fibrinopurulent ET performed under thoracic epidural anesthesia in fully awake, spontaneously ventilating patients.

*Address correspondence to Eugenio Pompeo: Department of Thoracic Surgery, Policlinico Tor Vergata University, Rome, Italy; Email: pompeo@med.uniroma2.it

Table 1. Relevant literature reports on VATS management of empyema thoracis.

First Author	Year	Study Design	Patients	Empyema Stage/Type	Success Rate
Ridley [7]	1991	Feasibility study	30	I	60%
Striffeler[8]	1996	Feasibility study	13	I/II	100%
O'Brien [9]	1994	Feasibility study	8	I/II (Post-traumatic)	100%
Sendt [10]	1995	Feasibility study	10	II/III	100%
Landrenau [11]	1996	Retrospective	76	II/III	83%
Mackinlay [12]	1996	Retrospective	33	II	90%
Wait [13]	1996	Randomized trial	11	II	91 %
Striffeler [14]	1998	Prospective	67	II/III	72 %
Scherer [15]	1998	Retrospective	17	II (Post-traumatic)	82 %
Lackner [16]	2000	Retrospective	17	II	86 %
Waller [17]	2001	Prospective	36	III	58 %
Cheng [18]	2002	Prospective	10	III	90 %
Bouros [19]	2002	Retrospective	20	CPE/I/II	85 %
Petrakis [20]*	2004	Retrospective comparison	20	I/II*	95%
			18	I/II-Immediate VATS	85%
Wurnig [21]	2006	Retrospective	130	II	88 %
Tajiri [22]	2006	Retrospective	30	II/*Early* III	90 %
Solaini [23]	2007	Retrospective	110	II/III	91 %
Drain [24]	2007	How-to-do-it	52	III	94 %
Chan [25]	2007	Retrospective	41	II	100%
Cardillo [26]	2009	Retrospective	185	*Chronic*	98 %
Shahin [27]	2009	Retrospective	52	III	81 %
Tong [28]	2010	Retrospective	326	II/III	89%
Tacconi [29]	2010	Retrospective (Awake VATS)	19	II/*Early* III	94 %

CPE: complex pleural effusion. *: this study compares results of VATS performed early or after conservative treatment by drainage placement and fybrinolytics instillation.

BASICS CONCEPTS ON EMPYEMA THORACIS

Epidemiology. It has been estimated that, in the United States, about 1.3 million individuals per year are hospitalized with pneumonia, and 40%-60% will develop a parapneumonic effusion [34-36]. Approximately, 5-10 % of these conditions evolve into a complicated pleural effusion or empyema requiring aggressive treatment [34]. In addition, though ET is usually regarded as an epidemiologically stable disease, some data suggest an increasing incidence of ET in both childhood and adulthood in North America and Europe [36-39].

It has been shown that bronchiectasis, rheumatoid arthritis, alcoholism, diabetes, and gastro-esophageal reflux facilitate the development of pneumonia and ET, whereas gender and race do not seem to affect it [34]. As far as mortality rate is concerned, despite the common perception that ET now has a relatively favorable outcome, some recent analyses have estimated the crude mortality rate to range between 7% and 10 % [34].

Etiology. Virtually, any microbiological species can be responsible for ET although aerobic infections are found in culture and smears in the vast majority of cases [34-36].

Amongst gram-positive bacteria, S*treptococci* and *Staphilococci* spp. are frequently found as the causative agent, while *Haemphilus Influentiae, Klebsiella* spp., *Pseudomonas aeruginosa,* and *Enterobacteriacee* are the most frequently involved gram-negative. *Streptococcus Milleri* (SM) [40-42] has been shown to electively colonize the pleural cavity, especially following major thoracic surgery, and accounts for up to 50% of all community-acquired pleural infections. SM-related empyemas are usually resistant to medical treatment and require aggressive surgery since a recurrence rate higher than 27% has been reported with conservative treatment alone. Pleural infections from Methicillin-Resistant *Staphilococcus aureus* (MRSA) may occur either as hospital- or community-acquired infection, the latter with more severe symptoms and clinical evolution (Fig. 1) [43, 44]. Due to the particular virulence and antibiotic resistance of MRSA, complications such as necrotizing fasciitis, osteomyelitis and sepsis are frequent and require early surgical management [44]. *Streptoccoccus Viridans* is most frequently found in young adults, and has been shown to be related to alcohol abuse [45].

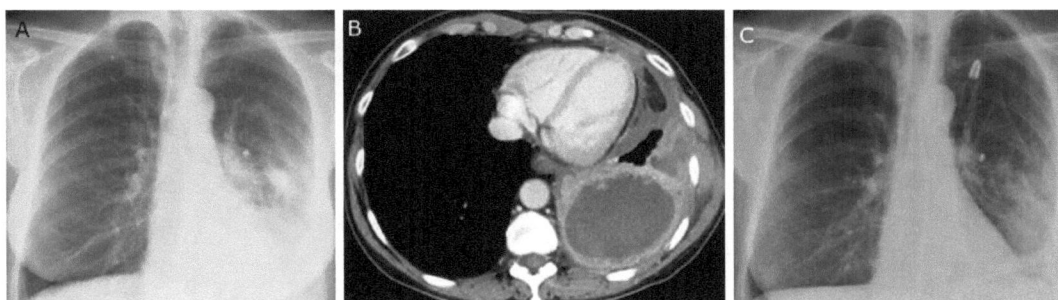

Fig. 1. Chest roengtenogram (A) and axial CT-scan (B) of a 57-years old male with multiple pleural loculations resulting from methicillin-resistant *Staphilococcus Aureus* empyema. Nearly complete lung re-expansion after awake VATS decortication (C).

Although isolated aerobic infections are considerably less frequent, concomitant anaerobic strains have been found in up to 74% of all ETs. Anaerobic infections are most frequently caused by *Fusobacterium* spp., *Prevotella* spp., *Petostreptococci,* and *Clostridium* spp., although an increasing incidence of *Acynetobacter*-positive cultures has been reported in recent updates on hospital-acquired infections [46].

Fungal ET are being increasingly reported [47], especially in immunocompromised or clinically deteriorated patients. In up to 80% of instances, the pleural infection is sustained by *Candida* spp., while *Aspergillus* spp. is reported less frequently. Regardless of the causative agent, fungal ET should be regarded as an extremely severe condition with a mortality rate higher than 70%.

Empyemas related to *Mycobacterium tuberculosis* are particularly worrying due to complex anatomic changes induced by the long acting infection, and are therefore usually regarded as a specific topic of thoracic surgery. Nonetheless, most of the ETs observed in patients with active tuberculosis are iatrogenic whilst today the presence of Koch's bacillus in cultures is rather infrequent.

Almost 1/3 of ETs are found to be sterile due to antibiotic therapy or incorrect laboratory practice. Nonetheless, a true non-infective empyema may exceptionally result as a complication of "smoked cocaine" abuse [48].

Classification. Traditionally, three different evolutional phases of ET are recognized, which are named as the *exudative stage*, the *fibrinopurulent stage*, and the *organizing stage*. These stages basically refer to the degree of desmoplastic reaction that is present in the pleural cavity and which is strictly related to the duration of the infection and the involved microorganism(s). This simple classification proves extremely useful from a surgical point of view, and is currently used in most institutions.

In 2000, The American College of Chest Physicians proposed a more comprehensive staging system, in order to better identify predictive factors of outcome [49, 50]. In this system, which is based on the characteristics of pleural fluid alongside the anatomic changes of the pleural cavity (Table **2**), the stages I-II correspond to the so-called *"simple parapneumonic effusion"*. These stages entail the early inflammatory answer of the visceral pleura to the underlying infection. The pleural fluid appears citrine due to scarce cellular and protein content, is free-flowing and usually occupies less than one-half of the hemithorax. Gram stains and cultures are usually negative and absence of biological activity is indicated by low lactate-dehydrogenase level, nearly normal pH and preserved glucose pool (>60 mg/dl). In most instances, a simple parapneumonic effusion may resolve with medical therapy alone, although evacuation may be useful for diagnostic purposes, to relieve symptoms and improve the effectiveness of medical therapy. The stage III indicates the *"complex parapneumonic effusion"*. This usually occurs 2-3 weeks later and is related to persistent inflammation, which increases vascular permeability leading to a spillover of protein and inflammatory cells. As a consequence, deposition of collagen occurs, ultimately resulting in fibrotic adhesions and septa, and thickening of the visceral pleura. The pleural fluid may be limpid or cloudy, depending on the amount of proteins and cells, although it may be sterile in many instances. A lower pH (<7.20) and glucose level (<60 mg/dl) indicate an increased bioactivity, which is related to the presence of bacteria and/or activated inflammatory cells. In this phase, conservative management is frequently ineffective due to the presence of multiple loculations and trapped lung (Fig. **1**).

Table 2. American college of chest physicians classification system for pleural effusions and ET.

Stage	Fluid Collection	pH	Cultures-Strains	Risk of Poor Outcome
I	Free flowing, < 1 cm on lateral decubitus position	Unknown	Unknown /Negative	Very low
II	Free flowing, < ½ of the involved hemithorax	>7.2	Negative	Low
III	Loculated ANR/OR ≥ 1/2 of the involved hemithorax, Pleural thickening	<7.2	Positive	Moderate
IV	Purulent	Any	Any	High

Adapted by Colice *et al.* [49].

Stage IV represents the ultimate evolution to true ET with presence of frank pus in the pleural cavity. It may develop as a consequence of bacterial spread towards the pleural fluid with subsequent leukocyte sequestration, apoptosis and fatty degeneration. Bacteria may colonize the pleural cavity from the underlying pulmonary infection, through repeated thoracenteses or as a consequence of ineffective drainage placement. In most instances, the pleural fluid is sketchy, smelly and culture-positive. Acute clinical presentation is characterized by fever, shortness of breath, fatigue and loss of weight, which advise expeditious treatment. If not properly managed, ET may evolve into severe complications.

Though ET usually encompasses a clinically "acute" condition, it may shift towards a chronic scenario in some instances (Fig. **2**). Pleural adhesions become thick, calcified or fleshy. The strong desmoplastic reaction can extend from the pleura to the lung tissue through the interlobular septa. In extreme stages, the fibrotic involvement of the parietal pleura may result in loss of expansibility of the chest. Chest-wall lymphoma may also occur as late-onset complication. In 1995, a further classification system has been proposed by Light and coworkers [51]. This includes 7 stages, amongst which stages 1-5 relate to various degrees of clinical severity of a parapneumonic effusion while acute and chronic pleural empyema are classified as stages 6 and 7, respectively. Although this system is considered accurate, the aforementioned classification systems remain the most employed ones in clinical practice.

Complications. Despite the advances in clinical management of ET, an unfavorable evolution may occur in up to 10 % of cases [52]. This is more commonly observed in clinically deteriorated individuals, in whom an aggressive treatment is often delayed or contraindicated.

The worst evolutional scenario entails the development of septic shock and multiorgan failure, which are fatal in nearly all instances.

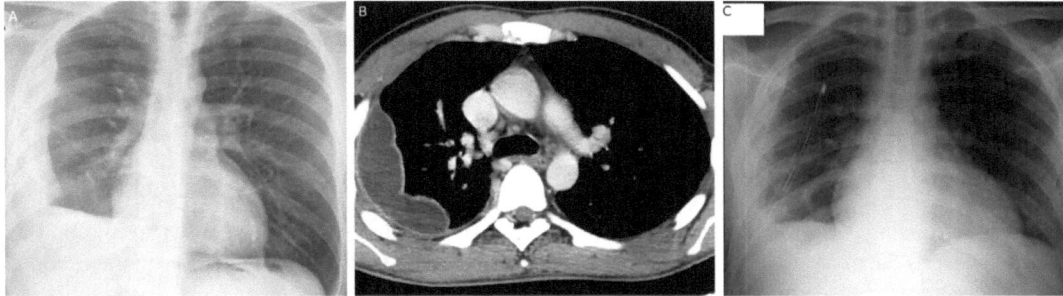

Fig. 2. A case of *chronic* empyema thoracis in a 72 years old patient with history of recurrent pleural effusion after repeated attempts of conservative treatment since 5 months (A). The pleural collection is limited to the lateral aspect of the right hemithorax due to thick adhesions (B). Decortication resulted in incomplete lung re-expansion (C) even though definitive resolution of chronic symptoms was achieved.

Local complications may vary in clinical severity depending on the extension and type of neighboring anatomic structures that are involved. The purulent cavity may drain outward through the chest wall *(empyema necessitatis)*, an event which can result in transient symptoms relief. In other cases, the purulent collection may infiltrate soft tissues without draining outward *(necrotizing fascitis)* [53], or drain toward the airways through a bronchial fistula.

Spread of pus to the neck through the medial cervical fascia may also occur in association with thrombosis of the internal jugular vein *(Lemièrre's syndrome)* [54]. Occasionally, phrenic nerve palsy and Bernard-Horner syndrome [55] have been described as late complications of ET.

AWAKE SURGERY FOR EMPYEMA THORACIS

Historical perspective. Since the Hippocratic era, ET has been considered as one of the most severe thoracic conditions. Nonetheless, the basic management strategy, which was based on sole drainage, remained substantially unchanged until World-War I, when the increasing incidence of empyema cases related to the swine-type influenza pandemics, stimulated a systematic investigational approach in this setting. In 1917, the U.S. Army surgeon William Gorgas first established the international Empyema Commission, in which eminent surgeons such as Evart Graham and Richard Bell [2-4, 56, 57] were actively involved. Brilliant observations based on a demanding daily clinical practice led these authors to establish some of the basic concepts of the modern management of ET. In particular, they stated that careful surgical treatment aimed at ensuring a complete re-expansion of the lung, together with postoperative physiotherapy and adequate caloric intake were the keys factors for a successful outcome. Nonetheless, one of the main problems Graham and colleagues were concerned by was the potentially hazardous consequences of iatrogenic pneumothorax while performing an open drainage, resulting in a mortality rate of up to 30%, in the presence of an associated active pneumonia. Considerable experimental evidence contributed to reinforce this concern. Indeed, Graham was able to demonstrate that, in dogs, the rise in intrapleural pressure consequent to air entry in the pleural cavity was transmitted to the contralateral side, leading to a life-threatening reduction in alveolar ventilation. In addition, they established that a pleural opening wider than 51.5 cm^2 could be lethal even in individuals with normal vital capacity [57, 58].

Starting from the mid 1920's, other surgeons including Berkley Moyinah and Pierre Duval, realized that, provided there was optimized pharmacological support, opening the thoracic cavity was no more hazardous or lethal than opening the abdomen. This revolutionary concept was based on previous observations carried out in the setting of "war surgery" such as the finding that soldiers with large, bilateral chest wounds could survive an open pneumothorax just as well as patients with ET receiving simultaneous bilateral thoracotomy did [58]. These observations, together with concomitant improvements in anesthesiology, represented milestones in the surgical management of ET.

A further advance was stimulated, at that time, by the increasing incidence of "chronic" empyemas of tubercular origin, which could benefit from the removal of the thickened visceral pleural to allow re-expansion of the trapped lung (namely, *pleural decortication*). This surgical procedure fell into disuse following the pioneering experiences of Delorme and Fowler in the late 1800s, and was then progressively re-advocated by Kergin [1], Tuffier [59], Mayo [60], and Gaensler [61].

It is worthy of note that the need for surgical management of ET also stimulated the development of minimally-invasive techniques in thoracic surgery. Indeed, the Irish physicians Francis Cruise and his pupil Samuel Gordon are credited as the precursors of thoracoscopy, which they first used in 1866 to detect "pleural granulations" in a single case of tubercular ET [62]. The original idea was subsequently revised and largely promoted by Hans Jacobaeus, who is nowadays acknowledged as the father of modern thoracoscopy [63]. Following Jacobaeus' pioneering experience, thoracoscopy was mainly employed as a diagnostic tool, while its therapeutic application was limited to pleural adhesiolysis performed to facilitate lung collapse in patients undergoing Forlanini's artificial pneumothorax for tuberculosis. In subsequent years, the increasing familiarity with the technique as well as the improved ergonomics of instrumentations, such as the *Coryllos thoracoscope,* led thoracoscopy to embrace a broader spectrum of indications, including diagnosis and treatment of acute pleural effusions. Interestingly, at that time, most of these minimally-invasive procedures were routinely performed under local anesthesia and spontaneous ventilation but remained relegated in a spurious context between thoracic surgery and interventional pneumology.

In recent years, VATS has gained acceptance as a valuable tool in the management of early-stage ET [64]. In addition, despite general-anesthesia with one-lung ventilation is still considered mandatory for successful VATS, an increasing number of surgeons have stressed the potential advantages of "awake" VATS approaches, in the belief that avoidance of ventilator-related lung injury [65, 66] would result in more physiological postoperative recovery and, ultimately, in an overall improvement in the quality of care.

Indications. Indications for awake VATS management of ET do not differ from those employed for the equivalent surgical procedures performed under general anesthesia and one-lung ventilation. They mainly encompass a diagnosis of exudative and/or fibrinopurulent ET on the basis of clinical history and radiologic imaging. In addition, selected patients with initial signs of organizing ET can also be considered for awake surgery, although the presence of extensive pleural calcifications and/or a history of pleural-pulmonary tuberculosis as well as any previous thoracic surgery procedure in the affected hemithorax should be regarded as general contraindications for VATS.

We electively reserve awake VATS for patients deemed at high-risk for general anesthesia (Table **3**). In addition, immunocompromised patients can benefit most from an awake surgical approach. This belief is reinforced also by our recent data showing that avoidance of general anesthesia may result in better perioperative maintenance of circulating lymphocytes and natural-killer cells as well as in reduced surgical stress hormone release [67, 68].

Table 3. Indications to awake decortication.

Presumptive diagnosis of fibrinopurulent ET.
Symptom duration <45 days.
Risk-factors to general anesthesia and OLV.
Age > 75 years.
Cardiac failure with LVEF < 50 %.
Advanced COPD.
ASA score $\geq$ 2.
Full patient cooperation.
No history of pleuro-pulmonary tuberculosis.
Absence of interstitial lung disease and PAPs < 35 mm Hg.
No lung lesions requiring resection.
Absence of coagulative disorders (INR<1.5).

ASA: American Society of Anesthesiology; INR: international normalized ratio; LVEF: left-ventricular ejection fraction, PAPs: systolic pulmonary arterial pressure.

Other relative contraindications for awake approach are represented by symptom duration longer than 45 days, ET related to bronchopleural fistula, esophageal injury or spreading from preexisting purulent collection sited in the neck or the abdomen. Finally, in the presence of concomitant lung lesions requiring resection, such as lung abscess, we prefer to employ general anesthesia with one-lung ventilation.

Unfavorable conditions for thoracic epidural catheterization such as spine deformities or previous spinal surgery should not preclude the awake surgical approach, since we have successfully employed paravertebral or intercostal blocks in these instances.

Preoperative workup. Accurate clinical history is mandatory to ascertain symptom duration, the first radiological evidence of pleural effusion and the number of attempted evacuation maneuvers.

Standard chest roentgenograms and multiplanar CT-scan should be routinely performed to precisely assess the extent and location of the pleural collection(s) as well as associated lesions involving the lung or other intrathoracic anatomic structures (Fig. **3**). Whenever one has the suspicion of an underlying tumor on the basis of laboratory findings, imaging or pleural cytology, total-body CT scan and [18]-fluorodeoxyglucoside positron-emission tomography should also be performed.

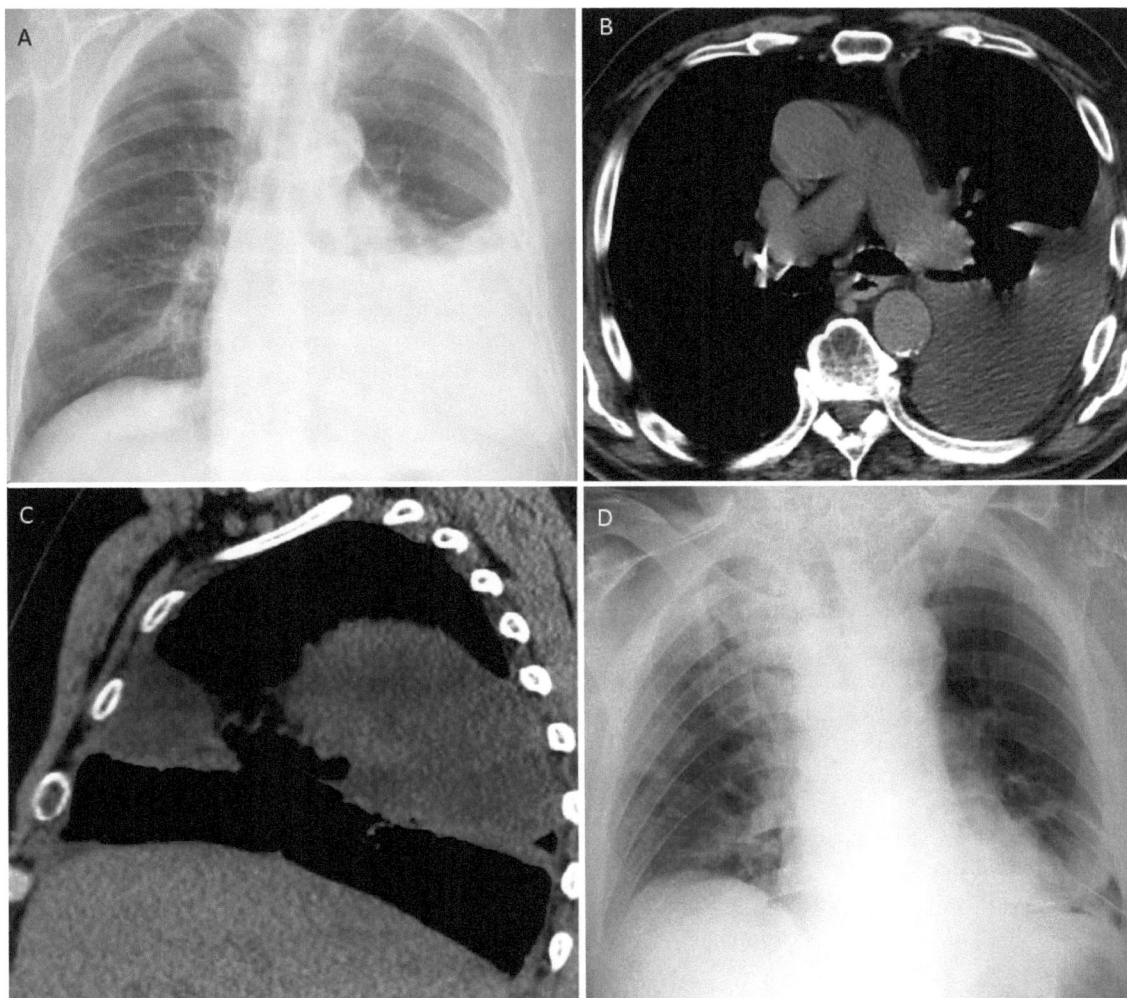

Fig. 3. A 48 years old Caucasian male with left pleural empyema resulting from *Streptococcus Pneumoniae*. Preoperative roentgenogram (A) and axial CT-scan (B). Multi-planar CT reconstruction allows a precise identification of fluid collections and shows their relationships with the underlying left diaphragmatic dome (C). Satisfactory postoperative result on postoperative day 2 (D).

In the event of loculated ET, ultrasonography can be useful to demark the limits of the pleural collection thus guiding the subsequent intraoperative trocar insertion.

Fiberoptic bronchoscopy should be performed in all instances, in order to rule out the presence of an unsuspected bronchial obstruction, foreign bodies or fluid outflow from the airways, which might cause inundation of the dependent lung in a lateral position.

Anesthesia technique. A thoracic epidural catheter is inserted at T4 level and continuous infusion of ropivacaine 0.5% plus sufentanil 1.66 µg/mL is started about 20 minutes prior to the operation at a rate of 5 mL/h. Meanwhile, the patient is placed in lateral decubitus with the hemithorax targeted for surgery in the dependent position, in order to attain optimal gravity distribution of the anesthetic drugs. Both warm-cold discrimination and pin-prick test are used to assess the effectiveness of anesthesia. If necessary, additional local injection of ropivacaine 0.5 % plus lidocaine 2 % is used to reinforce analgesia at the incision sites. In patients with unfavourable anatomy for epidural catheter, we prefer paravertebral blocks. During the operation, oxygen is delivered through a Venturi mask to keep arterial oxygen saturation above 90%. Creation of the surgical pneumothorax is usually well tolerated, although shortness of breath can sometimes be induced by an increased inspiratory load. The surgeon should always reassure the patient that this event has no adverse effects on main vital parameters and oxygenation, even though in anxious subjects a panic attack can sometimes develop. In these instances, light sedation with intravenous midazolam or propofol at subhypnotic dosage can be administered, without jeopardizing the patient's cooperation which is crucial to obtain re-expansion of the lung at the end of the procedure.

At the end of the operation, the patient is monitored in the recovery room and transferred to the ward as soon as possible. Intravenous fluids are then withdrawn and oral intake is allowed. In addition, the patient is immediately mobilized and ambulation permitted. Anticoagulant prophylaxis with low-molecular weight heparins is usually not administered due to the hypothetical risk of epidural hematoma.

The epidural catheter is removed after 24h and analgesia is switched to intravenous opioids. Unless pain control is suboptimal, non-steroidal anti-inflammatory drugs are avoided since they are thought to delay granulation of the pleural layers thus theoretically affecting air-leak duration.

Awake video-thoracoscopic decortication. Patients are placed in full lateral decubitus position with slight trunk elevation and forward rotation of the operating bed. A small antidecubitus mattress is placed below the dependent hemithorax to split the intercostal spaces. The operative field is prepped and draped to facilitate direct dialogue between the surgeon and the patient throughout the operation.

Three thoracoports are used. The camera trocar is placed at the level of 7th or 8th intercostals space, on the midaxillary line. Careful use of electrocautery and the fingertips can aid entering the pleural cavity in the presence of thickened parietal pleura. The surgeon should inform the patient that perception of pushing is normal and will not elicit pain. Once a 15-mm flexible trocar has been inserted, abundant spilling of fluid can occur if the purulent collection is watery and under pressure. The purulent fluid is then completely evacuated by mild aspiration, paying attention not to trigger coughing or discomfort to the patient.

A 30°-angled camera is then inserted, and careful inspection of the purulent cavity is accomplished. Adhesions lying in strict proximity with the cavity are frequently filmy and poorly vascularised due to inhibition of desmoplastic reaction, while they become thicker and fleshy more distantly [3]. Blunt debridment with an endoscopic swab and/or ring-shaped forceps is then started and fibrin coats are removed. Once the operative space has been widened (Fig. **4**), a second trocar is inserted 1-2 cm behind the posterior axillary line, in the 6th intercostal space. This position allows optimal adhesiolysis along the vertebral gutter that proves mandatory to ensure complete lung re-expansion. The third trocar is usually placed in the 4th intercostal space, on the anterior axillary line. Inserting the camera through the anterior access allows visualization of the costodiaphragmatic sinus. To this regard, it should be kept in mind that adhesions between the lower lobes and the diaphragm are usually more developed at the peripheral portion of the muscle, while they are filmy or absent at the level of the tendinous core.

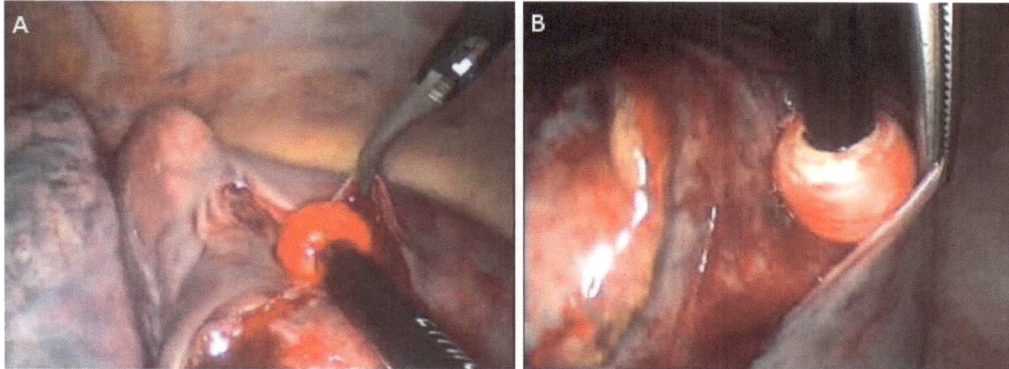

Fig. 4. Awake video-assisted pleural decortication. The thickened visceral pleura is dissected free at the level of the apical segment of left lower lobe (A) and the posterior-basal segment (B). Note the wide operative field, not dissimilar to that of an equivalent procedure performed under one-lung ventilation (**Video 1**).

Once the lung is mobilized, pleural decortication is begun by incising the thickened visceral pleura with electrocautery and progressively dissecting it free by using both cotton swabs and scissors (Fig. **4**). The quality of lung expansion is progressively tested during the ongoing procedure by asking the patient to inhale deeply and cough repeatedly.

Once pleural decortication is completed, the pleural cavity is irrigated with 1% solution of hydrogen-peroxide and then generously washed with saline, which also makes it possible to check the presence of air-leaks. At the end of the operation, one or two chest drainages are positioned, lung re-expansion is monitored under thoracoscopic vision and surgical wounds are sutured.

Single-trocar pleural debridement. Under favourable circumstances, debridement of the empyematous cavity can be accomplished by means of a single 20-mm trocar with a 30° angled camera and endoscopic instrumentation inserted coaxially. This approach is more likely when dealing with very early ET stages in which pleural adhesions and septa are usually scant and fibrous, so that they can be easily freed by blunt dissection alone. This situation can also occur in patients with jeopardized desmoplastic capacity because of age, malnutrition or concurrent steroid therapy (Fig. **5**).

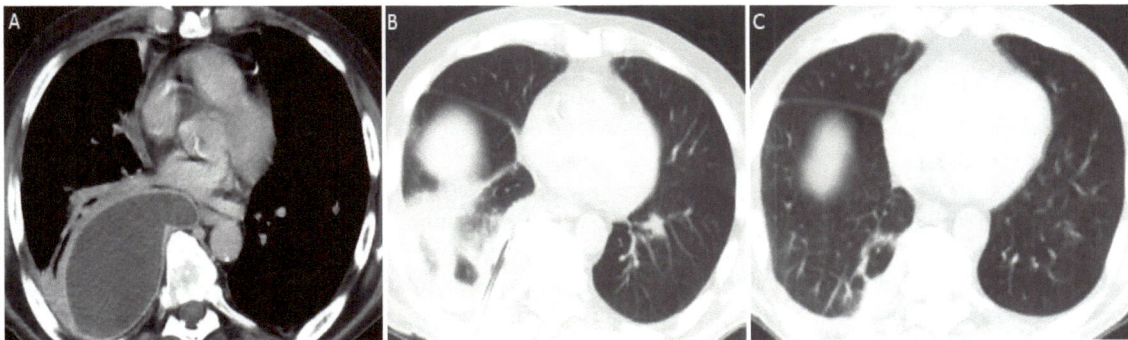

Fig. 5. Loculated empyema thoracis (A) resulting from *Acynetobacter* in a 72 years old patient with severe malnutrition. Awake videothoracoscopic debridemt trough a single-trocar approach resulted in complete drainage of the purulent collection (B). Irrigations with iodopovidone for 15 days. Complete resolution at 3 months follow-up (C).

Awake open decortication. Conversion to thoracotomy may be required whenever thick pleural adhesions prove unmanageable videothoracoscopically (Fig. **6**). In these instances, our preferred option is to employ a limited lateral, muscle-sparing, thoracotomy which can be performed without switching to general anesthesia and is usually well tolerated by the majority of patients. In selected instances, an even more limited thoracic incision, just sufficient to insert one hand inside the chest to allow manual palpation of intrathoracic structures, can be preferred while maintaining video-assistance.

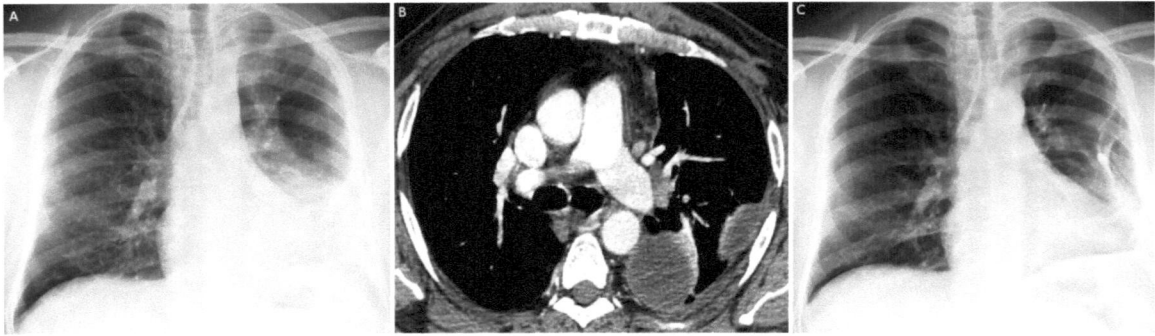

Fig. 6. Chest roentgenogram of a patient with chronic empyema resulting from *Mycobacterium Avium* infection (A). CT-scan (B) reveals white depositions on the thickened visceral pleura suggestive for calcifications. Awake pleural decortication was performed through muscle-sparing thoracotomy. Unfilled, residual pleural space resulting from persistent air-leaks is revealed at postoperative roentgenogram (C).

Thoracotomy in awake patients is not new. In 1950s, Buckingham and Crawford reported on more than 600 patients undergoing major thoracic operations, including anatomical lung resection as well as thoracoplasty for ET, performed with just thoracic epidural anesthesia and sedation [69, 70]. Impressively, for that time, the authors did state that inhaled anesthesia was performed only in a limited number of patients and mainly for experimental purposes. Other reports on this topic come from Djohar in the mid 1970s [71], and, more recently, from Al-Abdullatief and co-workers [72].

Postoperative management. Once the patient has been transferred to the ward, intravenous fluid administration is stopped and oral intake is immediately allowed. Chest drainage/s are positioned on -20/-25 cmH$_2$0 suction. The epidural catheter is left in place for 24h. Subsequently, the analgesia protocol entails continuous intravenous infusion of tramadole (200 to 300 mg/daily) *via* an elastomeric device. On postoperative morning 1 an intensive respiratory rehabilitation program is started and a chest roentgenogram is obtained. Removal of chest drains is carried out when the lung appears completely re-expanded on the chest roentgenogram, fluid loss is less than 200 mL/24 hours and pleural culture-gram stains are negative.

Complications. Some patients may experience transient intraoperative hypercarbia which is usually not associated with hypoxia. Hypoventilation and a rebreathing effect resulting from a sort of pendular ventilation induced by the pressure gradient existing between the pleural cavities are thought to be at the basis of this finding. Nonetheless, symptomatic hypercarbia is extremely rare and arterial PaCO$_2$ level usually returns towards normal values within 1-2 hours after the operation. Other minor complications are mostly related to epidural anesthesia and may include urinary retention requiring catheterization and transient hypotension.

Finally, it should be also kept in mind that epidural catheterization may potentially result in spreading of infection to the neural axis leading to epidural abscess as well as to the development of epidural hematoma. Fortunately, these severe complications are reported to occur in exceedingly rare instances and never occurred in our experience. Since long catheterization time has been hypothesized to facilitate the occurrence of these complications [73] we prefer early removal of the epidural catheter. Nonetheless, whenever the development of an epidural abscess is suspected by onset of lower-limb paresthesia, magnetic resonance imaging should be expeditiously carried out, since any delay may result in permanent invalidity.

COMMENT

The use of local/regional anesthesia for minimally invasive surgical management of ET is not a new. In 1987, Rusch and Mountain reported on a single-port thoracoscopic approach performed under just intercostals block and sedation in patients with loculated empyemas [31], while the employ of awake multiportal VATS has been first described by Smit and coworkers in 1998 [32]. More recently, Katlic and coworkers [33] reported on 74 patients with ET treated by VATS debridement under local anesthesia and deep sedation, although none of them received pleural decortication.

In 2010, our group reported on results of VATS decortication performed through thoracic epidural anesthesia alone in fully awake patients with fibrinopurulent ET [29]. In our experience, this procedure has proved safe and feasible, and resulted in a success rate of up to 95 %. This compares favorably with what is reported in selected literature for equivalent procedures performed under general anesthesia (Table **1**).

Technical feasibility proved satisfactory in most instances. We believe that this is due to some particular features of ET patients. In fact, the limited respiratory motion of the trapped lung results in optimal visualization, an adequate surgical field (Fig. **2**, Video **1**), and ergonomic dissection of the thickened visceral pleural plane (Fig. **3**). In addition, in patients with ET, opening of the pleural cavity and drainage of the fluid collections may immediately results in improved ventilation due to the reduced pressure exerted against both lungs, thus explaining the optimal patients' tolerance. It is worth noting that although in 21% of patients we converted the operation to a thoracotomy approach, this was easily accomplished without switching to general anesthesia.

As far as comparison of VATS versus nonsurgical management is concerned, in their revision of a prospective database entailing 104 patients with ET of different stages, Wozniak and coworkers [74] reported a failure rate of 19% in patients receiving VATS as opposed to 63% after just drainage placement, which was also associated with an increased mortality. Again, Wait and coworkers [75] reported a 91 % success rate and reduced hospital charges for VATS decortication in comparison to sole drainage positioning, followed by fibrinolytic instillation. Similar observation also come from Balci [76] and Lim [77], who reported a lower hospital stay in patients treated by early surgery versus those receiving conservative management.

CONCLUSION

On the basis of these observations, we believe that, apart from simple pleural effusions which can resolve definitively with conservative management, VATS should be considered as the standard of care in complex parapneumonic effusion and ET. All the pros of VATS in this setting are not jeopardized by performing the operation in spontaneously ventilating awake patients, including the possibility of conversion to open approach.

In summary, we believe that awake VATS should now be considered as a reliable option for management of complex parapneumonic effusions and ET. This novel surgical approach can prove particularly effective in early stages when definitive resolution of symptoms and complete reexpansion of the lung may be attained at the price of an acceptable surgical trauma.

REFERENCES

[1]   Kergin FG. The treatment of chronic pleural empyema. Ann R Coll Surg Engl 1995;17:271-90.

[2]   Keyes A. Remarks on the etiology, indications for treatment, behavior, and post-operative course of empyema thoracis. Ann Surg 1919;69:501-9.

[3]   Graham E. Principles involved in the treatment of acute and chronic empyema. Surg Gynecol Obstet 1924;38:466-70.

[4]   Mueller CB. Treatment of empyema. J Am Coll Surg 2005;201:158-9.

[5]   Light RW. Parapneumonic effusion and empyema. Proc Am Thorac Soc 2006;3:75-80.

[6]   Hamm H, Light RW. Parapneumonic effusion and empyema. Eur Respir J 1997;10:1150-6.

[7]   Ridley PD, Braimbridge MV. Thoracoscopic debridement and pleural irrigation in the management of empyema thoracis. Ann Thorac Surg 1991;51:461-4.

[8]   Striffeler H, Ris HB, Wursten HU, *et al.* Video-assisted thoracoscopic treatment of pleural empyema. A new therapeutic approach. Eur J Cardiothorac Surg 1994;8:585-8.

[9]   O'Brien J, Cohen M, Solit R, *et al.* Thoracoscopic drainage and decortication as definitive treatment for empyema thoracis following penetrating chest injury. J Trauma 1994;36:536-9.

[10]   Sendt W, Forster E, Hau T. Early thoracoscopic debridement and drainage as definitive treatment for pleural empyema. Eur J Surg 1995;161:73-6.

[11]   Landrenau RJ, Keenan RJ, Hazelrigg SR, Mack MJ, Naunheim KS. Thoracoscopy for empyema and hemothorax. Chest 1996;109:18-24.

[12]   Angelillo Mackinlay TA, Lyons GA, *et al.* VATS debridement versus thoracotomy in the treatment of loculated postpneumonia empyema. Ann Thorac Surg 1996;61:1626-30.

[13]   Wait MA, Sharma S, Hohn J, Dal Nogare A. A randomized trial of empyema therapy. Chest 1997;111:1548-51.

[14]   Striffeler H, Gugger M, Im Hof IV, *et al.* Video-assisted thoracoscopic surgery for fibrinopurulent pleural empyema in 67 patients. Ann Thorac Surg 1998;65:319-23.

[15]   Scherer LA, Battistella FD, Owings JT, Aguilar NM. Video-assisted thoracic surgery in the treatment of posttraumatic empyema. Arch Surg 1998;133:637-41.

[16]   Lackner RP, Hughes R, Anderson LA, Sammut PH, Thompson AB. Video-assisted evacuation of empyema is the preferred procedure for management of pleural space infections. Am J Surg 2000;179:27-30.

[17]   Waller DA, Rengarajan A. Thoracoscopic decortication: a role for video-assisted surgery in chronic postpneumonic pleural empyema. Ann Thorac Surg 2001;71:1813-6.

[18]   Cheng YJ, Wu HH, Chou SH, Kao EL. Video-assisted thoracoscopic surgery in the treatment of chronic empyema thoracis. Surg Today 2002;31:19-25.

[19]   Bouros D, Antoniou KM, Chalkiadakis G, *et al.* The role of video-assisted thoracoscopic surgery in the treatment of parapneumonic empyema after failure of fibrinolytics. Surg Endosc 2002;16:151-4.

[20]   Petrakis I, Kogerakis NE, Drositis IE, *et al.* Video-assisted thoracoscopic surgery for thoracic empyema: primarily, or after fibrinolytics therapy failure? Am J Surg 2004;187:471-4.

[21]   Wurnig PN, Wittmer V, Pridun NS, Hollaus PH. Video-assisted thoracic surgery for pleural empyema. Ann Thorac Surg 2006;81:309-13.

[22]   Tajiri M, Osawa H. Video-assisted thoracoscopic debridement for acute empyema; a low invasive surgery for acute empyema. Kyobu Geka 2006;59:S730-5.

[23]   Solaini L, Prusciano F, Bagioni P. Video-assisted thoracic surgery in the treatment of pleural empyema. Surg Endosc 2007;21:280-4.

[24]   Drain AJ, Ferguson JI, Sayeed R, *et al.* Definitive management of advanced empyema by two-windows video-assisted surgery. Asian Cardiovasc Thorac Ann 2007;15:238-9.

[25]   Chan DT, Sihoe AD, Chan S, *et al.* Surgical treatment for empyema thoracis: is video-assisted thoracic surgery "better" than thoracotomy? Ann Thorac Surg 2007;84:225-31.

[26]   Cardillo G, Carleo F, Carbone L, *et al.* Chronic postpneumonic pleural empyema: comparative merits of thoracoscopic versus open decortication. Eur J Cardiothorac Surg 2009;36:914-8.

[27]   Shahin Y, Duffy J, Beggs D, Black E, Majewski A. Surgical management of primary empyema of the pleural cavity: outcome of 81 patients. Interact Cardiovasc Thorac Surg 2010;10:565-7.

[28]   Tong BC, Hanna J, Toloza EM, *et al.* Outcomes of video-assisted thoracoscopic decortication. Ann Thorac Surg 2010;89:220-5.

[29]   Tacconi F, Pompeo E, Fabbi E, Mineo TC. Awake video-assisted pleural decortication for empyema thoracis. Eur J Cardiothorac Surg 2010;37:594-601.

[30]   Solér M, Wyser C, Bollinger CT, Perruchoud AP. Treatment of early parapneumonic empyema by "medical" thoracoscopy. Schweiz Med Wochenschr 1997;127:1748-54.

[31]   Rusch VW, Mountain C. Thoracoscopy under regional anesthesia for the diagnosis and management of pleural diseases. Am J Surg 1987;154:247-8.

[32]   Smit HJ, Schramel FM, Sutdeja TG, *et al.* Video-assisted thoracoscopy is feasible under local anesthesia. Diagn Ther Endosc 1998;4:177-178.

[33]   Katlic MR, Facktor M. Video-assisted thoracic surgery utilizing local anesthesia and sedation.: 384 consecutive cases. Ann Thorac Surg 2010;90:240-5.

[34]   Limsukon A, Soo Hoo GW. Parapneumonic Pleural Effusions and Empyema Thoracis. eMedicine Specialties. 2009 Sept 17. Available from http://emedicine.medscape.com/article/298485-overview.

[35]   Koegelember CF, Diaconi AH, Bolligeri CT. Parapneumonic pleural effusion and empyema. Respiration 2008;75:241-50.

[36]   Strange C, Sahn SA. The definitions and epidemiology of pleural space infections. Semin Respir Infect 1999;14:3-8.

[37]   Finley C, Clifton J, FitzGerald JM, Yee J. Empyema: an increasing concern in Canada. Can Resp J 2008;15:85-9.

[38] Bender JM, Ampofo K, Sheng X, *et al*. Parapneumonic empyema deaths during past century, Utah. Emerg Infect Dis 2009;15:44-8.

[39] Hendrickson DJ, Blumberg DA, Joad JP, *et al*. Five-fold increase in pediatric parapneumonic empyema since introduction of pnemococcal conjugate vaccine. Pediatr Infect Dis J 2008;27:1030-2.

[40] Porta G, Rodriguez-Carballeira M, Gomez L, *et al*. Thoracic infection caused by Streptocuccus Milleri. Eur Respir J 1998;12:357-62.

[41] Stelzmueller I, Biebl M, Berger N, *et al*. Relevance of group Milleri streptococci in thoracic surgery: a clinical update. Am Surg 2007;73:492-7.

[42] Kobashi Y, Mouri K, Yagi S, *et al*. Clinical analysis of cases of empyema due to Streptococcus milleri group. Jpn J Infect Dis 2008;61:484-6.

[43] Ahmed RA, Marrie TJ, Huang JQ. Thoracic empyema in patients with community-acquired pneumonia. Am J Med 2006;119:877-83.

[44] Divisi D, Imbriglio G, Crisci R. Videothoracoscopy in pleural empyema following methicillin-resistant Staphylococcus aureus (MRSA) lung infection. ScientificWorldJournal 2009;9:723-8.

[45] Liang SJ, Chen W, Lin YC, *et al*. Community-acquired thoracic empyema in young adults. South Med J 2007;100:1075-80.

[46] Civen R, Jousimies-Somer H, Marina M, *et al*. A retrospective review of anaerobic empyema and update of bacteriology. Clin Infect Dis 1995 20;S224-9.

[47] Ko SC, Chen KY, Hsueh PR, et al. Fungal empyema thoracis: an emerging clinical entity. Chest 2000;117:1672-8.

[48] Strong DH, Wescott JY, Biller JA, *et al*. Eosinophilic "empyema" associated with crack cocaine use. Thorax 2003;58:823-4.

[49] Colice GL, Curtis A, Deslauriers J, *et al*. Medical and surgical treatment of parapneumonic effusions: an evidence-based guideline. Chest 2000;118:1158-71.

[50] Manuel Porcel J, Vives M, Esquerda A, Ruiz A. Usefulness of the British Thoracic Society and the American College of Chest Physiscians guidelines in predicting pleural drainage of non-purulent parapneumonic effusions. Respir Med 2006;100:933-7.

[51] Light RW. A new classification of parapneumonic effusions and empyema. Chest 1995;108:2.

[52] Tsang KY, Leung WS, Chang VL, Lin AW, Chu CM. Complicated parapneumonic effusion and empyema thoracis: microbiology and predictors of adverse outcomes. Hong Kong Med J 2007;13:178-86.

[53] Tchervaniakov P, Svennevik E, Tzafetta K, Milton R. Necrotizing fasciitis following drainage of Streptococcus milleri empyema. Interact Cardiovasc Thorac Surg 2010;10:481-2.

[54] Hoehn KS, Capouya JD, Daum RS, *et al*. Lemierre-like syndrome caused by community-associated methicillin-resistant Staphylococcus aureus complicated by hemorrhagic pericarditis. Pediatr Crit Care Med 2010;11:e32-5.

[55] Westphal FL, De Lima LC, Menezes AQ, Sacramento e Silva DL. Claude Bernard-Horner syndrome resulting from pleural empyema. J Bras Pneumol 2006;32:176-9.

[56] Graham EA, Berck M. Principles versus details in the treatment of acute empyema. Ann Surg 1933;98:520-7.

[57] Graham EA, Bell R.D. Open pneumothorax: its relation to the treatment of empyema. Am J Med Sc 1918;46:839.

[58] Keyes EL. Bilateral empyema of the pleural cavities. Ann Surg 1931;93:1050-63.

[59] Tuffier T. The treatment of chronic empyema. Ann Surg 1920;72:266-87.

[60] Mayo CH, Beckman EH. Visceral pleurectomy for chronic empyema. Ann Surg 1914;59:884-90.

[61] Gaensler EA. The surgery for pulmonary tuberculosis. Am Rev Respir Dis 1982;125:73-84.

[62] Hoksch B, Birken-Bretsch H, Muller JM. Thoracoscopy before Jacobaeus. Ann Thorac Surg 2002;74:1288-90.

[63] Harzinger M, Hacker A, Langbein S, *et al*. Hans-Christian Jacobaeus (1879-1937): the inventor of human laparoscopy and thoracoscopy. Urologe 2006;45:1184-6.

[64] Suchar AM, Zureikat AH, Glynn L, *et al*. Ready for the frontline: is early thoracoscopic decortications the new standard of care for advanced pneumonia with empyema? Ann Surg 2006;72:688-92.

[65] Dhanireddy S, Altemeire WA, Matute-Bello G, *et al*. Mechanical ventilation induced inflammation, lung injury, and extra-pulmonary organ dysfunction in experimental pneumonia. Lab Invest 2006;86:790-799.

[66] Gothard J. Lung injury after thoracic surgery and one-lung ventilation. Curr Opin Anaesthesiol 2006;19:5-10.

[67] Vanni G, Tacconi F, Sellitri F, *et al*. Impact of awake videothoracoscopic surgery on postoperative lymphocyte responses. Ann Thorac Surg 2010;90:973-8.

[68] Tacconi F, Pompeo E, Sellitri F, Mineo TC. Surgical stress hormones response is reduced after awake videothoracoscopy. Interact Cardiovasc Thorac Surg 2010;10:666-71.

[69]   Crawford OB, Buckingham WW, Ottosen P, Brasher CA. Peridural anesthesia in thoracic surgery: a review of 677 cases. Anesthesiology 1951;12:73-84.

[70]   Buckingham WW, Beatty AJ, Brasher CA, Ottosen P. An analysis of 607 surgical procedures done under epidural anesthesia. Mo Med 1950;47:485.

[71]   Djohar A. Thoracotomy under local anaesthesia: personal experiences in 215 cases. Arch Chir Neerl 1976;28:233-41.

[72]   Al-Abdullatief M, Wahood A, Al-Shirawi N, *et al.* Awake anaesthesia for major thoracic surgical procedures: an observational study. Eur J Cardiothorac Surg 2007;346-50.

[73]   Wang LP, Hauerberg J, Schmidt JF. Incidence of spinal epidural abscess after epidural analgesia. A national 1-year survey. Anesthesiology 1999;91:1928-36.

[74]   Wozniak CJ, Paull DE, Moezzi JE, *et al.* Choice of first intervention is related to outcomes in the management of empyema. Ann Thorac Surg 2009;87:1525-30.

[75]   Wait MA, Sharma S, Hohn J, Dal Nogare, A. A randomized trial of empyema therapy. Chest 1997;111:1548-51.

[76]   Balci AE, Eren S, Ulku R, Eren MN. Management of multiloculated empyema thoracis in children: thoracotomy versus fibrinolytic treatment. Eur J Cardiothorac Surg 2002;22:595-8.

[77]   Lim TK, Chin NK. Empirical treatment with fibrinolysis and early surgery reduces the duration of hospitalization in pleural sepsis. Eur Respir J 1999;13:514-8.

CHAPTER 12

Awake Thymectomy

Isao Matsumoto, Makoto Oda and Go Watanabe[*]

Department of General and Cardiothoracic Surgery, Kanazawa University, Kanazawa, Japan

Abstract: Recently, several major thoracic procedures performed in awake patients have been reported. In order to reduce the adverse effects of general anesthesia and the cost, Thoracic Epidural Anesthesia (TEA) has been employed to perform such awake thoracic surgery procedures. Awake procedure under TEA can be performed even in endoscopic thymectomy. The postoperative recovery is fast, and surgery can be performed on patients in whom general anesthesia is difficult. Herein we discuss awake thymectomy procedure and perioperative management for patients and describe the techniques in detail.

Keywords: Awake thymectomy, thoracic epidural anesthesia, endoscopic surgery, robotic surgery, intraoperative pneumothorax.

INTRODUCTION

With recent advances in surgical and anesthesia techniques, surgery has become safer to perform, and the indications for surgery have expanded. The next steps needed are an expansion of surgical indications in cases where anesthesia management is difficult, and a reduction in complications. In addition, the need has arisen for healthcare professionals to meet patient and societal needs, aiming at faster rehabilitation and shorter hospital stays. Among these trends, surgery during which patients remain awake is increasing. The significance of patients remaining awake during surgery is that consciousness can be a useful monitor. A typical example in neurosurgery is an awake craniotomy [1]. When lesions are resected near speech areas, a decision on the extent of resection can be made while the patient speaks, thus being able to reliably preserve speech function. In the surgeries listed in Table **1**, by having patients remain awake during surgery, voluntary movements can be used to evaluate surgical results and reduce complications.

Table 1. General indications to awake surgery.

When consciousness needs to be monitored
Awake craniotomy in neurosurgery.
Awake tests in orthopedic surgery.
Incontinence tests in urologic surgery.
Early detection of water intoxication in urologic surgery.
Surgeries where evaluation of voluntary movement is important.
Cases in which general anesthesia should be avoided
Poor respiratory function when mechanical ventilation should be avoided.
Decreased cerebral blood flow.
Cardiovascular problems when general anesthesia is deemed to be a risk.

Meanwhile, for other reasons, there are times when general anesthesia should be avoided. In general anesthesia, because anesthetics are used systemically with mechanical ventilation, patients are in a nonphysiologic respiratory state. With mechanical ventilation, when intrathoracic pressure becomes positive, patients with emphysema are at risk for pneumothorax, and cardiac output and cerebral blood flow may decrease. Thus, there are patients in whom mechanical ventilation should ideally be avoided. Because

*Address correspondence to Go Watanabe: Department of General and Cardiothoracic Surgery, Kanazawa University, Kanazawa, Japan. Email: watago6633@gmail.com

mechanical ventilation may also be a risk factor for acute renal failure, it should also be avoided in patients with decreased renal function before dialysis has been started [2]. In some surgeries such as peripheral arterial surgery of the lower extremities, surgery under local anesthesia, compared to general anesthesia, has been reportedly associated with earlier hospital discharge, reduced complications, and higher bypass patency rates [3].

Recently, several major thoracic procedures performed in awake patients have been reported [4-6]. In order to reduce the adverse effects of general anesthesia and the cost, Thoracic Epidural Anesthesia (TEA) has been employed to perform such awake thoracic surgery procedures. For example, we demonstrated that TEA reduces incidence of postoperative atrial fibrillation in awake on-pump coronary artery bypass grafting (AOCAB) due to its inhibition of sympathetic activity without inhibiting vagal activity which has antiarrythmic effects [7]. The postoperative recovery is fast, and surgery can be performed on patients in whom general anesthesia is difficult.

AWAKE OPEN THYMECTOMY FOR MYASTHENIA GRAVIS

Myasthenia Gravis (MG) is a chronic autoimmune disease with antibodies directed against the acetylcholine receptor at the neuromuscular junction and characterized by progressive weakness and easy fatigability of voluntary skeletal muscles. Current treatment is based on enhancing neuromuscular transmission, suppression of the immune system, decreasing the levels of circulating antibodies, and thymectomy [8, 9]. Thymectomy is generally accepted as the standard treatment for MG patients, although there are no prospective randomized trials to support this.

There are many surgical thymectomy techniques for patients with MG: standard transsternal thymectomy, combined cervical exploration and transsternal thymectomy, transcervical thymectomy, video-thoracoscopic thymectomy including those performed by lifting the sternum [10-12], and endoscopic robotic thymectomy [13]. The most important surgical point when dealing with MG patients is whether complete extended thymectomy can be achieved by the particular procedure. Masaoka and colleagues [14] demonstrated that it is important to resect not only thymic tissue but also mediastinal fatty tissue because thymic tissue is present in both intracapsular thymic tissue and extracapsular mediastinal fatty tissue. Thus complete resection influences the remission rates and long-term outcomes [14].

When an extended thymectomy is performed for MG, the patient's postoperative respiratory insufficiency can always be a potential problem. Current general anesthesia requires volatile anesthetic agents and sometimes muscle relaxants for tracheal intubation and anesthetic maintenance. Anesthesia of patients with MG requires special attention, particularly to the use of muscle relaxants. Patients with MG are usually sensitive to the effects of nondepolarizing muscle relaxants, and volatile anesthetic agents accelerate those effects. Furthermore, the potential interaction of anticholinesterases (administered as therapeutic agents for MG) with both the depolarizing and nondepolarizing muscle relaxants is also a problem. In order to stabilize postoperative respiratory function in MG patients, pain control using epidural anesthesia has been reported to be useful [15,16]. Recently, intubation techniques using combined epidural and intravenous anesthesia, without muscle relaxants, have also been employed [17]. Although such innovative anesthesia procedures have been reported for patients with MG, almost all of them are intravenous or epidural techniques and after all use volatile agents and tracheal intubation [18,19]. The respiratory insufficiency introduced by such agents and the complications due to endotracheal tube placement can continue postoperatively and may require reintubation or prolonged intubation.

We believe that high TEA without tracheal intubation is a less invasive anesthesia procedure for MG patients, and it can be used when performing transsternal extended thymectomy, thereby avoiding general anesthesia and intubation. This procedure has raised our expectation of a rapid recovery and no postoperative respiratory muscle weakness due to muscle relaxants and volatile anesthetic agents. Moreover, it causes none of the laryngopharyngeal or laryngotracheal iatrogenic complications associated with general anesthesia because this method does not require tracheal intubation and extubation.

Since 2003, we have performed AOCAB [20]. We have also developed several innovative techniques for AOCAB such as awake subxyphoid minimally invasive direct coronary artery bypass grafting [21]. These techniques have been introduced in surgery for patients with MG. By performing awake thymectomy, the invasiveness of intubation and mechanical ventilation, and the use of muscle relaxants can be avoided. The procedures of awake thymectomy have been reported in our previous report [22] and the details of the techniques are described herein. We were given advice by Dr. Tsunehisa Tsubokawa (Department of Anesthesiology, Kanazawa University) regarding the techniques for TEA. These techniques can also be applied to anterior mediastinal non-invasive tumors.

Indications. Candidates for awake thymectomy are nonthymomatous MG patients with Osserman I and II and Myasthenia Gravis Foundation of America (MGFA) class I, II, and some III diseases. In addition patients with non-invasive thymoma of less than 3 cm in size are also well suited for the operation. Criteria for exclusion include a thymoma that is in contact with the lung (especially the left lung) or is seen by computed tomography or magnetic resonant imaging to be invasive type. The operation is also contraindicated in patients whose thoracic respiration accounts for a large proportion of their voluntary respiration. Severe respiratory function strongly influenced by palsy of the intercostal muscles may make it impossible for the patient to breathe voluntarily.

Requirements for awake thymectomy include: (1) indication for epidural anesthesia; (2) scheduled completion of surgery within 3 hours; and (3) informed consent from the patient for awake thymectomy. In addition, awake thymectomy is strongly recommended in patients who are poor candidates for mechanical ventilation, including patients in whom using muscle relaxants would be expected to prolong respiratory muscle weakness, patients with cerebral hypoperfusion (*e.g.*, history of stroke, severe stenosis on carotid ultrasound), and patients with severe emphysema.

Conversely, awake thymectomy should not be performed: (1) if epidural anesthesia is contraindicated due to anticoagulant drugs or a bleeding diathesis; (2) when multiorgan resection is required due to advanced thymoma, or prolonged surgery is necessary; (3) in patients with excessive sputum; and (4) in patients not consenting to awake thymectomy.

Anesthesia by TEA. Premedication is usually avoided. An anticholinesterase is administered on the morning of surgery. Basic monitoring (blood pressure, electrocardiography, pulse oximetry, temperature) is used for patients undergoing the operation. The means for direct blood pressure measurements and gas monitoring in the radial artery are established. An epidural catheter is inserted through a Tuohy needle at the level of T1-2 on the day of surgery. To test the effect and proper placement and to achieve somatosensory and motor block at the T1-8 level, the catheter is directed cephalad and advanced 4 cm into the epidural space. Then 10 mL of an epidural anesthesia solution (50 ml of 2% lidocaine hydrochloride and 5 ml of fentanyl citrate 0.05 mg/mL) is administered as a bolus.

It is important to monitor for the development of Horner syndrome because it means that the anesthesia has reached the C6 level. Patients breathe only by diaphragmatic respiration after the anesthesia. If the anesthesia reaches the C4 level, diaphragmatic respiration may be inadequate, and the patient is not able to breathe voluntarily. The motor block level is estimated by an Epidural Scoring Scale for Arm Movements (ESSAM) [23]. Sensory response is determined with pinprick sensation and cold discrimination. In the operating room, continuous epidural infusion of the epidural anesthesia solution (lidocaine hydrochloride and fentanyl citrate) is started at a rate of 15 to 25 mL/hr. In order to avoid excessive cephalad spread of the drug, we do not use an intraoperative bolus dose of the drug for epidural administration. With continuous infusion, this excessive spread does not occur.

In general, when using epidural anesthesia in surgery, the incidence of epidural hematoma is 1/150,000 [24]. In addition, when administering heparin within 1 hour after puncture, compared to heparin administration after 1 hour, the risk of hematoma is increased at least 10 times, so caution is advised [25].

The effects of epidural anesthesia on hemodynamics during surgery are few, without significant changes in heart rate, blood pressure, cardiac output, or systemic vascular resistance [26]. Central venous pressure tends to gradually increase during surgery, but this is probably due to fluid administration. The reasons for such hemodynamic stability include stabilization of cardiac function by blockade of sympathetic cardiac branches, preservation of function of sympathetic nerves distributed in venous capacitance vessels in the lower half of the body, and the modulatory effects of epidural anesthesia [7].

Surgical procedure. The patient is positioned in the supine position, and a pillow is secured under the shoulders. First- or second—generation antibiotic is administered intravenously prior to operation. A median sternotomy is performed. If it is not enough to block an edge level sensation completely, the patient is given an additional dose of local anesthetics at the xiphoid process or at the level of the jugular notch.

Standard extended thymectomy, including the thymus and the surrounding mediastinal fatty tissue en bloc, is performed. The area from bilateral cardiophrenic angles near the diaphragm inferiorly to the innominate vein (including pretracheal fatty tissue superiorly) and laterally to the phrenic nerve is dissected. The thymus and the fatty tissue are carefully separated from the mediastinal pleura. If the fatty tissue is strongly adherent to the pleura, both tissues are resected and the pleura sutured. When mediastinal fatty tissue is connected to the intrapleural fatty tissue beyond the pleura, both fatty tissues are resected together with the mediastinal pleura. After downward traction on the inferiorly mobilized thymus and fat, we can see the bilateral thymus-thyroid ligaments and dissect them at the cervical site. The thymic veins are ligated or transected with an ultrasonically activated device or bipolar vessel sealing system.The phrenic nerves must be treated extra carefully to avoid any damage. A drainage tube is placed on the anterior mediastinum, and the sternum is closed as usual.

Intraoperative management. Throughout the operation patients breathe room air or naso-oral oxygen (2-3 l/min), and they can talk to a nearby nurse and anesthesiologist.

With an extended thymectomy the pleura can easily be injured when fatty tissue near a phrenic nerve is dissected. Therefore most pleural injury is incurred on the lower pole near the diaphragm. Commonly, the pleura of the right lower pole are easily injured, and unilateral pneumothorax occurs. In left-sided pneumothorax, the site of injury often cannot be identified. On electrocardiogram, a low QRS amplitude may be a sign that a pneumothorax has developed. In addition, when a pneumothorax occurs, diaphragmatic movement is greater, and the patient's breathing can become irregular.

However, there is usually no problem even if unilateral pneumothorax occurs. In our experiences [22], hemodynamics and the respiratory state are not severely changed by unilateral pleural injury alone. In contrast, bilateral pneumothorax causes low SaO_2 and PaO_2, thus positive-pressure ventilation is required. If necessary, positive-pressure ventilation with an Ambu bag or laryngeal mask can be performed under a sedative state. However, to be prepared for emergency, in all cases we must prepare tracheal tubes preoperatively.

When dealing with operations of non-myasthenic patients, if sedation is required, a 0.07 to 0.10 mg/kg dose of midazolam can be administered together with low-dose sevoflurane inhalation by maintaining the bispectral index at 70 to 80. Patients can respond when necessary, but have no memories of intraoperative events. Whether mild sedation for intraoperative restlessness or respiratory discomfort exacerbates the symptoms of MG and whether it undermines the advantages of awake thymectomy in MG patients requires further investigation in a larger number of cases.

Postoperative management. When surgery is completed, even if there are no abnormalities, for example, on blood gas analysis, patients may be restless. This may be due to local anesthetic toxicity. Postoperatively, a continuous infusion of 0.2% ropivacaine is continued for 48 hours, and then the catheter is removed. About 50% of epidural hematomas develop when epidural catheters are removed, so clotting function should be normal when the catheter is removed. After the operation, fentanyl citrate (0.01 mg/ml physiological saline), 0.02 mg/hr, is administrated through the epidural catheter for postoperative pain management for 6 hours to 2 days. Patients can walk, drink and eat on the day of surgery. Moreover, they can be discharged on postoperative day 1 to 3 without complications.

AWAKE ENDOSCOPIC THYMECTOMY

Awake procedure under TEA can be performed even in an endoscopic thymectomy [27]. In the management of anterior mediastinal mass lesions, the transsternal approach has been the standard surgical procedure. However, endoscopic approaches have been developed to avoid a sternotomy, provide a cosmetic advantage and reduce the pain [11, 28]. There are several endoscopic surgical approaches for anterior mediastinal lesions including the thoracoscopic approach, the transcervical approach, and the infrasternal approach [29]. The infrasternal approach allows the surgeon to view and treat the whole thymus without even requiring one-lung ventilation, and is less painful than a thoracoscopic procedure performed through the chest wall. As described in the previous section we have successfully performed extended thymectomies in awake patients with MG [22]. Originally, the use of the infrasternal approach for thymectomy procedures was developed to eliminate the need for one-lung ventilation. We have expanded the use of awake surgery under TEA in endoscopic thymectomy by using sternal lifting [27]. This procedure is less invasive than awake thymectomy with median sternotomy. It can provide a cosmetic advantage and reduce the pain compared with the sternotomic procedure while still allowing the patient to eat, drink, and walk on the day of surgery.

Thoracic epidural anesthesia. In the same manner as awake thymectomy with median sternotomy, premedication is avoided. Basic monitoring (blood pressure, electrocardiography, pulse oximetry, temperature, gas monitoring) is used. Except for minor differences, awake TEA is performed according to the method that we have described in the previous section [22]. Because it is not necessary to perform median sternotomy in endoscopic thymectomy *via* infrasternal approach, the area for anesthesia slightly differs. An epidural catheter is inserted at the level between T3 and T4 on the day of surgery. A mixture containing 1 % ropivacaine hydrochloride hydrate (20 mL), 2 % lidocaine hydrochloride (20 mL), and fentanyl citrate 0.05 mg/mL (5 mL) is prepared. Anesthesia is started at a dosage of 20 ml/hour, which is gradually reduced and maintained at 5 to 10 mL/hour, and the area from the levels between T1 and T12 is anesthetized. In this procedure, patients breathe only by diaphragmatic respiration throughout the operation. After the operation, fentanyl citrate (0.01 mg/mL physiological saline), 0.02 mg/h, is administered for 1 day through the epidural catheter for postoperative pain management. Throughout the operation patients breathe room air or naso-oral oxygen (2-3 L/min), and they can talk to a nearby nurse and anesthesiologist (Fig. **1**).

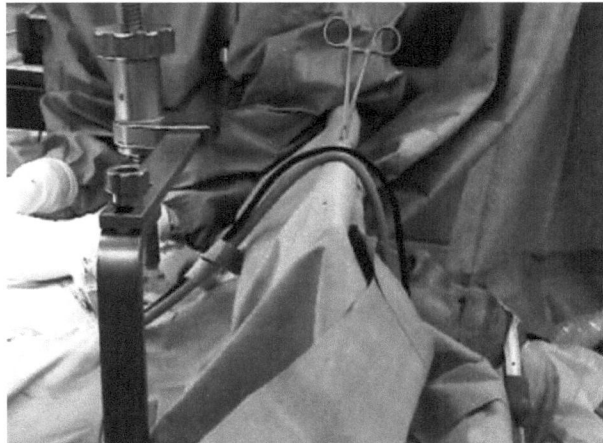

Fig. 1. The sternum is lifted and the operation is performed through an incision that is made just below the xiphoid process.

Surgical technique. After inducing awake TEA, the patient is treated in a supine position. An arc-shaped, 4-cm incision is made just below the xiphoid process as an access incision. After opening the retrosternal space, the sternum is lifted using a lifting device (VarioLift®, B. Braun Aesculap, Tuttlingen, Germany), and thymectomy is performed through this incision. As shown in Fig. **2**, first a lifting device is attached to the bed. The sternum can be lifted or lowered by winding or unwinding the adjuster. The sternum can be lifted by 3.0 - 4.0 cm, giving a wide operative field. Setting up the device is very easy and takes only a few minutes. A 30-degree angled telescope is inserted through a trocar placed below the surgical wound. The thymus is exposed, avoiding pleural damage, and the thymus including the tumor is dissected free from the pericardium using a grasping forceps and ultrasonically activated device or bipolar vessel sealing system (Fig. **3**). After the innominate vein is identified, the thymus is resected. The resected specimen is removed through the access incision. A drainage tube is placed in the anterior mediastinal space through a trocar wound. The surgical wound is shown in Fig. **4**.

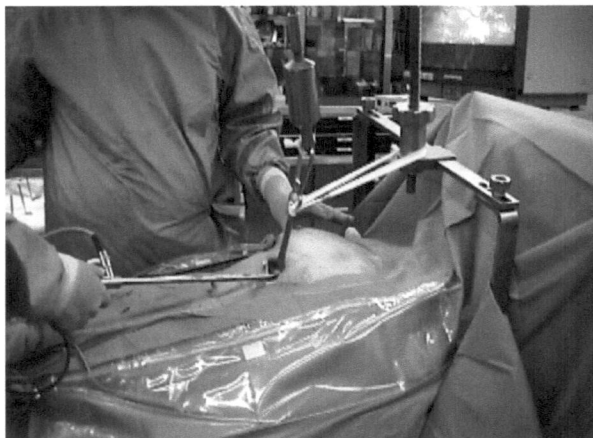

Fig. 2. The thymus is exposed after opening the retrosternal space.

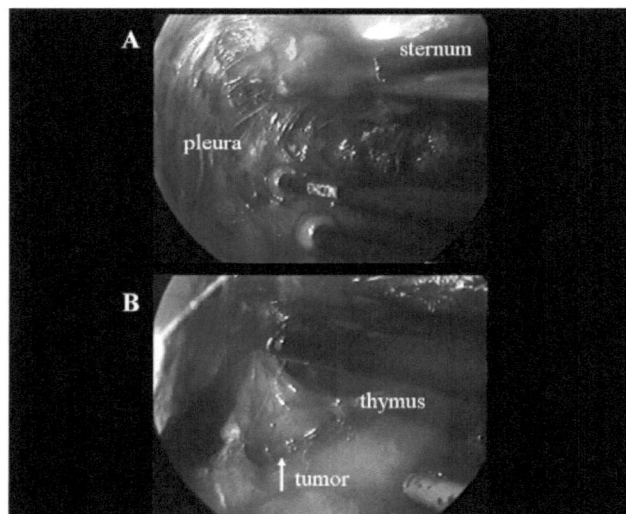

Fig. 3. A: The thymus is exposed after opening the retrosternal space. B: The thymus including the tumor is dissected.

Sternum lifting device. Wide exposure of the retrosternal space is still an issue in endoscopic thymectomy, especially when using an infrasternal approach. We employ a double-arm frame device to lift the anterior chest wall. Although the commonly used lifting devices with a single-arm frame [28, 29] are suitable for abdominal wall use, when applied to the sternum, their effect is minimal as they do not permit a sufficient view. Because the lifting arms of such systems are directly attached to the bed, they fail to support the lifted sternum and instead tilt sideways. In contrast, as the double-arm frame firmly supports the lifting arm, the sternum can be easily lifted, giving a wide operative field. Although the force of retraction by a device with a double-arm frame is very strong, the sternum suffers much less injury because the lifting height can be easily manipulated manually with the adjuster. Ten patients have undergone endoscopic thymectomy at our institution using the lifting device and none of the patients suffered sternal injuries.

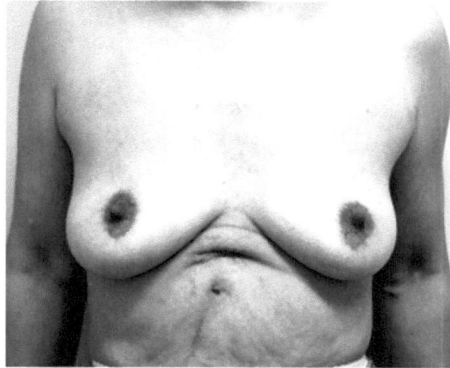

Fig. 4. Surgical wounds of the patient, showing satisfactory cosmesis.

AWAKE ROBOTIC ENDOSCOPIC THYMECTOMY

If this endoscopic procedure is performed robotically (*e.g.*, using the da Vinci surgical system), the existing lifting systems may interfere with placement of the robotic surgical arm units. So far, we have developed some innovative techniques and devices to lift the sternum for robotic endoscopic thymectomy under general anesthesia [30, 31]. In order to perform awake thymectomy, the procedure must be achieved through the infrasternal wound alone without manipulation through intercostal space. Therefore we have developed a new Automatic Sternal Lifting System (ASLS, Fig. **5**) recently. ASLS is assembled with a sternum-lifting hook, a lifting arm, and an actuator. The sternum-lifting hook and the lifting arm are movable and can be set to desired angle and length, and their positions can be adjusted to the sternum of the patient. ASLS is raised and lowered by means of a remote control, with a maximum stroke of 150 mm and a maximum load of 60 kg. The lifting and lowering speed can be set from 0 to 100 mm/s, and the lifting speed can be set to either a low-speed or high-speed mode. We set low-speed elevation to 3 mm/s, high-speed elevation to 10 mm/s, and lowering to 15 mm/s. As the actuator mechanically self-locks because it moves along a screw and nut construction, even if the power is cut, it will not drop.

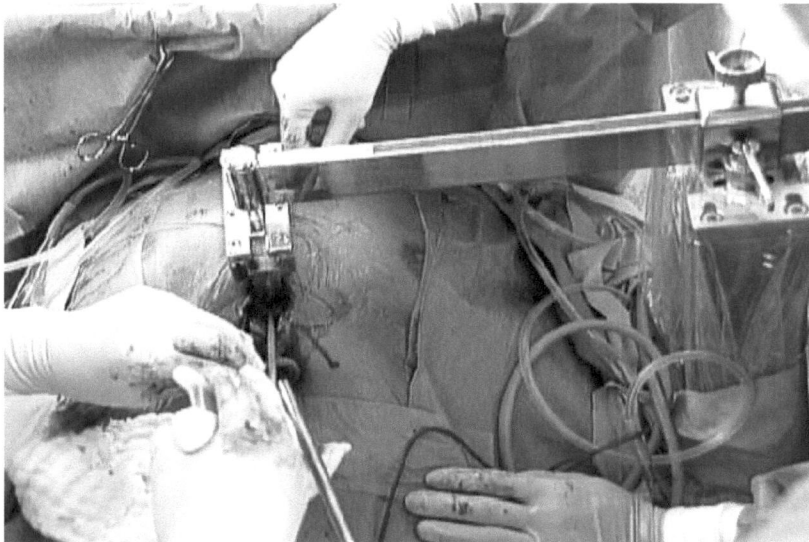

Fig. 5. A new automatic sternal lifting system.

ASLS is designed so it does not interfere with the operation of daVinci surgical system when set up together. In respect to thymectomy, when using ASLS, it is possible to perform thymectomy through the infrasternal wound alone without manipulation through intercostal space even for robotic surgery. We intend to apply ASLS for awake robotic endoscopic thymectomy after comfirming the safety of ASLS in an endoscopic thymectomy through the infrasternal approach under general anesthesia. ASLS can be also suitable for harvesting internal thoracic artery in coronary artery bypass grafting, making it possible to avoid median stertonomy.

Management for intraoperative pneumothorax during awake thymectomy. When performing awake thoracic surgery *via* sternum, pneumothorax caused by pleural damage is the biggest obstacle [32]. Pneumothorax prevents spontaneous breathing and causes respiratory distress. It has been hypothesized that an increase in carbon dioxide stimulates the medulla oblongata to induce the sensations associated with respiratory distress or that paradoxical thoracic movement and restricted lung dilatation stimulate the brainstem and motor area to cause the sensations associated with respiratory urgency. Subsequently, patients suffer and experience tachypnea. The thoracic movements associated with tachypnea further complicate the surgical procedures. Various surgical techniques have been reported for the treatment of such pneumothorax [20, 22, 32]. If the pleura was injured and opened, Karagoz and colleagues [32] and we [20, 22] have been dealing with pneumothorax by suturing the pleura and then performing drainage of the thoracic cavity or widely opening the chest. However, suturing is very difficult because the damaged pleura are both very thin and always moving due to respiration. When it is difficult to repair the pleural defect with sutures, wet gauze is temporarily placed on the defect to prevent air from entering the thoracic cavity by a suction instrument. These treatments of blocking or repairing the injured pleura and applying intrathoracic air suctioning usually prevent respiratory distress. If air enters the thoracic cavity through other pleural defects, a large wet towel is pressed against the pleural defect, and thoracic drainage is performed. There is a small possibility that dyspnea or low oxygen saturation develops, but if such symptoms do occur, they can be controlled by opening the mediastinal pleura and applying assisted positive Bag-valve-mask ventilation under light sedation with midazolam. According to Karagoz and colleagues, endotracheal intubation was required in 4 of 137 patients (2.9%) in AOCAB [32]. At our institution, respiratory assistance was needed due to pneumothorax in 15 of 43 patients and endotracheal intubation was required in 2 patients (4.7%) in AOCAB [20]. Therefore, it is necessary to develop other effective surgical method for treating pneumothorax, in order to safely perform awake thoracic surgery *via* the sternum, we have developed a novel technique to close the pleura [20]. We use a so-called rub-and-spray method using polyglycolic acid (PGA) nonwoven fabric and fibrin glue [33]. Some fibrinogen solution is rubbed on the edge of the pleural defect and then the PGA fabric is placed and the fibrinogen and thrombin solutions are sprayed (Fig. **6**). This pleural repair method achieves a strong closure with sufficient durability. In the field of thoracic surgery, fibrin glue proved useful to achieve hemostasis during surgery or prevent air leakage from the pulmonary parenchyma [34-36]. Pressure testing for air leakage confirmed that the strongest technique is the rub-and-spray method combining PGA fabric and fibrin glue [33]. With the rub-and-spray method, by rubbing fibrinogen into PGA fabric, fibrinogen deeply penetrates the fabric and then by spraying fibrinogen and thrombin solutions, polymerization within the framework of PGA fabric becomes strong and even. Microscopic experiments also confirmed that the rub-and-spray method achieves the deepest penetration of fibrin glue into the fabric and the surface is covered most evenly [33].

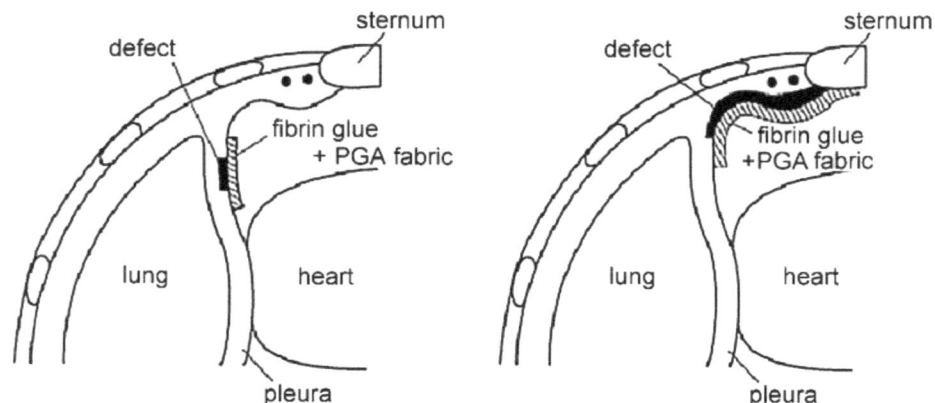

Fig. 6. We use a so-called rub-and-spray method using polyglycolic acid (PGA) nonwoven fabric and fibrin glue.

Our method is highly resistant to moisture, respiratory movements and chronological degradation in the short term. The PGA fabric and fibrin glue are very flexible and pliable and since suturing is not required, repair is safely achieved on the moving thin pleura regardless of the defect size in not only flat areas, but also rough uneven areas. During surgery, since the PGA fabric alone is permeable, it can be successfully applied regardless of airflow through the defect due to respiratory movements. PGA is bioabsorbable, but it can be easily removed at the end of surgery. In addition, this method may also be useful for visceral pleural repair.

The limitations of this technique are that, even after nanofiltering, the infection risk of fibrin glue cannot be completely eliminated [37] and that PGA fabric and fibrin glue are expensive. However our method can be potentially useful for performing other forms of awake thoracic surgery [5, 6, 22, 27, 32] or reconstruction of the thorax. We believe that this technique can be also useful in awake endoscopic thymectomy.

Further investigations are needed, however, to confirm the clinical efficacy of the present method.

CONCLUSION

Awake thymectomy is useful to reduce the adverse effects of general anesthesia and the cost for patients with MG or anterior mediastinal lesions. Awake procedure under TEA can be performed even in endoscopic or robotic thymectomy. The postoperative recovery is fast, and surgery can be performed on patients in whom general anesthesia is difficult. Currently, application of awake thymectomy is limited to low risk patients. Techniques must be developed further and established for wider applications of awake thymectomy.

REFERENCES

[1]   Conte V, Baratta P, Tomaselli P, *et al.* Awake neurosurgery: an update. Minerva Anestesiol 2008;74:289-92.

[2]   Kuiper JW, Groeneveld AB, Slutsky AS, Plötz FB. Mechanical ventilation and acute renal failure. Crit Care Med. 2005;33:1408-15.

[3]   Christopherson R, Beattie C, Frank SM, *et al.* Perioperative morbidity in patients randomized to epidural or general anesthesia for lower extremity vascular surgery. Perioperative Ischemia Randomized Anesthesia Trial Study Group. Anesthesiology 1993;79:422-34.

[4]   Pompeo E, Mineo TC. Awake operative videothoracoscopic pulmonary resections. Thorac Surg Clin 2008;18:311-20.

[5]   Mineo TC. Epidural anesthesia in awake thoracic surgery. Eur J Cardiothorac Surg 2007;32:13-9.

[6]   Al-Abdullatief M, Wahood A, Al-Shirawi N, *et al.* Awake anaesthesia for major thoracic surgical procedures: an observational study. Eur J Cardiothorac Surg 2007;32:346-50.

[7]   Yashiki N, Watanabe G, Tomita S, *et al.* Thoracic epidural anesthesia for coronary bypass surgery affects autonomic neural function and arrythmias. Innovations 2005;2:83-7

[8]   Drachman DB. Medical progress: myasthenia gravis. N Engl J Med 1994;330:1797-1810.

[9]   Baraka A. Anesthesia and critical care of thymectomy for myasthenia gravis. Chest Surg Clin N Am 2001;11:337-61.

[10]   Pompeo E, Tacconi F, Massa R, *et al.* Long-term outcome of thoracoscopic extended thymectomy for nonthymomatous myasthenia gravis. Eur J Cardiothorac Surg 2009;36:164-9.

[11]   Magee MJ, Mack MJ. Surgical approaches to the thymus in patients with myasthenia gravis. Thorac Surg Clin. 2009;19:83-9.

[12]   Murai H, Uchiyama A, Mei FJ, *et al.* Long-term effects of infrasternal mediastinoscopic thymectomy in myasthenia gravis. J Neurol Sci 2009;287:185-7.

[13]   Ashton RC Jr, McGinnis KM, Connery CP, *et al.* Totally endoscopic robotic thymectomy for myasthenia gravis. Ann Thorac Surg 2003;75:569-71.

[14]   Masaoka A, Yamakawa Y, Niwa H, *et al.* Extended thymectomy for myasthenia gravis patients: a 20-year review. Ann Thorac Surg. 1996;62:853-9.

[15]   Akpolat N, Tilgen H, Gürsoy F, Saydam S, Gürel A. Thoracic epidural anaesthesia and analgesia with bupivacaine for transsternal thymectomy for myasthenia gravis. Eur J Anaesthesiol 1997;14:220-3.

[16] Hübler M, Litz RJ, Albrecht DM. Combination of balanced and regional anaesthesia for minimally invasive surgery in a patient with myasthenia gravis. Eur J Anaesthesiol 2000;7:325-8.

[17] Bagshaw O. A combination of total intravenous anesthesia and thoracic epidural for thymectomy in juvenile myasthenia gravis. Paediatr Anaesth 2007;17:370-4.

[18] Tripathi M, Srivastava K, Misra SK, Puri GD. Peri-operative management of patients for video assisted thoracoscopic thymectomy in myasthenia gravis. J Postgrad Med 2001;47:258-61

[19] Della Rocca G, Coccia C, Diana L, *et al.* Propofol or sevoflurane anesthesia without muscle relaxants allow the early extubation of myasthenic patients. Can J Anaesth 2003;50:547-52.

[20] Kato Y, Matsumoto I, Tomita S, Watanabe G. A novel technique to prevent intra-operative pneumothorax in awake coronary artery bypass grafting: biomaterial neo-pleura. Eur J Cardiothorac Surg 2009;35:37-41.

[21] Watanabe G, Yamaguchi S, Tomiya S, Ohtake H. Awake subxyphoid minimally invasive direct coronary artery bypass grafting yielded minimum invasive cardiac surgery for high risk patients. Interact Cardiovasc Thorac Surg 2008;7:910-2.

[22] Tsunezuka Y, Oda M, Matsumoto I, Tamura M, Watanabe G. Extended thymectomy in patients with myasthenia gravis with high thoracic epidural anesthesia alone. World J Surg. 2004;28:962-5.

[23] Abd Elrazek E, Scott NB, Vohra A. An epidural scoring scale for arm movements (ESSAM) in patients receiving high thoracic epidural analgesia for coronary artery bypass grafting. Anaesthesia 1999;54:1104-9.

[24] Vandermeulen EP, Van Aken H, Vermylen J. Anticoagulants and spinal-epidural anesthesia. Anesth Analg. 1994;79:1165-77.

[25] Horlocker TT, Wedel DJ, Rowlingson JC, *et al.* Regional anesthesia in the patient receiving antithrombotic or thrombolytic therapy: American Society of Regional Anesthesia and Pain Medicine Evidence-Based Guidelines (Third Edition). Reg Anesth Pain Med 2010; 35:64-101.

[26] Kessler P, Aybek T, Neidhart G, *et al.* Comparison of three anesthetic techniques for off-pump coronary artery bypass grafting: general anesthesia, combined general and high thoracic epidural anesthesia, or high thoracic epidural anesthesia alone. J Cardiothorac Vasc Anesth. 2005;19:32-9.

[27] Matsumoto I, Oda M, Watanabe G. Awake endoscopic thymectomy *via* an infrasternal approach using sternal lifting. Thorac Cardiovasc Surg 2008;56:311-3.

[28] Sakamaki Y, Kido T, Yasukawa M. Alternative choices of total and partial thymectomy in video-assisted resection of noninvasive thymomas. Surg Endosc 2008;22:1272-7.

[29] Kido T, Hazama K, Inoue Y, Tanaka Y, Takao T. Resection of anterior mediastinal masses through an infrasternal approach. Ann Thorac Surg 1999;67:263-5.

[30] Ishikawa N, Sun YS, Nifong LW, *et al.* A new retractor system for thoracoscopic thymectomy using the anterior chest wall-lifting method. Surg Endosc 2007;21:140-1.

[31] Ishikawa N, Sun YS, Nifong LW, *et al.* Thoracoscopic robot-assisted extended thymectomy in human cadaver. Surg Endosc 2009;23:459-61.

[32] Karagoz HY, Kurtoglu M, Bakkaloglu B, *et al.* Coronary artery bypass grafting in the awake patient: three years' experience in 137 patients. J Thorac Cardiovasc Surg. 2003;125:1401-4.

[33] Minato N, Shimokawa T, Katayama Y, *et al.* New application method of fibrin glue for more effective hemostasis in cardiovascular surgery: rub-and-spray method. Jpn J Thorac Cardiovasc Surg 2004;52:361-6.

[34] Dresdale A, Bowman FO Jr, Malm JR, *et al.* Hemostatic effectiveness of fibrin glue derived from single-donor fresh frozen plasma. Ann Thorac Surg. 1985;40: 385-7.

[35] Kawamura M, Gika M, Izumi Y, *et al.* The sealing effect of fibrin glue against alveolar air leakage evaluated up to 48 h; comparison between different methods of application. Eur J Cardiothorac Surg. 2005;28:39-42.

[36] Hanks JB, Kjaergard HK, Hollingsbee DA. A comparison of the haemostatic effect of Vivostat patient-derived fibrin sealant with oxidised cellulose (Surgicel) in multiple surgical procedures. Eur Surg Res. 2003; 35:439-44.

[37] Tateishi J, Kitamoto T, Mohri S, *et al.* Scrapie removal using Planova virus removal filters. Biologicals. 2001;29:17-25.

CHAPTER 13

Awake Thoracoscopic Biopsy of Anterior Mediastinal Masses

Eugenio Pompeo[*], **Alessandra Picardi**[†], **Maria Cantonetti**[†] **and Tommaso Claudio Mineo**

Departments of Thoracic Surgery and [†]*Onco-Hematology, Policlinico Tor Vergata University, Rome, Italy*

Abstract: Anterior mediastinal masses can develop due to a number of conditions, most of which require prompt pathologic diagnosis to initiate appropriate treatment.

Diagnosis can be achieved by surgical and non-surgical methods but Video-Assisted Thoracic Surgery (VATS) through general anesthesia is frequently preferred due to its minimal invasiveness and optimal diagnostic yield. One limitation of VATS includes the need for general anesthesia and one-lung ventilation, which can induce life-threatening adverse effects, particularly in patients with bulky masses

In order to reduce general anesthesia-related operative risks, we employed a VATS biopsy approach performed by just thoracic epidural or local anesthesia in fully awake, spontaneously ventilating patients.

This surgical method allows a wide visual control of mediastinal compartments, an accurate assessment of the disease extension and achievement of multiple biopsy specimens from different sites of the mass, eventually resulting in excellent diagnostic yield. In addition, adequate surgical management of associated intrathoracic conditions including drainage of pleural-pericardial effusions or pleural-pulmonary biopsy is possible when necessary.

We believe that this novel and globally less invasive surgical option might thus be included within the framework of the most reliable methods currently available to achieve a rapid diagnosis and adequate surgical management in patients with undetermined anterior mediastinal masses.

Keywords: Anterior mediastinum, mediastinal tumor, VATS, awake anesthesia, lymphoma.

Undetermined anterior mediastinal masses with radiological features of benign cysts, mature teratomas or early stage thymomas commonly lead to direct surgical resection whereas the presence of poorly demarcated masses requires a biopsy to rule out pathologic diagnosis and decide the appropriate treatment strategy [1].

Amongst the various surgical and non-surgical methods which are currently available for this purpose, Video-Assisted Thoracic Surgery (VATS) has often been employed due to its mini-invasive nature and optimal visualization of mediastinal compartments [2-4]. In addition, VATS allows drainage of associated pleural-pericardial effusions and biopsy of neighboring structures to be simultaneously performed.

One limitation of VATS is the need for general anesthesia and one-lung ventilation, which can be followed by life-threatening adverse events such as severe airway obstruction and even cardiovascular collapse, particularly in patients with bulky anterior mediastinal masses [5-7].

In an attempt to minimize general-anesthesia-related risks, we adopted a VATS approach entailing use of just thoracic epidural or local anesthesia in fully awake, spontaneously ventilating patients [8].

The aim of this chapter is to describe indications, technical details and results of this mini-invasive surgical option.

[*]**Address correspondence to Eugenio Pompeo:** Department of Thoracic Surgery, Policlinico Tor Vergata University, Rome, Italy;
E-mail: pompeo@med.uniroma2.it

CLINICAL FINDINGS

Anterior mediastinal lesions can be discovered incidentally by routine chest roentgenograms although about 2/3 of patients have symptoms. Severity of symptoms and their characteristics largely depends on the biological behaviour of the mass, its location and size, as well as the coexistence of associated systemic disease or of specific paraneoplastic syndromes. Chest pain, cough and dyspnea are the most commonly reported symptoms. In the presence of bulky masses or aggressive malignant disease invading or compressing adjacent structures, hoarseness, Horner's syndrome, diaphragmatic paralysis, and superior vena cava syndrome can occur and are generally associated with a poor prognosis. Systemic symptoms due to release of hormones and antibodies are rarely present. Antiacetylcholine receptor antibodies should always be measured in patients with a thymic mass because occult myasthenia gravis may be associated with thymoma. On the other hand, hypokalemia, high-serum cortisol, and Adrenocorticotropic Hormone (ACTH) levels are seen in some patients with thymic carcinoid tumors. Ectopic thyroid tumors may be associated with thyreotoxicosis. Young adult men with an anterior mediastinal mass should have determinations of levels of α-fetoprotein and β-hCG since either one or both can be elevated in the presence of a non-seminomatous germ cell tumor. In particular, gynecomastia is present in over 50% of patients with coriocarcinoma and is likely to be due to β-hCG production. In some patients, serum-soluble interleukin-2 receptors may be elevated in the presence of mediastinal lymphoma [1].

Age at onset is also an important factor when dealing with an anterior mediastinal mass. In childhood, germ cell tumors and lymphomas account for the most frequent etiology whereas in adults, thymic tumors, lymphomas and mature germ cell tumors are more frequently discovered.

IMAGING

The imaging work-up plays a pivotal role in deciding which lesion can be directly operated on with resectional purposes and which, instead, mandates initial histo-phenotypic characterization.

Whenever an undetermined mediastinal mass is disclosed at chest radiography (Fig. **1**, **Video 1**), Computed Tomography (CT), Magnetic Resonance Imaging (MRI) [9, 10] and Positron Emission Tomography (PET)[11, 12] are commonly employed for precise assessment of the lesion's characteristics and its relationship with adjacent structures (Fig. **2**). In fact, although thymomas, thymic carcinomas, seminomas, nonseminomatous germ cell tumors, and lymphomas can be quite similar in their imaging study appearance, there are some differential radiological features that can help orient the diagnosis and which should be kept in mind.

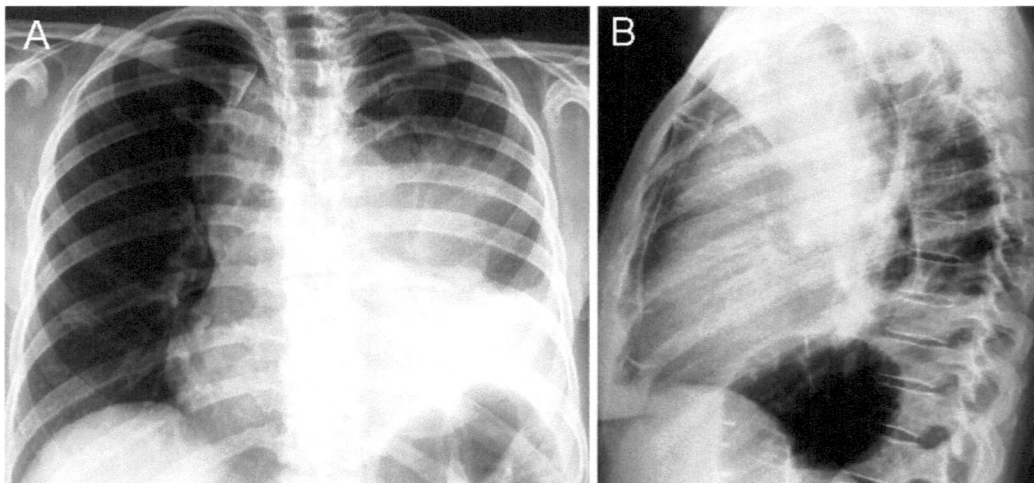

Fig. **1.** Standard chest roentgenogram in postero-anterior (A) and lateral (B) views disclosing an undetermined, bulky, anterior mediastinal mass associated with left-sided pleural effusion.

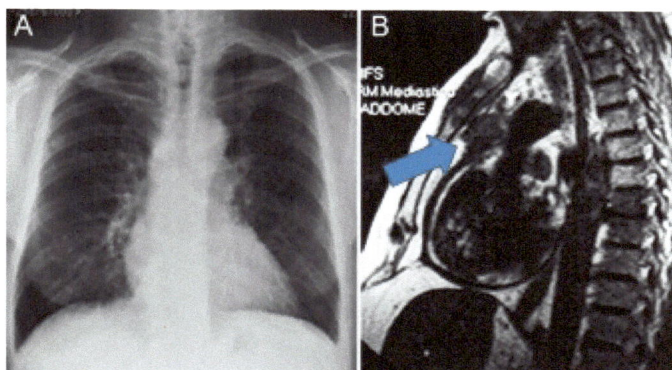

Fig. 2. At standard chest roentgenogram (A), a slight bulging of the right-sided mediastinal profile suggests the presence of an anterior mediastinal mass, which is better delineated by MRI in sagittal view (B, arrow).

Solid tumors. Thymic carcinoma include a heterogeneous group of aggressive tumors characterized by early local invasion and widespread metastases occurring predominantly in middle-aged males [13, 14]. On CT, they typically present as a large anterior mediastinal mass with lobulated or poorly defined margins. Homogeneous or heterogeneous soft tissue attenuation can be variable depending on the presence of necrosis whereas foci of calcification can be found in 10%-40% of cases [14-16]. Occasionally, invasive thymomas and poorly differentiated carcinoids can be associated with local invasion and distant metastases, showing radiologic findings similar to those of thymic carcinoma. In this respect, MRI can prove useful to identify a plane of cleavage with surrounding vascular structures whereas PET can help in differentiating thymoma from thymic carcinoma, which shows a higher median fluedoxydglucose (FDG) uptake (Fig. **3**) [17].

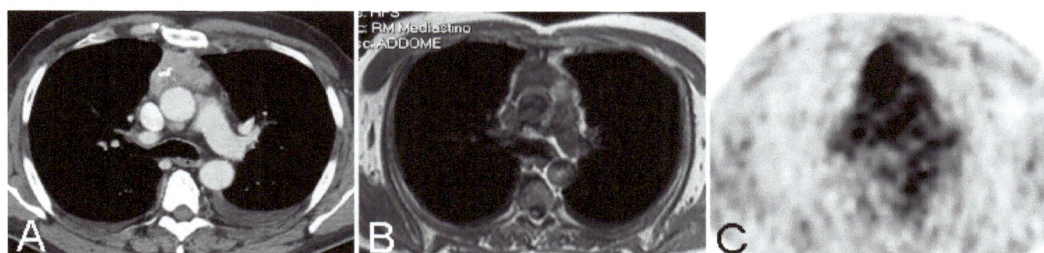

Fig. 3. A poorly defined mediastinal mass with eccentric calcification at CT scan (A) with no signs of vascular invasion at MRI (B) and elevated FDG uptake at PET scan (C). After awake biopsy, histology examination showed a thymic carcinoma.

Mediastinal germ cell tumors are uncommon and occur predominantly within the anterior mediastinum. They frequently present as a huge mass with local compression and usually affect young adults between 20 and 40 years of age.

About 80% of germ cell tumors are benign teratomas which typically present as rounded/lobulated, well defined anterior mediastinal masses ranging in size between 5 and 25 cm [18, 19]. On CT they usually have a multiloculated, cystic appearance with walls of variable thickness that usually enhance after IV contrast administration. The combination of soft tissue, fluid, calcium and fat attenuation is highly specific and allows an easy presumptive diagnosis. Focal calcification is present in 20%-80% of cases whereas areas of fat attenuation occur in 50% of instances.

More than 90% of malignant germ cell tumors occur in men. They present as bulky irregular masses with inhomogeneous areas due to necrosis and hemorrhage and can be associated with invasion of adjacent structures and pleural-pericardial effusions. They include teratocarcinomas, seminomas and non-seminomatous dysembriomas such as tumors of the endodermal sinus or yolk sac, choriocarcinomas and the mixed variants.

PET has found a niche in the evaluation of these metabolically active tumors. In particular, FDG PET was shown to be accurate in the initial staging of germ cell tumors and in detecting unsuspected metastatic disease [20].

In rare instances, anterior mediastinal masses disclosed at standard radiography or CT can reveal a thymolipoma [21, 22], an idiopathic sclerosing mediastinitis [23], a plasmocytoma [24] or other benign lesions (Fig. **4**). In childhood, true hyperplasia of the thymus can also occasionally present as an asymptomatic anterior mediastinal mass [25].

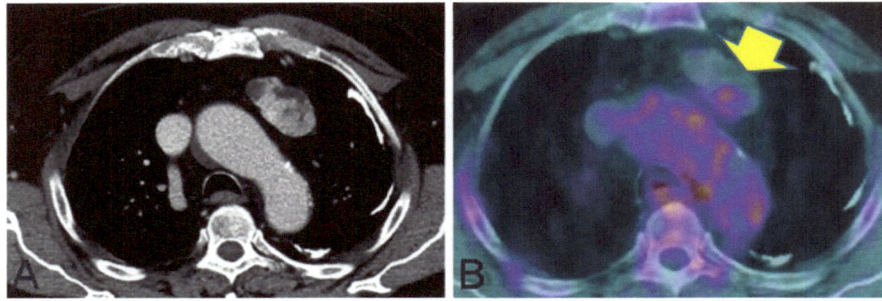

Fig. 4. CT findings (A) and low FDG-uptake at PET scan (B) of mediastinal ectopic goitier (arrow) in a patient treated by left artificial pneumothorax for tuberculosis 40 years before.

Lymphoproliferative disorders. The mediastinum may be the primary site of disease, like in Hodgkin's Lymphoma (HL) and Non-Hodgkin's (NHL) primary mediastinal B-cell lymphoma, or it may be involved as part of systemic disease. Hodgkin's disease is more common and tends to more frequently involve the thymus with radiological appearance of a bulky anterior mediastinal mass [26, 27]. Associated involvement of contiguous nodal stations is characteristic of HL, being observed in nearly 90% of cases [26, 28]. An anterior mediastinal mass is disclosed by simple chest radiograph in about 60% of patients (Fig. **1**). On CT scan, the enlarged thymus can maintain its normal shape or may appear with convex borders or lobulated contours. In HL both the enlarged thymus and lymph nodes commonly have a homogeneous density on CT and demonstrate slight enhancement after intra-venous administration of contrast. However, cystic areas reflecting central necrosis have been described in more than 20% of patients [29]. NHL also manifests as a bulky anterior mediastinal mass, but compared to HL there is often heterogeneous CT attenuation due to areas of necrosis (Fig. **5**) [30].

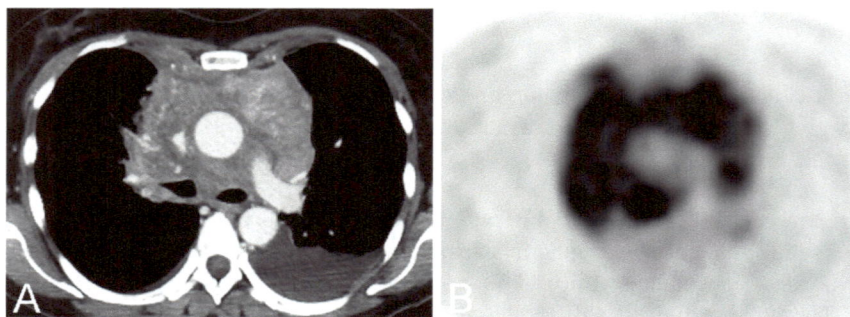

Fig. 5. Contrast-enhanced CT scan (A) shows a non-homogeneous, bulky, anterior mediastinal mass. The lesion had an elevated FDG-uptake at PET scan (B). At awake surgical biopsy this proved to be a NHL.

Lymphomas may spread beyond the lymph nodes invading mediastinal structures and the chest wall [31, 32]. However, in contrast to invasive carcinoma, lymphoma is only rarely associated with invasion of the phrenic nerve and diaphragmatic paralysis [32]. Intrathoracic lymphoma is almost always associated with extrathoracic disease that facilitates a correct diagnosis; however, in about 5% of cases, the mediastinum is the sole localization, a feature that renders a differential diagnosis with other anterior mediastinal masses more difficult [26].

Frequently, a residual mass is found after treatment for mediastinal lymphoma. CT and MRI have an important role in the evaluation of these masses. An increase in size on follow-up studies is currently one of the most common features of recurrent lymphoma though it may sometimes be due to rebound thymic hyperplasia. Additionally, a decrease in size of the mass does not rule out the presence of viable tumor cells [33-37]. In this respect, MRI is superior to CT in the detection of foci of viable tumor cells within residual masses, with a sensitivity ranging from 45% to 90% and a specificity of 80% to 90% [38-40].

Increased uptake of FDG on PET scans is highly predictive for the presence of active disease [41-43]. Indeed PET has virtually replaced gallium scanning in the pretreatment work-up of lymphoma and recently proved to be 90% sensitive and 90% specific when employed in the initial staging of lymphoma [44]. It is also worth noting that PET can change the staging and/or management of lymphomas in up to 20% of patients. Furthermore, in lymphoma patients, PET can have a great impact in the assessment of response to therapy and to guide decisions about further treatment since it was shown to be more accurate than CT by reducing the number of false positive findings (Fig. **6**) [45]. Finally, PET can also prove extremely useful for guiding biopsy of the most suspicious areas corresponding to those with higher FDG uptake [46].

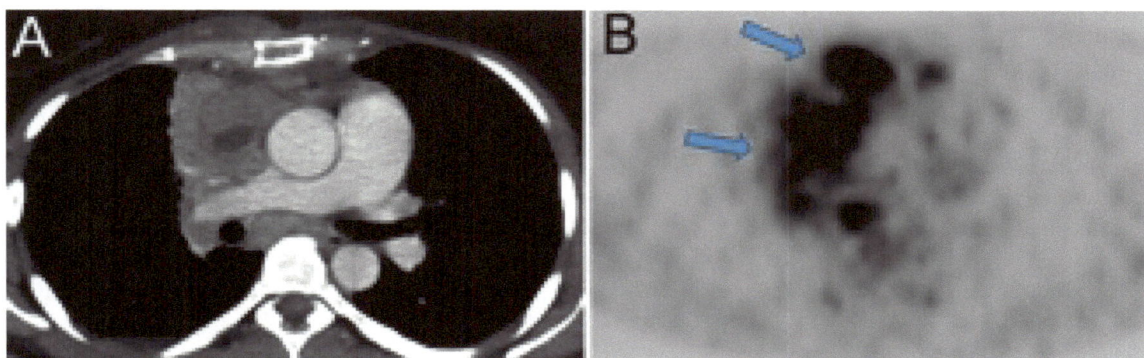

Fig. 6. Post-radiochemotherapy CT scan (A) of a patient with HL showing persistence of a anterior mediastinal mass with elevated FDG-uptake at PET scan (B, arrows). Histology confirmed a residual disease.

AWAKE VATS BIOPSY

Background. Local anesthesia with spontaneous ventilation has been advocated as the safest type of anesthesia to be used in the surgical management of patients with bulky mediastinal masses although, so far, this type of approach has been anecdotally reported in the literature. In 1970, Ward [47] first reported on the use of mediastinoscopy under local anesthesia and emphasized the easy feasibility and some particular advantages of this procedure, although standard mediastinoscopy is not suitable for biopsy of anterior mediastinal masses. In 1977, Arom and colleagues [48] proposed insertion of the mediastinoscope through a subxiphoid incision to allow exploration and biopsy of anterior mediastinal compartments. In 1987, Sibert and colleagues [49] reported on a patient with a bulky mediastinal mass and superior vena cava syndrome undergoing thoracotomy with awake intubation and spontaneous ventilation. In 1998, Watanabe and coworkers [50] compared the results of awake anterior mediastinotomy versus percutaneous needle biopsy, achieving a higher diagnostic accuracy with the awake surgical method.

In 2002, Rendina and colleagues [51] employed an optical mediastinoscope inserted through a parasternal incision under local anesthesia to biopsy anterior mediastinal lesions reporting a 100% diagnostic yield with no mortality and minimal morbidity. More recently, awake VATS has been reported for management of pericardial effusion [52, 53], complex anterior mediastinal masses [54] and even for thymectomy [55, 56].

Indications. Indications to awake mediastinal biopsy are detailed in Table **1** and include the radiological finding of a recently developed, undetermined, anterior mediastinal mass; patient acceptance of the awake procedure with signed informed consent, exclusion of severe anxiety or psychic disorders and no history of previous pleural disease or previous thoracic surgery on the side chosen for the awake VATS procedure.

Table 1. Indication to awake VATS biopsy for anterior mediastinal masses.

Radiographic evidence of an undetermined, poorly demarcated, anterior mediastinal mass or any other mass not amenable to surgical resection.
Radiographic evidence of an undetermined anterior mediastinal mass with associated intrathoracic conditions requiring surgical management.
Previous non-conclusive non-surgical biopsy findings or need for large samples for adequate immuno-histochemistry characterization.
No peripheral lymphadenopathy or skin lesions.
Patients with a mixed anterior/middle mediastinum mass amenable to mediastinoscopy but at high-risk for general anesthesia.
No severe anxiety or other psychic disorders.
No evidence of fibrous pleural adhesions or history of pleurodesis or previous thoracic surgery on the side chosen for the awake VATS.
Written informed consent for the awake procedure.

Anesthesia. We routinely employ either thoracic epidural catheterization or local anesthesia. As a rule, when the surgical procedure is performed in an urgent setting due to unstable or critical clinical conditions of the patient, local anesthesia is preferred since it is more rapid to perform and it is mostly well accepted by patients.

However, in the presence of complex mediastinal masses with associated conditions requiring multiple pleural/pulmonary biopsy or pericardial fenestration we prefer to perform the procedures through epidural anesthesia whenever possible, due to the wider intrathoracic analgesia assured by this type of anesthesia.

Venous and radial artery catheterization is carried out in the operating room. Premedication is limited to mild sedation with midazolam in selected instances.

For local anesthesia, 60 mL of a 50% mixture of lidocaine 2% and ropivacaine 7.5% is prepared immediately before starting the operation.

In rare instances, when using local anesthesia, the biopsy of the mediastinal mass, can elicit some pain. Additional irrigation of the mediastinal pleura with lidocaine can thus be required. If additional pleural biopsy is deemed necessary due to the presence of associated pleural lesions, transparietal subpleural injection of local anesthetic can be performed perilesionally.

Thoracic epidural anesthesia is carried out with an epidural catheter placed at T4-T5 level *via* a loss-of-resistance technique and the degree of thoracic analgesia that is achieved is assessed by both warm-cold and pin-prick discrimination tests.

Perioperatively, fluids are given at a minimum rate while assuring adequate urinary output. If necessary, oxygen is administered *via* a Venturi mask to keep arterial oxygen saturation above 90%. Intraoperatively, the patient must be alerted that creation of the surgical pneumothorax following insertion of the trocar can result in some difficulty during spontaneous ventilation, although oxygen saturation remains satisfactory as the patient her/him-self can personally observe in the anesthesiologist monitor. Panic attacks triggered by anxiety or mild dyspnea can occasionally develop and can be easily controlled by increasing sedation slightly with remifentanyl or sub-hypnotic boluses of propofol. Low-volume classical music can be played in the operating room and has been shown to reduce anxiety and the need for pharmacological sedation during awake surgical procedures [57].

Should conversion to general anesthesia prove necessary, orotracheal intubation is usually performed without changing the patient's position. In such instances, both videolaryngoscopy and a fiber-optic bronchoscopy can prove useful to aid faster and easier intubation of the patient placed in the semilateral decubitus position.

Surgical technique. The side for the VATS approach is chosen on the basis of the main bulge of the mass as well as of the associated intrathoracic conditions requiring surgical management. As for every type of awake VATS procedure, one chest tube with its water seal chamber is kept ready on the nurse's table to allow immediate drainage of the pleural cavity and interruption of the procedure whenever deemed necessary. Care is also devoted to placing the patient in a comfortable position and to prep and drape the operating field in order to maintain her/his face free, thus facilitating spontaneous breathing and the patient's interaction with the surgical staff (Fig. **7**). We also consider maintenance of a friendly and empathetic environment in the operating room very important to maximize patients' perioperative well being. The patient is placed in the semilateral decubitus position with mild trunk elevation and the arm adducted. We believe that the semilateral decubitus position as well as the avoidance of muscle relaxation during the operation may both contribute to reduce risks of compression of the airways by the mass. One 20-mm-flexible trocar is inserted in the 6th or 7th intercostal space, on the anterior axillary line. A 30-degree, 10-mm camera is used to facilitate both oblique vision of the anterior mediastinum and co-axial surgical maneuvering (Figs. **7, 8**). One or more supplemental trocars can be inserted whenever deemed helpful to facilitate more complex surgical maneuvers such as pericardial fenestration or wedge resection of a pulmonary nodule. In most instances, instrumental retraction of the lung is not necessary to reach the anterior mediastinum, since with the patient lying in the semilateral position, the lung tends to fall posteriorly by gravity. The mediastinal pleura is incised by scissors or electrified hook, and multiple biopsies of the most representative target sites are then taken under direct vision. To avoid electrocautery artifacts, coagulation must be minimized during the procedure (Fig. **8**). Hemostasis is then revised and clips are placed to mark the bioptic area. At the end of operation, one chest tube is placed to water seal and the patient is asked to cough repeatedly to aid lung re-expansion.

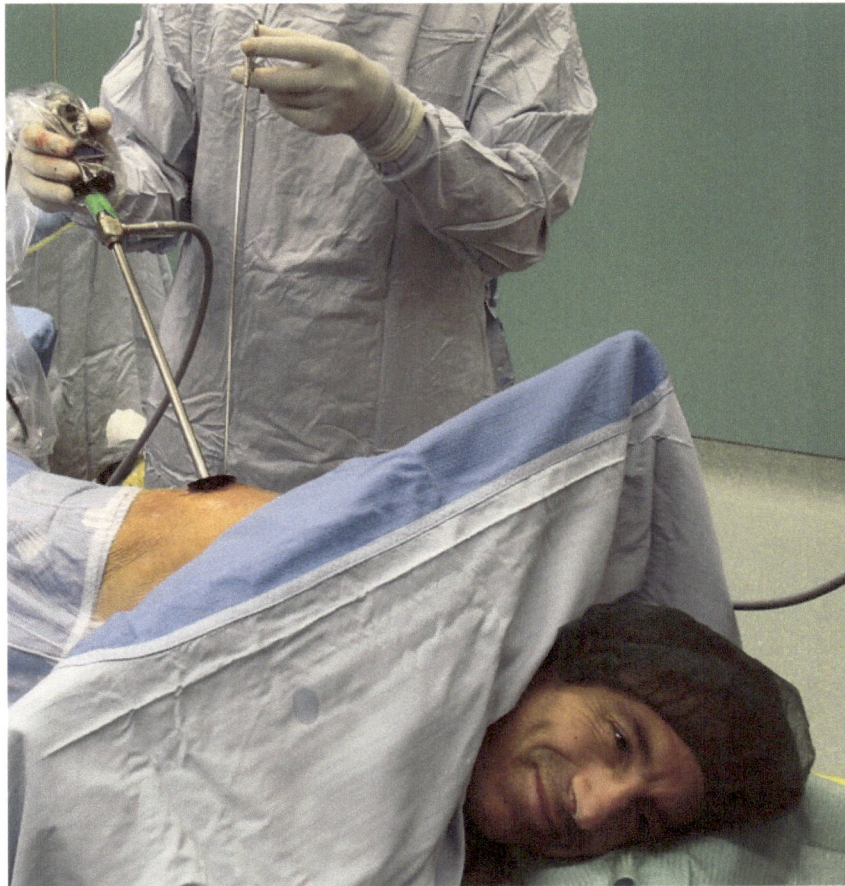

Fig. 7. Intraoperative view of a fully awake and cooperative patient placed in comfortable semilateral position during biopsy for undetermined mediastinal mass.

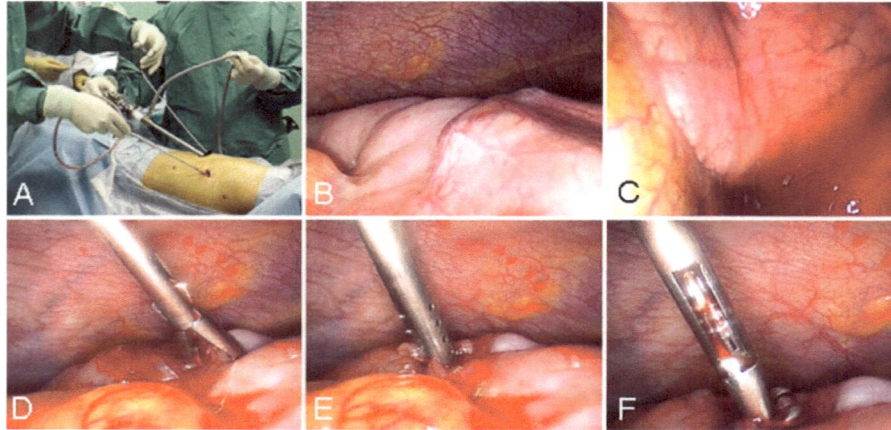

Fig. 8. External view showing an awake mediastinal biopsy with pericardial fenestration performed through a two-trocars access (A). Intraoperative view of an anterior mediastinal mass (B) with associated pleural-pericardial effusion (C). Multiple biopsy samples of the mass are easily taken during the awake surgical procedure (D-F)(Video 1).

In patients operated *via* thoracic epidural analgesia, the epidural catheter is left in place for 24h. Postoperative care is made according to a fast track policy. Following a brief stay in the recovery room the patient is rapidly transferred to the ward where oral fluid intake and walking is immediately allowed. Patients are normally discharged the day after surgery although some patients have recently been operated on in an ambulatory setting.

CONCLUSION

In the authors' hands, awake VATS biopsy of anterior mediastinal masses was safely feasible and resulted in an excellent diagnostic yield.

These features contrast with previously reported results of surgical biopsy carried out through general anesthesia that have been associated with difficult weaning, prolonged mechanical ventilation and a morbidity rate as high as 20% [5-7].

Theoretical concerns about an awake surgical approach might include the risk of ventilatory impairment induced by the surgical pneumothorax, loss of airway patency and compression of the dependent lung by the mediastinal mass. However, clinical experience with this surgical method has shown that most concerns were unfounded, as already suggested by the highly satisfactory results that we observed with other procedures including awake lung volume reduction surgery [58] and awake lung resection [59].

Anterior mediastinotomy has been the most commonly used surgical alternative to VATS [60, 61]. However, we believe that compared to the awake approach, limitations of anterior mediastinotomy include a less than ideal visualization of the anterior mediastinum, suboptimal scarring, potential delay in starting salvage radio-chemotherapy and the need for additional surgical access for management of associated intrathoracic conditions.

The pros and cons of awake VATS biopsy must be balanced against the choice of non-surgical methods, including CT-guided fine-needle aspiration or core-biopsy whose diagnostic accuracy has been less satisfactory and might translate into significant diagnostic delay.

In a large retrospective review of patients with mediastinal lymphomas undergoing CT-guided biopsy, the diagnostic yield was only 82.5% [62]. Furthermore, in a prospective study comparing anterior mediastinotomy versus CT-guided biopsy for bulky mediastinal masses, the latter resulted in a diagnostic yield of less than 45% [63]. Finally, in another study assessing the accuracy of CT-guided needle biopsy in restaging residual lymphomas after treatment, this method resulted in a 75% failure rate [64].

For these reasons, the use of a non-surgical biopsy method with less than optimal diagnostic accuracy as the first choice can increase the risk of diagnostic delay if a subsequent surgical biopsy becomes necessary. This diagnostic strategy can prove particularly dangerous in critically ill patients with bulky masses.

We believe that the advantages of awake VATS include a wide visual control during tumor sampling, accurate assessment of the disease extension, and an excellent diagnostic yield (Table **2**).

Table 2. Proposed advantages and disadvantages of the main non-surgical and surgical methods.

	Accuracy	Safety	Cost	Advantages	Disadvantages
Non-surgical methods					
CT-guided FNA	++	+++	++	Mini-invasive	Limited sampling
CT-guided CB	++	++	++	Mini-invasive	Limited sampling
Ultrasonography-guided FNA	++	++	+	Mini-invasive	Limited sampling
EUS/EBUS*	++	++	+	Fast procedure, cost saving	Limited sampling
Surgical methods					
Thoracotomy	+++	+	+++	Highest diagnostic yield	OLV needed, surgical trauma
Extended mediastinoscopy	+++	+	++	Limited traumatism	Risk of vascular injury
Anterior mediastinotomy	+++	+	++	Limited traumatism	Narrow operating field
VATS	+++	++	+++	Possibility of managing associate thoracic conditions	OLV needed
Awake VATS	+++	++	++	Possibility of managing associate thoracic conditions	Still under evaluation

CB: core biopsy; EBUS: endo-bronchial ultrasound-guided sampling, EUS: endoscopic ultrasound sampling; FNA: fine-needle aspiration; OLV: one-lung ventilation; VATS: video-assisted thoracic surgery.

This surgical approach can prove particularly useful in presence of mediastinal localization of lymphoproliferative disorders, in which pathologists appreciate the possibility of analyzing multiple biopsy specimens to allow a precise histo-phenotypic characterization. In addition, awake VATS offers the possibility of concomitant management of associated intrathoracic conditions.

In conclusion, awake VATS biopsy of undetermined anterior mediastinal masses is a promising surgical option that makes it possible to safely achieve pathologic diagnosis with minimal surgical trauma.

REFERENCES

[1]   Date H. Diagnostic strategies for mediastinal tumors and cysts. Thorac Surg Clin 2009;19:29-35.

[2]   Sugarbaker DJ. Thoracoscopy in the management of anterior mediastinal masses. Ann Thorac Surg 1993;56:653-6.

[3]   Roviaro G, Varoli F, Nucca O, Vergani C, Maciocco M. Videothoracoscopic approach to primary mediastinal pathology. Chest 2000;117:1179-83.

[4]   Yim AP. Video-assisted thoracoscopic management of anterior mediastinal masses. Preliminary experience and results. Surg Endosc 1995;9:1184-8.

[5]   Goh MH, Liu XY, Goh YS. Anterior mediastinal masses: an anaesthetic challenge. Anaesthesia 1999;54:670-4.

[6]   Azizkhan RG, Dudgeon DL, Buck JR, *et al.* Lifethreatening airway obstruction as complication to the management of mediastinal masses in children. J Pediatr Surg 1985;20:816-22.

[7]   Bechard P, Le´tourneau L, Lacasse Y, *et al.* Perioperative cardiorespiratory complications in adults with mediastinal mass. Anesthesiology 2004;100:826-34.

[8] Pompeo E, Tacconi F, Mineo TC. Awake video-assisted thoracoscopic biopsy in complex anterior mediastinal masses. Thor Surg Clin 2010;20:225-33.

[9] Remy-Jardin M, Duyck P, Remy J, *et al.* Hilar lymph nodes: Identification with spiral CT and histologic correlation. Radiology 1995;196:387-94.

[10] Remy-Jardin M, Remy J, Mayo JR, Müller NL. Acquisition, injection, and reconstruction techniques. In: Remy-Jardin M, Remy J, Mayo JR, Müller NL, Eds. CT Angiography of the chest. Philadelphia, Lippincott Williams & Wilkins, 2001; pp. 1-14.

[11] Puri V, Meyers BF. Utility of Positron Emission Tomography in the Mediastinum: Moving Beyond Lung and Esophageal Cancer Staging. Thorac Surg Clin 2009;19:7-15.

[12] Truong MT, Erasmus JJ, Munden RF, *et al.* Focal FDG uptake in mediastinal brown fat mimicking malignancy: a potential pitfall resolved on PET/CT. Am J Roentgenol 2004;183:1127-32.

[13] Rosado de Christenson ML, Galobardes J, Moran CA. Thymoma: radiologic-pathologic correlation. Radiographics 1992;12:151-68.

[14] Suster S, Rosai J. Thymic carcinoma: a clinicopathologic study of 60 cases. Cancer 1991; 67:1025-32.

[15] Strollo DC, Rosado de Christenson ML, Jett JR. Primary mediastinal tumors. Part 1: Tumors of the anterior mediastinum. Chest 1997; 112:511-22.

[16] Do YS, Im JG, Lee BH, *et al.* CT findings in malignant tumors of thymic epithelium. J Comput Assist Tomogr 1995;19:192-7.

[17] Sasaki M, Kuwabara Y, Ichiya Y, *et al.* Differential diagnosis of thymic tumors using a combination of 11C-methionine PET and FDG PET. J Nucl Med 1999;40:1595-601.

[18] Brown LR, Aughenbaugh GL. Masses of the anterior mediastinum: CT and MR imaging. Am J Roentgenol 1991;157:1171-80.

[19] Moeller KH, Rosado de Christenson ML, Templeton PA. Mediastinal mature teratoma: Imaging features. AJR Am J Roentgenol 1997;169:985-90.

[20] Hain S, O'Doherty M, Timothy A, *et al.* Fluorodeoxyglucose PET in the initial staging of germ cell tumours. Eur J Nucl Med 2000;27:590-4.

[21] Yeh HC, Gordon A, Kirschner PA, Cohen BA. Computed tomography and sonography of thymolipoma. AJR Am J Roentgenol 1983;140:1131-3.

[22] Faerber EN, Balsara RK, Schidlow DV, *et al.* Thymolipoma: computed tomographic appearances. Pediatr Radiol 1990;20:196-7.

[23] Miyata T, Takahama M, Yamamoto R, Nakayama R, Tada H. Sclerosing mediastinitis mimicking anterior mediastinal tumor. Ann Thorac Surg 2009;88:293-5.

[24] Luh S, Lai Y, Tsai C, Chang-Yang Tsao T. Extramedullary plasmacytoma: report of a case manifested as mediastinal mass and multiple pulmonary nodules and review of literature. World J Surg Oncol 2007;5:123.

[25] Pompeo E, Cristino B, Mauriello A, Mineo TC. Recurrent massive hyperplasia of the thymus. Scand Cardiovasc J 1999;33:306-8.

[26] Filly R, Blank N, Castellino R. Radiographic distribution of intrathoracic disease in previously untreated patients with Hodgkin's disease and non-Hodgkin's lymphoma. Radiology 1976;120:277.

[27] Castellino RA, Blank N, Hoppe RT, Cho C: Hodgkin's disease: Contributions of chest CT in the initial staging evaluation. Radiology 1986;160:603-5.

[28] Cobby M, Whipp E, Bullimore J, *et al.* CT appearances of relapse of lymphoma in the lung. Clin Radiol 1990; 41:232-8.

[29] Wernecke K, Vassallo P, Rutsch F, *et al.* Thymic involvement in Hodgkin disease: CT and sonographic findings. Radiology 1991;181:375-83.

[30] Shaffer K, Smith D, Kirn D, *et al.* Primary mediastinal large-B-cell lymphoma: radiologic findings at presentation. AJR Am J Roentgenol 1996; 167:425-30.

[31] Bergin CJ, Healy MV, Zincone GE, Castellino RA. MR evaluation of chest wall involvement in malignant lymphoma. J Comput Assist Tomogr 1990;14:928-32.

[32] Fisher AM, Kendall B, Van Leuven BD: Hodgkin's disease: a radiological survey. Clin Radiol 1962;13:115-27.

[33] Webb WR. MR imaging of treated mediastinal Hodgkin disease. Radiology 1989;170:315-6.

[34] Rahmouni A, Tempany C, Jones R, *et al.* Lymphoma: monitoring tumor size and signal intensity with MR imaging. Radiology 1993;188:445-51.

[35] Fisher AM, Kendall B, Van Leuven BD: Hodgkin's disease: A radiological survey. Clin Radiol 1962;13:115-27.

[36] North LB, Fuller LM, Sullivan-Halley JA, Hagemeister FB. Regression of mediastinal Hodgkin disease after therapy: Evaluation of time interval. Radiology 1987;164:599-602.

[37] Rahmouni A, Divine M, Lepage E, *et al.* Mediastinal lymphoma: quantitative changes in gadolinium enhancement at MR imaging after treatment. Radiology 2001;219:621-8.

[38] Devizzi L, Maffioli L, Bonfante V, *et al.* Comparison of gallium scan, computed tomography, and magnetic resonance in patients with mediastinal Hodgkin's disease. Ann Oncol 1997;8:S53-S6.

[39] Hill M, Cunningham D, MacVicar D, *et al.* Role of magnetic resonance imaging in predicting relapse in residual masses after treatment of lymphoma. J Clin Oncol 1993;11:2273-8.

[40] Gasparini MD, Balzarini L, Castellani MR, *et al.* Current role of gallium scan and magnetic resonance imaging in the management of mediastinal Hodgkin lymphoma. Cancer 1993;72:577-82.

[41] Jerusalem G, Beguin Y, Fassotte MF, *et al.* Whole-body positron emission tomography using 18F-fluorodeoxy-glucose for posttreatment evaluation in Hodgkin's disease and non-Hodgkin's lymphoma has higher diagnostic and prognostic value than classical computed tomography scan imaging. Blood 1999;94:429-33.

[42] Jerusalem G, Warland V, Najjar F, *et al*: Whole-body 18F-FDG PET for the evaluation of patients with Hodgkin's disease and non-Hodgkin's lymphoma. Nucl Med Commun 1999;20:13-20.

[43] Moog F, Bangerter M, Diederichs CG, *et al*: Lymphoma: role of whole-body 2-deoxy-2-(F-18)fluoro-d-glucose (FDG) PET in nodal staging. Radiology 1997;203:795-800.

[44] Facey K, Bradbury I, Laking G, *et al.* Overview of the clinical effectiveness of positron emission tomography imaging in selected cancers. Health Technol Assess 2007;11:267.

[45] Juweid ME, Wiseman ME, Vose JM, *et al.* Response assessment of aggressive non-Hodgkin's lymphoma by integrated International Workshop Criteria and fluorine-18-fluorodeoxyglucose positron emission tomography. J Clin Oncol 2005;23:4652-61.

[46] Cheson BD, Pfistner B, Juweid ME, *et al.* Revised response criteria for malignant lymphoma. J Clin Oncol 2007;25:579-86.

[47] Podoloff DA, Advani RJ, Allred C, *et al.* NCCN task force report: positron emission tomography (PET)/computed tomography (CT) scanning in cancer. J Natl Compr Canc Netw 2007;5:S1-S22.

[48] Ward P. Mediastinoscopy under local anesthesia. A valuable diagnostic technique. Calf Med 1970;112:15-22.

[49] Arom KV, Franz JL, Grover FL, *et al.* Subxiphoid anterior mediastinal exploration. Ann Thorac Surg 1977;24:289-90.

[50] Sibert KS, Biondi JW, Hirsch NP. Spontaneous respiration during thoracotomy in a patient with mediastinal mass. Anesth Analg 1987;66:904-7.

[51] Watanabe M, Takagi K, Aoki T, *et al.* A comparison of biopsy through a parasternal anterior mediastinotomy under local anesthesia and percutaneous needle biopsy for malignant anterior mediastinal tumors. Surg Today 1998;28:1022-6.

[52] Rendina EA, Venuta F, De Giacomo T, *et al.* Biopsy of anterior mediastinal masses under local anesthesia. Ann Thorac Surg 2002;74:1720-2.

[53] Katlic MR. Video-assisted thoracic surgery utilizing local anesthesia and sedation. Eur J Cardiothorac Surg 2006;30:529-32.

[54] De Bellis P, Delfino R, Robbiano F, *et al.* High epidural thoracic anesthesia for pericardial surgery. Minerva Anestesiol 2005;71:595-9.

[55] Al-Abdullatief M, Wahood A, Al-Shirawi N, *et al.* Awake anaesthesia for major thoracic surgical procedures: an observational study. Eur J Cardiothorac Surg 2007;32:346-50.

[56] Matsumoto I, Oda M, Watanabe G. Awake endoscopic thymectomy *via* an infrasternal approach using sternal lifting. Thorac Cardiovasc Surg 2008;56:311-3.

[57] Lepage C, Drolet P, Girard M, *et al.* Music decreases sedative requirements during spinal anesthesia. Anesth Analg 2001;93:912-6.

[58] Pompeo E, Mineo TC. Two-year improvement in multidimensional body mass index, airflow obstruction, dyspnea and exercise capacity index after nonresectional lung volume reduction surgery in awake patients. Ann Thorac Surg 2007;84:1862-9.

[59] Pompeo E, Mineo D, Rogliani P, *et al.* Feasibility and results of awake thoracoscopic resection of solitary pulmonary nodules. Ann Thorac Surg 2004;78:1761-8.

[60] Steiger Z, Chaundhry S, Wilson RF. The use of anterior mediastinotomy to assess intrathoracic lesions. Am Surg 1981;47:251-3.

[61] Martigne C, Velly JF, Clerc P, *et al.* Value and current role of anterior mediastinotomy in the diagnosis of mediastinal diseases. Apropos of a series of 100 cases. Ann Chir 1989;43:171-3.

[62] Agid R, Sklair-Levy M, Bloom AI, *et al.* CT-guided biopsy with cutting-edge needle for the diagnosis of malignant lymphoma: experience of 267 biopsies. Clin Radiol 2003;58:143-7.

[63] Fang W, Xu M, Chen G, *et al.* Minimally invasive approaches for histological diagnosis of anterior mediastinal masses. Chin Med J 2007;120:675-9.

[64] Gossot D, Girard P, de Kerviler E, *et al.* Thoracoscopy or CT-guided biopsy for residual intrathoracic masses after treatment of lymphoma. Chest 2001;120:289-94.

Awake Thoracic Surgery, 2012, 177-190

CHAPTER 14

Awake Thoracoscopic Sympathectomy

Maria Elena Cufari, Eugenio Pompeo[*], Tommaso Claudio Mineo and Vincenzo Ambrogi

Department of Thoracic Surgery, Policlinico Tor Vergata University, Rome, Italy

Abstract: Video-Assisted Thoracic Surgery (VATS) sympathectomy is a safe and effective procedure for treatment of facial, palmar and axillary hyperhidrosis. It can be more rarely used in other conditions. Awake thoracic surgery with epidural anesthesia and spontaneous ventilation has been employed to perform many surgical procedures including VATS sympathectomy.

This chapter describes the anatomy of the nerve with the most frequent abnormalities, the indications and contraindication for both sympathectomy and awake surgery, the method for awake anesthesia, a detailed step-by-step description of the surgical technique and postoperative management as well as an analysis of benefits and potential side-effects of awake VATS sympathectomy.

Patient selection, choice of the level of sympathectomy and adequate information about anesthesia and side effects of the operation are extremely important for the good result of the procedure.

Awake VATS sympathectomy may be considered a globally minimally invasive approach combining avoidance of general anesthesia-related adverse effects with maximum patient satisfaction.

Keywords: Sympathectomy, VATS, awake thoracic surgery, hyperhidrosis, local anesthesia, thoracic epidural anesthesia.

INTRODUCTION

Sympathectomy is defined as the surgical interruption of the thoracic sympathetic chain. Although palmar hyperhidrosis represents the major indication for sympathectomy, it is also commonly employed to treat a variety of conditions, which include facial flushing, Raynaud's phenomenon, acrocyanosis, arterial insufficiency, Buerger's disease, causalgia, and thoracic outlet syndrome [1]. Transection of the major splanchnic branches of the thoracic sympathetic chain is also used in the management of untreatable pancreatic chronic pain [2]. In addition, sympathectomy was advocated to treat specific cardiac disorders such as angina pectoris and long QT syndrome although these latter indications are now mostly discarded [1].

Video-Assisted Thoracic Surgery (VATS) is currently considered the gold-standard for sympathectomy, and has virtually replaced open surgical approaches [3].

General anesthesia with one lung ventilation has been the most employed type of anesthesia in this setting although it may be associated with a number of adverse effects that may increase the morbidity rate.

Awake anesthesia has recently been employed to perform various thoracic surgery procedures including bullectomy in spontaneous pneumothorax, resection of pulmonary nodules and solitary metastases, lung volume reduction, coronary artery bypass and thymectomy [4]. Following these preliminary experiences, thoracic epidural or local anesthesia in fully awake patients has also been employed for VATS sympathectomy [5].

This chapter describes the indications and contraindications, surgical technique, benefits and potential

***Address correspondence to Eugenio Pompeo:** Department of Thoracic Surgery, Policlinico Tor Vergata University, Rome, Italy; Email: pompeo@med.uniroma2.it

complications of VATS sympathectomy performed through epidural or local anesthesia in awake patients.

ANATOMY AND PHYSIOLOGY

The thoracic sympathetic nerves are part of the autonomic nervous system. They prepare the body in stress conditions ("fight-or-flight" situations) and provide sensorimotor innervation to the visceral organs of the chest. The sensory component is responsible for visceral pain detection while the motor component innervates structures such as the vascular smooth muscle, *erector pili* muscles, and sweat glands of the skin, the heart and the lungs.

Sympathetic nerves originate from the lateral horn of the spinal cord and extend from the first thoracic segment to the second or third lumbar segments. These nerves initially run inside the spinal nerves, but a few centimeters outside the vertebral column they diverge to meet the relative ganglion, which is sited on another plane, immediately underneath the parietal pleura, according to a metameric distribution. Connections between spinal nerve and sympathetic ganglia are established through the *rami communicantes* (Fig. **1**). The preganglionic sympathetic fibers arrive at the chain *via* white *rami communicantes* of the ventral primary rami of spinal nerves T1 to L2. Postganglionic sympathetic fibers depart *via* gray *rami communicantes* directed at all spinal cord segments.

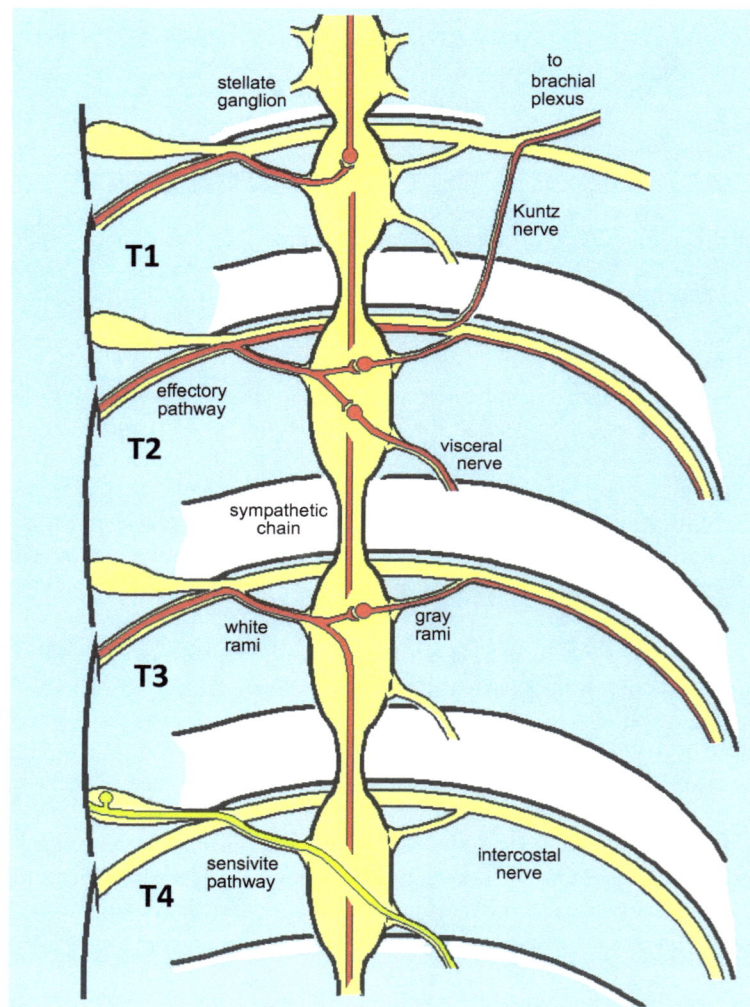

Fig. 1. Schematic view of the sympathetic chain. Effectory (red) and sensitive (green) pathways are shown. Kuntz nerve is visible laterally to the sympathetic chain. It creates a connection between the first and second ventral ramus of the intercostal nerve, proximally to the point where the former provides a large branch to the brachial plexus.

Sympathetic ganglia are located along a paravertebral line and are connected each other by a longitudinal thick band of neural fibers delineating an elongated, white-colored structure called the sympathetic chain, which orthogonally crosses the intercostal spaces.

The first thoracic ganglion may be fused with the lower cervical ganglion to originate a unique anatomical structure denominated the stellate ganglion. The stellate ganglion is present in 90% of instances on the right and in 94% on the left side [6]. At the level of the stellate ganglion, the oculosympathetic pathway projects postganglionic axons to the eye to innervate the dilator of the iris, the Muller muscle of the eyelid and regulates the sweat glands of the face. Its interruption causes the Horner syndrome.

Supplementary and inconstant neural fibers were studied by Kuntz in 1927 [7]: these branches are sited laterally to the sympathetic chain and create a connection between the first and second ventral ramus of the intercostal nerve, proximally to the point where the former provides a large branch to the brachial plexus (Fig. **2**).

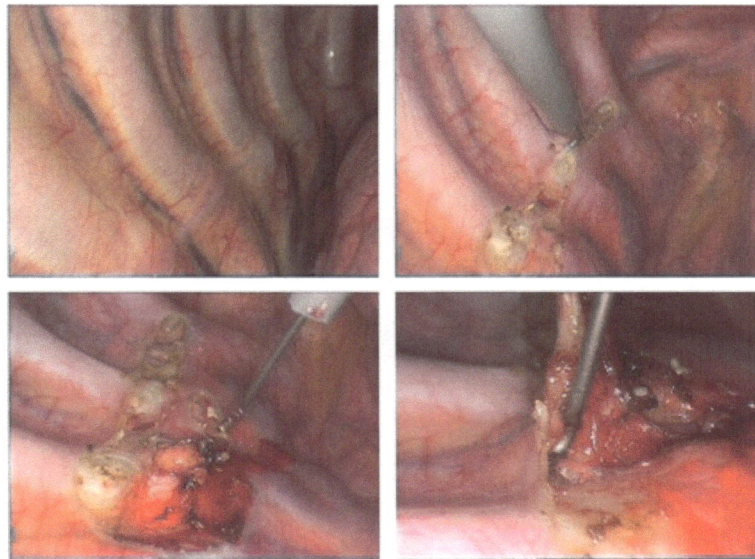

Fig. 2. Intraoperative steps of awake sympathectomy. Left upper: identification of the sympathetic chain; right upper: opening of the pleura lateral to the chain by the hook; left lower: opening of the pleura medial to the chain; right lower: caudal dissection of the chain.

Thus, these fibers may reach the brachial plexus without passing through the sympathetic chain. The distribution of these neural pathways has enormous clinical significance because the presence of valid bridging fibers may unable the therapeutic effects of a limited ganglionectomy. Additional sympathetic connections between the second and third up to the fifth intercostal nerves are also described [8].

HISTORY

Early surgical approaches to sympathectomy were anterior, as described by Jonnesco, Leriche, Royle, Gask and Fontaine in the early 1930s, while in 1929 Adson and Brown proposed a posterior approach [9-11]. The operation consisted of a preganglionic sympathectomy as reported by Telford in 1935 [12] or a second thoracic ganglionectomy by Goetz and Marr [13]. In 1948 Goetz proposed the inclusion of the third and fourth thoracic ganglia as well.

More recently, in 1985, Urschel and Razzuk [14] introduced another approach based on bilateral paravertebral incisions in prone position performed by resection of the second rib, and sympathectomy of the T1, T2 and T3 ganglia.

Another alternative was the transaxillary transpleural approach, which until few years ago was the most commonly employed because of the superior visualization of the sympathetic chain and the feasibility of a more extensive sympathectomy. A further surgical option proposed by Urschel in 1993 entailed extrapleural sympathectomy through transaxillary first rib resection [15].

The first endoscopic approach to the thoracic sympathetic trunk was described by Hughes in 1942 [16]. The sympathetic trunk was approached through an endoscope placed in the third intercostal space along the anterior axillary line with the patient in the supine position [17].

The endoscopic technique regained importance with the introduction of better illumination, improved optics, and video-magnification. The first reports of VATS sympathectomy were by Lin [18], Kao [19] and Edmondson *et al.* [20] in the early '90s, who used general anesthesia and one-lung ventilation.

Since then, VATS sympathectomy has become the gold-standard for the treatment of palmar hyperhidrosis. The first series on VATS sympathectomy through Thoracic Epidural Anesthesia (TEA) and spontaneous ventilation for palmar hyperhidrosis was reported by our group in 2005 [5].

INDICATIONS FOR SURGERY

For decades, sympathectomy remained the gold standard for treatment of peripheral occlusive vascular disease. In the early 1960s, with the development of specific vascular surgery techniques, sympathectomy ceased to be the main treatment for this disease.

Currently, the most frequent indication for thoracic sympathectomy is represented by hyperhidrosis of the face, armpit and upper extremities. Other indications include [21] certain arteriospastic disorders such as Raynaud's disease and acrocyanosis; occlusive arteriolar disorders with Raynaud's phenomenon due to sclerodermia and cryoproteinemia; microembolism including intrarterial drug injections; thrombangiitis obliterans; some rare cases of atherosclerosis; occupational digital thrombosis and cold injuries; some neurological disorders such as post-traumatic sympathetic dystrophy, causalgia, vibration tools syndrome; chronic pancreatic pain syndromes [2]. Table **1** reports the ideal levels of resection for each specific pathology.

Table 1. Indications for sympathectomy and ideal level of resection [22].

Indication	Level of Thoracic Sympathectomy
Facial hyperhidrosis	T2 ganglia
Facial blushing	T2 ganglia
Arm and hand hyperhidrosis	T3-T5 ganglia
Axillary hyperhidrosis	T2-T4 ganglia
Trunk hyperhidrosis	T3-T9 ganglia
Chest pain syndrome	Communicantes rami from T2/3 to T8/9 ganglia
Chronic pancreatic pain	Communicantes rami T4-T10 ganglia
Angina pectoris	Sympathetic cardiac rami and aortic ganglia
Long QT syndrome	From the lower third of stellate ganglion to T5

Hyperhidrosis. Hyperhidrosis is a dysregulation of the neural sympathetic control of the eccrine sweat glands, which leads to excessive sweating [23]. Excessive sweating starts in childhood or adolescence and continues throughout life. It is caused by regional increased activity of the sympathetic nervous system. The thoracic sympathetic chain is involved in the neural control of upper extremities sweating, but may also involve face, trunk and plantar surfaces.

The use of topic drugs (*i.e.* aluminum chloridre), oral medications (*i.e.* psychotropics, beta-blockers and cholinergic) or iontophoresis does not provide long-lasting effects. On the contrary, thoracic sympathectomy can provide dramatic and durable benefits. In our experience, palmar hyperhidrosis is the most common indication for awake VATS sympathectomy.

The recent introduction of Botulinum toxin-A local injection seemed to limit the role of thoracic sympathectomy. Botulinum injection has proved quite effective and more easily acceptable to patients. Nevertheless, the preference of one technique over another should also take into consideration the duration of the benefit since from the effect of a botulinum injection lasts only about 6-12 months [24] whereas the effects of sympathectomy are nearly-definitive. According to these features, the overall procedure-related economic cost should also be considered since the apparently lower cost of botulinum must be counterbalanced by the need for iterative injections [24].

Sympathetic maintained pain or causalgia. Causalgia is a common indication for sympathectomy in the US although quantifying pain before and after surgery has not proved easy. Before inclusion in the surgical program, the patient should be tested with stellate ganglion block, using an intravenous injection of phentolamine. VATS thoracic sympathectomy should be reserved only for desperate cases with crippling pain [25].

Arterial insufficiency. The skin capillaries of the hand are constantly influenced by sympathetic nerve activity. Therefore VATS sympathectomy will result in increased skin circulation in the hands leading to increased temperature which lasts for about 6 months. In patients with occlusion of palmar and/or digital arteries, ulceration of the fingertips may occur. The cause of such distal vascular disease may be traumatic, atherosclerotic, or may develop as a side effect of treatment with cytostatic drugs. By abolishing the sympathetic innervation to the hand, it is possible to improve the skin circulation and thus allows the ulcerations to heal definitively [26].

Raynaud's Syndrome. Raynaud's vasospastic disease may also be positively affected by VATS sympathectomy. Immediately after surgery, operated patients will be commonly cured as shown by their warm and dry hands. However, after 6 months, signs of recurrence may reappear and after one year almost all patients return to a clinical status, which is only slightly better than the preoperative one. This is not due to regeneration of the nerve but to hypersensivity of the noradrenergic receptors regulating the pre-capillary sphincters, which reacts to very small amounts of circulating cathecolamines [27].

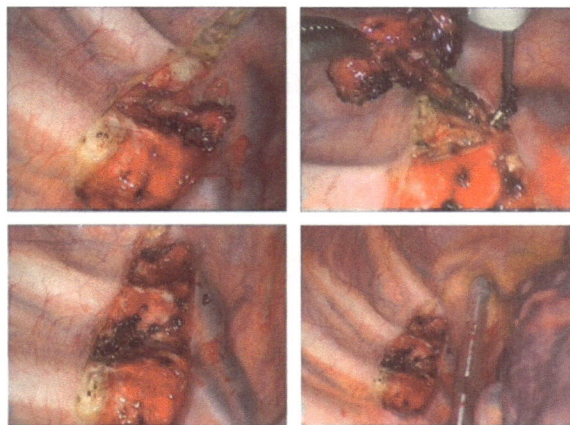

Fig. 3. Intraoperative steps of awake sympathectomy. Left upper: caudal interruption of the sympathetic chain; the nerve lies horizontally along the intercostal space; right upper: cranial dissection of the sympathetic chain which is pulled by endoscopic forceps introduced through the camera port; left lower: the operative field after chain removal; right lower: chest drainage positioning.

PREOPERATIVE WORKUP

Before undergoing the awake surgical procedure, a routine preoperative assessment is always carried out including standard laboratory tests, electrocardiogram, blood gas analysis and spirometry [28]. The radiological study includes full-length standing posteroanterior and lateral chest radiographs.

The psychologic profile of the patient and acceptance to undergo an awake procedure should also be evaluated in order to predict the mandatory cooperation required with this surgical approach.

The patient should be warned about the main physiologic consequences induced by creation of a surgical pneumothorax in awake conditions that can result in minimal ventilatory disturbances intraoperatively. At the same time, adequate information about the risk of compensatory sweating should be also provided.

Since the vast majority of patients undergoing awake VATS sympathectomy have both axillary and palmar hyperhidrosis, precise subjective and objective evaluations should be performed at baseline and then repeated postoperatively to adequately assess results. Subjective sweating changes can be assessed by specific questionnaires such as the Hyperhidrosis Quality of Life questionnaire® [29] and the Dermatology Life Quality Index® [30]. These questionnaires are not only focused on palmar hyperhidrosis but also on occurrence of postoperative compensatory sweating changes. In order to determine the impact of sweating on physical and psychosocial activities, the general health status can also be evaluated by generic questionnaires (Short Form-36® [31] and the Nottingham Health Profile® [32]). An objective assessment can be performed by the Minor's iodine starch test [33] and the pad glove weight test [34]. The temperature of the forefinger measured by a fluoroptic thermometer in a 20°C room represents another effective objective test which can easily be repeated.

ANESTHESIA AND SURGERY

Indications to awake sympathectomy. The most frequent indication for awake VATS sympathectomy is palmar and axillary hyperhidrosis. This technique may be adopted for both young and healthy subjects and all patients who have an increased risk for general anesthesia. We now propose epidural or loco-regional anesthesia as the first option, reserving general anesthesia as a further reliable alternative.

The first contraindication for awake VATS sympathectomy is the psychologic inability of the patient to tolerate an awake procedure. In spite of a formal signed consensus, the presence of severe anxiety or other neurological disturbances potentially jeopardizing the patient's full cooperation should mandate to prefer general anesthesia. In our experience, these conditions are more frequently encountered in younger patients.

In some instances, intercostal blockade by local anesthesia can be preferred to epidural anesthesia because the latter carries a potential risk of spinal hematoma. Also, placement of a thoracic epidural catheter may be difficult in patients with congenital or acquired spinal deformities in whom intercostal blockade should always be preferred.

All other contraindications are similar to those applied for any type of VATS procedure. The presence of diffuse adhesions or a pleurodesis in the upper thorax is an absolute and yet quite uncommon contraindication due to the young age of most surgical candidates. In the presence of a coagulopathy, medical treatment should be preferred due to the surgery-related risk of bleeding [35].

Thoracic epidural anesthesia. In the operating room, venous and radial artery catheters are inserted. Premedication is usually not necessary unless selective minimal sedation with midazolam is considered worthwhile. The technique of TEA requires an epidural catheter placed at the T4 to T5 level *via* a loss-of-resistance technique. Warm-cold and pin-prick discrimination tests can be used to assess the degree of thoracic analgesia.

Perioperatively, fluids are given at a minimum rate to ensure adequate urinary output. If necessary, oxygen is administered *via* a Venturi mask to keep arterial oxygen saturation above 90%. Before creation of the surgical pneumothorax, the patient must be warned that this maneuver can render spontaneous ventilation less comfortable although oxygen saturation is easily maintained at a satisfactory level. In rare instances, panic attacks triggered by anxiety or mild dyspnea can develop although they can be mostly controlled without conversion to general anesthesia, by simply increasing sedation with subhypnotic boluses of propofol (0.5-1 mg/Kg).

Due to the preferable semi-prone decubitus of the patient, the conversion to general anesthesia requires a slight change of the patient's position to lateral. In such instances, videolaryngoscopy and a fiberoptic bronchoscopy can be useful to aid faster and easier tracheal intubation [35].

Local anesthesia. When local or locoregional anesthesia is employed, sole intercostal block can be performed by local injection of a 50% mixture of lidocaine 2% and ropivacaine 7.5 mg/mL. For this purpose, at least 5 mL of this solution is injected at the site chosen for insertion of each trocar.

Supplementary local anesthesia is then locally delivered during the procedure because incision of the parietal pleura may elicit pain. This second step is accomplished under thoracoscopic vision and entails infiltration of the intercostal space from T2 to T4 directly from inside with the same anesthetic mixture. Anesthesia should be delivered medially to the sympathetic chain close to the inferior margin of the rib in order to create a space between the parietal pleura and the endothoracic fascia while avoiding vascular damage. The maneuver may separate the sympathetic chain from the surrounding structures thus simplifying the subsequent dissection. The effect of neural block due to the diffusion of the anesthesia to the other metameric levels is transient. In addition, with TEA patients maintain spontaneous breathing throughout the procedure and supplementary oxygen is administered by means of a facemask whenever required [35].

SURGICAL TECHNIQUE

A calm environment and maximal staff cooperation are mandatory prerequisites for the success of an awake procedure. Diffusion of relaxing music may be of a great help as well as frequent colloquial expressions and encouragements. The patient is placed in a semi-prone position for each side/procedure with the ipsilateral arm abducted and mild anti-Trendelenburg inclination (Fig. **4**). We routinely prefer the right chest as the first side to approach but the choice may change according to the variable clinical findings. Physiologic monitoring includes electrocardiogram, pulse oxymetry, hand temperature by means of a finger probe.

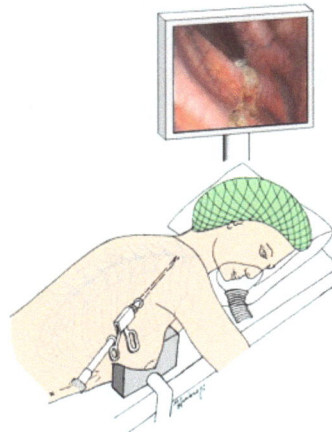

Fig. 4. Operative setting of right awake sympathectomy. The patient is placed in a semi-prone position and by a two-ports access, the camera and operative instruments are introduced.

Two ports are created respectively in the submammary line along the fifth intercostal space, anterior to midaxillary line, and the second at the third intercostal space on the midaxillary line. The former trocar is used to introduce a 30-degree, 10-mm thoracoscope while dissection is performed through the other port by a hook or dissection forceps. These two ports should be quite distant from each other to allow adequate movements of the dissector avoiding knitting effects. A thinner thoracoscope of 5-7 mm in diameter can be alternatively employed although this should be inserted more cephalad to avoid risk of damage while forcing it excessively to allow an upwards oblique vision.

Intraoperative maintenance of a certain lung ventilation does not usually jeopardize surgical maneuvering since in the semi-prone position the partially collapsed lung lies far down from the apex. Cough or deep inspirations may temporarily hamper adequate visualization requiring interruption of surgical maneuvers for a few seconds. Whenever visualization of the sympathetic chain proves difficult, a third small anterior port should be created for cotton-swab insertion working as a lung retractor.

Single-port VATS sympathectomy through an operative thoracoscope with dissection and suction devices can be an alternative option [36, 37] that may prove less time-consuming and less painful.

During VATS, thoracic sympathetic chains are readily visualized in each hemithorax in their posterior paravertebral location. The sympathetic chain appears as an elongated, white-colored structure, which is often visible underneath the parietal pleura, running parallel to the vertebral column and just lateral to the heads of the thoracic ribs. Although the location of the sympathetic chain is generally constant, its width and size can be variable; the cephalad caudal course of the chain can be straight or somewhat meandering.

Proper identification of the chain level is determined by counting the ribs from an intrathoracic approach at the time of surgery. Commonly, each ganglion is located within the intercostal space; hence, the second thoracic ganglion is found below the second rib in the second intercostal space. Some surgeons prefer a ganglion-oriented approach rather than a rib-oriented approach.

Some anatomical variations can be present and must be taken into consideration. In 7% of cases, the second thoracic ganglion cannot be identified [8]. In another 5%, it can be fused with the stellate ganglion and in 2.5% of instances, it may lie over the neck of the second rib or across the first intercostal space [6].

Due to the inconstant presence of a sympathetic ganglia at the corresponding rib, the International Sympathetic Surgery Society adopted the rib number (indicated as R) to describe the level of the procedure instead of the spinal root or the ganglia. This Society indicated by consensus a clear distinction between the definition of sympathectomy that includes either resection or division of the sympathetic chain, and that of sympathicotomy entailing division only without removal of the chain.

Planning the level and type of resection represents the major points of thoracic sympathectomy. The level of sympathectomy may change according to the pathology and the risk of complications. The ideal levels for each specific pathology have been already shown in Table **1**. They can be restricted to two or even one metamerus in order to decrease the probability and the entity of compensatory sweating.

Total ablation of the sympathetic chain is considered the classic procedure, but various lesser operations have been proposed, including simple interruption of the chain over and under the ganglion without removal, removal of the sole *rami communicantes* (ramicotomy) or clamping of the nerve with surgical clips [38, 39]. All partial techniques may result in a higher failure rate in resolving sweating but lower compensatory sweating effects.

For facial sweating or blushing, division of the chain above the second rib by endoscopic scissors can be considered sufficient. The operation can be limited to simple sympathicotomy without resection of the second ganglion. In experienced hands, separation at the lower third of the stellate ganglion can also be accomplished without causing a Horner's Syndrome [40].

In the case of palmar hyperhidrosis, the chain should be isolated at the second and third ribs and cut both cranially and caudally with or without its removal. In theory, the interruption should include T2 and T3 but not T4 in order to decrease compensatory sweating [40]. According to this purpose, the sole ramicotomy of the second and third ganglion has also been described [40]. In a similar manner, for axillary hyperhidrosis, cranial incision at the third rib level and caudal at the fourth rib level with or without ablation of the chain is performed. Interruption of the T3 and T4 sympathetic roots would result in a mild compensatory sweating. Milanez de Campos *et al.* [41] have recently proposed the division at the third rib level with the isolation of the fourth thoracic ganglia.

Once the sympathetic chain is anatomically identified and the level of resection is decided, there are several viable options for performing sympathectomy. The operation usually begins with the incision of the parietal pleura. As a first step, the *rami communicantes* are interrupted using diathermy. Subsequent mobilization of the chain from the posterior plane is performed by encircling it with an endoscopic hook. Cranial transection of the chain should always be performed by cold scissors to avoid the risk of retrograde heat injury to the stellate ganglion. Instead, caudal division can be safely performed by cautery to reduce bleeding. While performing this maneuver, one should take care not to injure the underlying costal periosteum as this can trigger postoperative intercostal burn. In addition, dissection should proceed avoiding damaging or abruptly retracting intercostal vessels. In fact, their avulsion from the aorta or azygos-hemiazygos vein can cause significant bleeding that may be difficult to control through such a minimal access. The presence of a Kuntz nerve should be carefully searched for and, if present, divided in all instances to prevent relapses.

Technological tools for chain division or destruction include electrocautery, harmonic scalpel, laser, and most recently, clipping [38, 39, 42]. This last method has the theoretic advantage of reversibility by simple removal of the clips whenever the post-sympathectomy side effects become intolerable [43]. In the case of resection, the specimen should always be sent for histological examination in order to confirm the presence of sympathetic nerves and the extent of the resection that also proves useful for medical-legal purposes.

No additional sedative medication or intravenous analgesic agents are usually given to the patient throughout the procedure. Lung re-expansion is obtained by asking the patient to cough and inhale deeply while keeping trocar incisions closed with gauzes, and is controlled under thoracoscopic vision. No chest drain is usually positioned after the procedure. A temporary 24Ch thoracic drain connected to mild suction may sometimes be inserted for few hours.

Once one side is completed, the operation can be interrupted or may proceed for treatment of the contralateral side. The opportunity to perform a one-stage bilateral sympathectomy or rather a staged unilateral treatment has been comprehensively discussed in the literature [44]. The majority of surgeons prefers a one-stage bilateral approach but the reason for this choice has been mainly attributed to the avoidance of repeated general anesthesia. We now usually prefer a staged approach to better evaluate the results and occurrence of compensatory sweating before deciding to operate the contralateral side.

POSTOPERATIVE CARE

Following a short surveillance period in the recovery room, patients are transferred to the ward, and drinking, walking and eating are rapidly allowed. Whenever necessary, analgesic medication is administered. Patients undergoing awake VATS sympathectomy are usually discharged the same day of surgery once a routine postoperative chest roentgenogram has excluded the presence of residual pneumothorax, which can be found in less than 10% of the cases [5]. In some peculiar cases, the discharge may be postponed to the day after the operation.

Mild physical activities can be started immediately after discharge and gradually increased thereafter. It would be desirable for each patient to freely express written personal satisfaction degree about the chosen type of anesthesia and the effects of the procedure. This represents an important standpoint to ameliorate the technique and refine indications. All patients are examined before discharge for evidence of bradycardia or Horner's syndrome.

COMPLICATIONS AND SIDE EFFECTS

Postoperative complications are mainly surgery-related rather than anesthesiology-related. Uncommon minor complications include [45, 46] pneumothorax, bleeding, infections, paresthesias, and incisional pain (Table **2**). One of the most disturbing and yet unusual complications is the development of a Horner's syndrome due to stellate ganglion damage [47]. Other rare complications can be represented by chylothorax and esophageal or lung injury [48].

Table 2. Frequency of complications after sympathectomy [28].

Complication	Frequency (%)
Severe compensatory sweating	20 to 80
Depression in heart rate	10
Horner's syndrome	5
Incisional pain	2
Paresthesias	1
Pneumothorax	1
Bleeding and infection	1
Chylothorax or esophageal and lung injury	<1

The most common postoperative adverse event is the onset of compensatory sweating [49]. It may progressively affect the non-operated limb or other districts like the scalp, trunk, groin and feet. Compensatory sweating is usually moderate and temporary, but in some unpredictable instances it may become significant and even more intolerable than the pre-sympathectomy hyperhidrosis [50]. Milanez de Campos *et al.* [51] found an almost direct relationship between the post-sympathectomy extent of compensatory sweating and body mass index. This is probably related to the lower heat-dispersion observed in obese subjects who have a lower body-surface/body-volume.

Patients must always be clearly warned about this risk and full written informed consent to sympathectomy should be obtained before this type of surgery [52]. Severity of compensatory sweating may be decreased by reducing the number of the metameri to be resected or performing only partial denervations like ramicotomy [53].

A certain postoperative reduction in heart rate is expected in all patients. This is a possible major cause of postoperative dysfunction and should be cautiously monitored. Patients with resting heart rate below 50 to 60 beats per minute should undergo an electrocardiogram [54-56].

COMMENT

VATS sympathectomy is a surgical procedure aimed at treatment of a non-life-threatening condition. The risk of complications and any potential discomfort should therefore be minimized. According to this premise, the possibility to employ an awake VATS seems to be logical and desirable in this setting.

As far as the preferred type of surgical technique is concerned, questions have been raised as to the validity and effectiveness of different types of sympathectomies [57, 58] and their comparative merits with respect to other non-surgical treatment options [59, 60].

Since the most common indication for thoracic sympathectomy is represented by hyperhidrosis, one of the major issues when establishing indications for surgical treatment is represented by the difficulty in quantifying the severity of the disease. For this purpose, different tests and specific questionnaires have been developed [61]. However, the great part of this decision-making process is strictly related to patient acceptance and degree of satisfaction towards both anesthesia and surgery.

A large number of studies have shown positive satisfaction rates after sympathectomy for hyperhidrosis ranging from 85% to 95%[62]. The major reason of dissatisfaction can be attributed to the occurrence of excessive compensatory sweating [63]. As previously mentioned, this unpleasant and yet frequent complication may be limited in extent by reducing the number of resected ganglia to two [64] or by performing partial denervations like ramicotomy [65]. Unfortunately, these procedures, and especially the latter one, weaken the effects of sympathectomy. One valid option can be represented by the initial unilateral treatment. In this way, the surgeon can better evaluate the contralateral compensatory effects and predict the final results achievable once the bilateral operation is completed.

VATS sympathectomy under general anesthesia and a single-lumen endotracheal intubation is a well established procedure, although adverse-effects related to general anesthesia should not be underestimated. Theoretically, one-lung ventilation represents the easiest way for the surgeon to operate in a widely visible and immobile operative field. However, the physiological impact of general anesthesia and one-lung ventilation is well known and several adverse effects can derive from its use [66, 67]. Many of these are related to complete exclusion of one lung from ventilation and use of intermittent positive pressure ventilation, which can cause an increment in shunt fraction and right ventricle work [68].

On the other hand, with an awake procedure, some physiological discomfort can be created by the surgical pneumothorax although this proved well tolerated by the majority of patients, particularly when dealing with fit and healthy, young or even adolescent subjects, as those suffering from hyperhidrosis often are [4].

Although no randomized controlled study matching awake versus conventional VATS sympathectomy has been carried out so far, we believe that the use of TEA or local anesthesia in this setting can offer several advantages [4, 5]. Immediate relief of symptoms and significant improvement in quality of life can be obtained with low morbidity regardless of the type of anesthesia that is chosen, although awake patients have shown less anesthesia-related adverse effects, a shorter in-operating room time and a faster resumption to common daily life activities. These characteristics facilitated our fast-track surgery program that allowed patients to be managed within a one-day surgery setting, thus also reducing overall procedure-related costs.

In addition, patient satisfaction evaluated by a direct interview 24 hours after procedures was significantly better in the awake group [5]. Furthermore, it is worth noting that following unilateral awake VATS sympathectomy, patients undergoing completion of the bilateral treatment more commonly prefer another awake procedure.

One limitation can be represented by the difficulty of operating in an awake patient due to a restricted and precarious operative field, cooperating with the patient and refraining from inappropriate comments [69]. The surgeon and the staff should be very well trained in VATS and familiar to working as a single team. Though relatively simple and rapid, awake sympathectomy should not be attempted without appropriate training.

CONCLUSION

In conclusion, awake VATS sympathectomy proved to be a feasible and safe procedure in selected patients and might succeed in combining maximal patient satisfaction, minimal morbidity and low costs.

REFERENCES

[1]　Claes G. Indication for endoscopic thoracic sympathectomy. Clin Auton Res 2003;13:16-9.

[2]　Worsey J, Ferson PF, Keenan RJ, Julian TB, Landreneau RJ. Thoracoscopic pancreatic denervation for pain control in irresectable pancreatic cancer. Br J Surg 1993; 80: 1051-1052.

[3]　Daniel TM. Thoracoscopic sympathectomy. Chest Surg Clin N Am 1996; 6: 69-83.

[4]　Mineo TC. Epidural anesthesia in awake thoracic surgery. Eur J Cardio-thorac Surg 2007; 32:13-9.

[5]　Elia S, Guggino V, Mineo D, *et al.* Awake one stage bilateral thoracoscopic sympathectomy for palmar hyperhidrosis: a safe outpatient procedure. Eur J Cardio-thorac Surg 2005;3:12-17.

[6]　Singh B, Moodley J, Randall PK, *et al.* Pitfalls in thoracoscopic sympathectomy: mechanism for failure. Surg Laparosc Endosc Percutan Tech 2001;6:364-7.

[7]　Kuntz A. Distribution of the sympathetic rami to the brachial plexus: its relation to sympathectomy affecting the upper extremity. Arch Surg 1927; 15: 871-7.

[8]　Chung IH, Oh CS, Koh KS, *et al.* Anatomic variations of the T2 nerve root (including the nerve of Kuntz) and their implications for sympathectomy. J Thorac Cardiovasc Surg 2002;123:498-501.

[9]   Leriche R. De l'elongation et de la section des nerfs perivasculaires dans certains syndromes douloureux d'origine arterielle et dans quelques troubles trophiques. Lyon Chir 1913;10:378-382.

[10]   Adson AW, Brown GE. Treatment of Raynaud's disease by lumbar ramisection and ganglionectomy and perivascular sympathetic neurectomy of the common iliacs. JAMA 1925; 84:1908-10.

[11]   Adson AW, Brown GE. Raynaud's disease of the upper extremities; successful treatment by resection of the sympathetic cervicothoracic and second thoracic ganglions and the intervening trunk. JAMA 1929;92:444-9.

[12]   Telford ED. The technique of sympathectomy. Br J Surg 1935;23:448-50.

[13]   Goetz RH, Marr JAS. The importance of the second thoracic ganglion for the sympathetic supply of the upper extremities- two new approaches for its removal. Clin Proc 1944;3:102-14.

[14]   Urschel HC, Razzuk MA. Posterior thoracic sympathectomy. In Malt RA, Ed. Surgical techniques illustrated: a comparative atlas. Philadelphia, WB Saunders, 1985; pp. 615-8.

[15]   Urschel HC. Dorsal sympathectomy and management of thoracic outlet syndrome with VATS. Ann Thorac Surg 1993;56:717-20.

[16]   Hughes J. Endothoracic sympathectomy. J R Soc Med 1942;35:585-6.

[17]   Kux M. Thoracic endoscopic sympathectomy in palmar and axillar hyperhidrosis. Arch Surg 1978;113:264-6.

[18]   Lin CC. A new method of thoracoscopic sympathectomy in hyperhidrosis palmaris. Surg Endosc 1990;4:224-6.

[19]   Kao MC. Video endoscopic sympathectomy using a fiberoptic CO_2 laser to treat palmar hyperhidrosis. Neurosurg 1992;30:131-5.

[20]   Edmondson RA, Banerjee AK, Rennie JA. Endoscopic transthoracic sympathectomy in the treatment of hyperhidrosis. Ann Surg 1992;215:289-93.

[21]   Hashmonai M, Schein M. Upper thoracic sympathectomy- open approaches. In: Paterson-Brown S, Garden J, Eds. Surgical Laparoscopy. London, W.B. Saunders, 1994; pp. 587-603.

[22]   Wittmoser R. Die thorakoskopische operation des rechten unteren brustsympathicus. Med Bilddienst (BD) Roche 1954;6:79

[23]   Cinà CS, Cinà MM, Clase CM. Endoscopic thoracic sympathectomy for hyperhidrosis: technique and results. J Min Access Surg 2007;3:132-40.

[24]   Ambrogi V, Campione E, Mineo D, et al. Bilateral thoracoscopic T2 to T3 sympathectomy versus botulinum injection in palmar hyperhidrosis. Ann Thorac Surg 2009; 88:238-45.

[25]   Samuelsson H, Claes G, Drott C. Endoscopic electrocautery of the upper thoracic sympathetic chain for treatment of sympathetic mantained pain. Eur J Surg 1994;160:55-57.

[26]   Claes G, Drott G, Gothberg G. Thoracoscopic sympathicotomy for arterial insufficiency. Eur J Surg 1994;160:63-4.

[27]   Adson AW, Brown GE. The treatment of Raynaud's disease by resection of the upper thoracic and lumbar sympathetic ganglia and trunks. Surg Gynecol Obstet 1929;48:577-603.

[28]   Krasna MJ. Thoracoscopic sympathectomy. Thorac Surg Clin 2010;20:323-30.

[29]   Milanez De Campos JR, Kauffman P, et al. Quality of life, before and after thoracic sympathectomy: report on 378 operated patients. Ann Thorac Surg 2003;76:886-91.

[30]   Finlay AY, Khan GK. Dermatology Life Quality Index (DLQI)-a simple practical measure for routine clinical use. Clin Exp Dermatol 1994;19:210-6.

[31]   Brazier JE, Harper R, Jones NM, et al. Validating the SF-36 Health Survey Questionnaire: new outcome measure for primary care. BMJ 1992;18:160-4.

[32]   Wiklund I. The Nottingham Health Profile: a measure of health related quality of life. Scand J Prim Health Care 1990;1:S15-S8.

[33]   Sato KT, Richardson A, Timm DE, Sato K. One-step iodine starch method for direct visualization of sweating. Am J Med Sci 1988;295:528-31.

[34]   Kalkan MT, Aydemir EH, Karakoc Y, Korpinar MA. The measurement of sweat intensity using a new technique. Tr J Med Sci 1998;28:515-7.

[35]   Pompeo E, Tacconi F, Mineo TC. Awake video-assisted thoracoscopic biopsy in complex anterior mediastinal masses. Thorac Surg Clin 2010;20:225-33.

[36]   Chen YB, Ye W, Yang WT, et al. Uniportal versus biportal video-assisted thoracoscopic sympathectomy for palmar hyperhidrosis. Chin Med J 2009;122:1525-28.

[37]   Murphy MO, Ghosh J, Khwaja N, et al. Upper dorsal endoscopic thoracic sympathectomy: a comparison of one- and two-port ablate techniques. Eur J Cardiothorac Surg 2006;30:223-7.

[38] Lin CC, Mo LR, Lee LS, *et al.* Thoracoscopic T2 sympathetic block by clipping. A better and reversible operation for treatment of hyperhydrosis palmaris: experience with 326 cases. Eur J Surg 1998;580:S13-S6.

[39] Sugimura H, Spratt EH, Compeau CG, Kattail D, Shargall Y. Thoracoscopic sympathetic clipping for hyperhidrosis: Long term results and reversibility. J Thorac Cardiovasc Surg 2009;137:1370-8.

[40] Weksler B, Luketich JD, Shende MR. Endoscopic thoracic sympathectomy: at what level should you perform surgery? Thorac Surg Clin 2008;18:183-91.

[41] Milanez de Campos JR, Kauffmann P, Wolosker N *et al.* Axillary hyperhidrosis. T3/T4 versus T4 thoracic sympathectomy in a series of 276 cases. J Laparoendoscop Adv Surg Tech 2006;16:598-63.

[42] Hashmonai M, Assalia A, Kopelman D. Thoracoscopic sympathectomy for palmar hyperhidrosis. Ablate or resect? Surg Endosc 2001;15:435-41.

[43] Neumayer C, Zacherl J, Holak G, *et al.* Limited endoscopic thoracic sympathetic block for hyperhidrosis of the upper limb. Reduction of compensatory sweating by clipping T4. Surg Endosc 2004;18:152-6.

[44] Awad MS, Elzeftawy A, Mansour S, Elshelfa W. One stage bilateral endoscopic sympathectomy under local anesthesia: is a valid, and safe procedure for treatment of palmer hyperhidrosis? J Minim Access Surg 2010;6:11-5.

[45] Plas EG, Fugger R, Herbst F, *et al.* Complication of endoscopic thoracic sympathectomy. Surgery 1995;118:493-5.

[46] Dumont P. Side effects and complications of surgery for hyperhidrosis. Thorac Surg Clin 2008;18:193-207.

[47] Singh B, Moodley J, Allopi L, Cassimjee HM. Horner syndrome after sympathectomy in the thoracoscopic era. Surg Laparosc Endosc Percutan Tech 2006 Aug;16:222-5.

[48] Heckmann M. Complications in patients with palmar hyperhidrosis treated with transthoracic endoscopic sympathectomy. Neurosurg 1998;42:1403-4.

[49] Libson S, Kirshtein B, Mizrahi S, Lantsberg L. Evaluation of compensatory sweating after bilateral thoracoscopic sympathectomy for palmar hyperhidrosis. Surg Laparosc Endosc Percutan Tech 2007;17:511-513.

[50] Licht PB, Pilegaard HK. Severity of compensatory sweating after thoracoscopic sympathectomy. Ann Thorac Surg 2004;78:427-31.

[51] Milanez de Campos JR, Wolosker N, Takeda FR, *et al.* The body mass index and level of resection. Predictive factors for compensatory sweating after sympathectomy. Clin Auton Res 2005;15:116-120.

[52] Leseche G, Castier Y, Thabut G, *et al.* Endoscopic transthoracic sympathectomy for upper limb hyperhidrosis: limited sympathectomy does not reduce postoperative compensatory sweating. J Vasc Surg 2002;37:124-8.

[53] Dumont P, Denoyer A, Robin P. Long-term results of thoracoscopic sympathectomy for hyperhidrosis. Ann Thorac Surg 2004;78:1801-7.

[54] Inbar O, Leviel D, Shwartz I, Paran H, Whipp BJ. Thoracic sympathectomy and cardiopulmonary responses to exercise. Eur J Appl Physiol 2008;104:79-86.

[55] Papa MZ, Bass A, Schneiderman J, *et al.* Cardiovascular changes after bilateral upper dorsal sympathectomy. Short and long-term effects. Ann Surg 1986; 204: 715-8.

[56] Noppen M, Dendale P, Hagers Y *et al.* Changes in cardiocirculatory autonomic function after thoracoscopic upper dorsal sympathicolysis for essential hyperhidrosis. J Auton Nerv Syst 1996; 60: 115-20.

[57] Inan K, Goksel OS, Uçak A, *et al.* Thoracic endoscopic surgery for hyperhidrosis: comparison of different techniques. Thorac Cardiovasc Surg 2008;56:210-3.

[58] Baumgartner FJ. Surgical approaches and techniques in the management of severe hyperhidrosis. Thorac Surg Clin 2008;18:167-81.

[59] Reisfeld R, Berliner KI. Evidence-based review of the nonsurgical management of hyperhidrosis. Thorac Surg Clin 2008;18:157-66.

[60] Gee S, Yamauchi PS. Nonsurgical management of hyperhidrosis. Thorac Surg Clin 2008; 18:141-55.

[61] Solish N, Wang R, Murray CA. Evaluating the patient presenting with hyperhidrosis. Thorac Surg Clin 2008;18:133-40.

[62] Swan MC, Paes T. Quality of life evaluation following endoscopic transthoracic sympathectomy for upper limb and facial hyperhydrosis. Ann Chir Gynaecol 2001;90:157-9.

[63] Almeida de Araùjo CA, Azevedo IM, Fernandes Ferreira MA, *et al.* Compensatory sweating after thoracoscopic sympathectomy: characteristics, prevalence and influence on patient satisfaction. J Bras Pneumol 2009;35:213-20.

[64] Dumont P, Hamm A, Skrobala D, Robin P, Toumieux B. Bilateral thoracoscopy for sympathectomy in the treatment of hyperhidrosis. Eur J Cardiothorac Surg 1997;11:774-5.

[65]   Oliveira HA, Ximenes M, Filho FB, *et al.* Experimental selective sympathicotomy (ramicotomy) and sympathetic regeneration. Interact Cardio Vasc Thorac Surg 2009; 9:411-5.

[66]   Fredman B, Olsfanger D, Jereikin R. Thoracoscopic sympathectomy in the treatment of palmar hyperhydrosis: anaesthetic implications. Br J Anaesth 1997;79:113-9.

[67]   Conacher ID. Anaesthesia for thoracoscopic surgery. Best Pract Res Clin Anaesthesiol 2002;16:53-62.

[68]   Whitehead T, Slutsky AS. The pulmonary physician in critical care. Ventilatory induced lung injury. Thorax 2002;57:635-42.

[69]   Katlic MR, Facktor MA. Video-assisted thoracic surgery utilizing local anesthesia and sedation: 384 consecutive cases. Ann Thorac Surg 2010;90:240-5.

CHAPTER 15

Video-Assisted Thoracic Surgery Utilizing Local Anesthesia and Sedation

Mark Katlic[*]

Department of Surgery, Sinai Hospital,Baltimore, MD, USA

Abstract: Video-Assisted Thoracic Surgery (VATS) is usually performed with general anesthesia and endotracheal intubation. There are risks to such anesthesia and some operations may not require general anesthesia or intubation. Presently at our institution all stable patients with large unilateral pleural effusion, Stage I and II empyema, pericardial effusion with coexisting pleural effusion, diffuse lung disease, or multiple lung nodules are offered local anesthesia and sedation. No patient is excluded based on age or comorbidity.

Details of the technique are presented in this chapter. All operations are performed in the operating room with the patient in full lateral position.

Of 384 consecutive patients reported in 2010, no patient required intraoperative intubation or epidural or nerve block analgesia. No patient required conversion to thoracotomy. Diagnosis was achieved, without need for additional procedure, in all cases of biopsy; 2 patients (3% of 74) required a subsequent procedure for empyema. No patient had awareness or memory of the operation. There were 10 complications (3%) and no deaths due to operation.

VATS utilizing local anesthesia/sedation is well tolerated, safe, and valuable for an increasing number of indications.

Keywords: Video-assisted thoracic surgery, local anesthesia.

The history of video-assisted thoracic surgery (VATS) utilizing local anesthesia and sedation is the history of VATS itself. Both Jacobaeus [1] and Bethune [2] performed thoracoscopy under local anesthesia, the former to allow the lung to collapse (for the accepted treatment of tuberculosis) and the latter to prevent it (selectively adhere one lobe for later open removal of its neighboring lobe). The arrival of safe general anesthesia, fiberoptic telescopes, and sophisticated instruments allowed modern VATS procedures, including pulmonary lobectomy, thymectomy, and esophagectomy.

General anesthesia and endotracheal intubation, however, are not necessary for every type of operation and there are risks to such anesthesia.

Surgeons have performed VATS utilizing less than general anesthesia, chiefly for pleural disease. Twenty years ago Rusch [3] employed multiple intercostal blocks and a standard rigid mediastinoscope for pleural problems in 46 patients. Similar nerve block analgesia was used with fiberoptic equipment a decade later to treat malignant pleural effusion [4] and spontaneous pneumothorax [5] and more recently for thoracic sympathectomy [6]. Current techniques of awake thoracic surgery are presented in other chapters of this book. In Saudi Arabia Al-Abdullatief [7] employs epidural analgesia for a variety of awake thoracic operations, as does Macchiarini [8] for upper airway surgery. In Italy local anesthesia and sedation have been utilized for pleural disease [9]; and Pompeo and Mineo [10-15] have performed a broader range of procedures with "awake thoracoscopic surgery" (epidural analgesia, spontaneous ventilation).

Encouraged by the results treating pleural disease with VATS under local anesthesia and success creating an unanticipated pericardial window in a patient undergoing surgery for a malignant pleural effusion we broadened our indications for this technique [16].

*Address correspondence to Mark Katlic:** Department of Surgery, Sinai Hospital, Baltimore, MD, USA; Email: mkatlic@lifebridgehealth.org

Eugenio Pompeo (Ed)

TECHNIQUE

Selection Criteria. Patients are not selected for this technique if any of the following pertains: hemodynamic instability, patient already intubated and ventilated, anticipated need for decortication, solitary pulmonary nodule, need for mediastinal dissection, or pericardial effusion without coexisting large pleural effusion. All patients with large unilateral pleural effusion, empyema, pericardial effusion with coexisting pleural effusion, diffuse lung disease, or multiple pulmonary nodules are offered local anesthesia and sedation (Table **1**). No patient is excluded based on age or comorbidity.

Table 1. Major indications to local anesthesia/sedation or general anesthesia in VATS.

General Anesthesia	Local Anesthesia/Sedation
Hemodynamic instability	Hemodynamic stability
Patient already intubated/ventilated	Large unilateral pleural effusion
Empyema, decortication anticipated	Empyema/Chronic hemothorax
Solitary pulmonary nodule	Diffuse lung disease, multiple nodules
	Pericardial effusion with coexisting pleural effusion

General. Patients are sedated with an individualized combination of midazolam, fentanyl, and propofol; ketamine has been effective as has a continuous infusion of propofol (starting at about 120 micrograms/kg/min and increasing as needed). Supplemental oxygen is administered *via* face mask and oxygen saturation, electrocardiogram, and blood pressure are monitored. End-tidal carbon dioxide can be monitored *via* a catheter tucked into an oral airway. Flexible bronchoscopy is carried out when indicated, then the patient is turned into full lateral position. Local anesthesia (1% xylocaine, 10 to 30cc depending on number of incisions) is infiltrated into skin, then 1-3 two centimeter incisions are made. Intercostal muscle and pleura are infiltrated under direct vision or palpation through the skin incision.

Contingency plans for intubation or conversion to thoracotomy (never used) include immediate placement of a chest tube through one incision and occlusive dressings to others, followed by turning the patient supine for intubation. Alternatively, a laryngeal mask airway can be placed with the patient in lateral position depending upon circumstances.

Elective patients are discharged the same or next day, usually with a Heimlich valve attached to the chest tube. The chest tube is removed in the office as appropriate.

Pleural Disease. One port is employed, with cup biopsy forceps and possible talc insufflation catheter passed along the outside wall of the short trocar (Endopath®, Ethicon) (Fig. **1**). When necessary, *e.g.*, for multiloculated empyema, a second site without trocar allows introduction of other instruments in order to disrupt adhesions (**Video 1**; **Video 2**; **Video 3**).

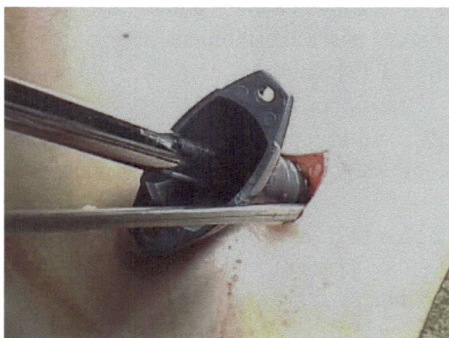

Fig. 1. Single-trocar technique. One port is used to insert several instruments.

Lung Biopsy. Three incisions allow introduction of telescope *via* trocar, grasping ring forceps, and endoscopic stapling device. Finger palpation is performed as needed. Pleural adhesions can be divided bluntly or with scissors or cautery. Typically, two or three wedge biopsies are performed with targeted areas of lung identified from preoperative Computed Tomogram (CT) scans (**Video 4**).

Pericardial Window. If a pleural effusion co-exists, and the lung is thereby "accustomed" to being collapsed, two sites will suffice, with grasper being passed alongside the telescope and an anterior site for #15 scalpel blade then endoscopic scissors. If necessary a third anterior-superior site allows the lung to be further retracted superiorly with a grasper or blunt instrument. Only hemodynamically stable patients are offered this approach. Arterial line monitoring is not employed (**Video 5**).

RESULTS

Results of our technique in 384 consecutive patients were recently reported. The medical records of all patients undergoing VATS utilizing local anesthesia and sedation at our system's three hospitals between 6/1/02 and 6/1/09 were retrospectively reviewed. The authors or residents under supervision performed all procedures. Unsuccessful attempts at this technique were eligible for inclusion but there were none. No patient was excluded based on age or comorbidity. All procedures were performed in the operating room with patients in full lateral position; no patient had endotracheal intubation or epidural or nerve block analgesia.

One hundred twenty six of these procedures in 115 patients were previously reported [16]. The Geisinger Health System Institutional Research Review Board approved this research.

Three hundred fifty-three patients ranged in age from 21 to 100 years (mean 67, median 69) and in size from 40 to 172 kg. There were 189 men and 164 women. At the time of the procedure American Society of Anesthesiologists Physical Status Class were: 1 (none), 2 (29 patients), 3 (225 patients), 4 (130 patients).

Diagnoses (Table **2**) included malignant pleural effusion 142 (Fig. **2**), benign pleural effusion 98, empyema 74 (Fig. **3**), lung disease 40 (Figs. **4** and **5**), chronic hemothorax 13, pericardial effusion 7 (Fig. **6**), mesothelioma 4, chylothorax 2, lung abscess 2, mediastinal mass 1, pneumothorax 1. The 384 procedures included drainage of pleural effusion/pleural biopsy 243 (183 with talc insufflation, 60 without talc), drainage of empyema 74, lung biopsy 41, evacuate chronic hemothorax 13, pericardial window 7, treat chylothorax 2, drain lung abscess 2, biopsy mediastinal mass 1, treat pneumothorax 1. Mean operating time for all procedures was 28 minutes (range 8-111 minutes). No patient required intraoperative intubation or epidural or nerve block analgesia.

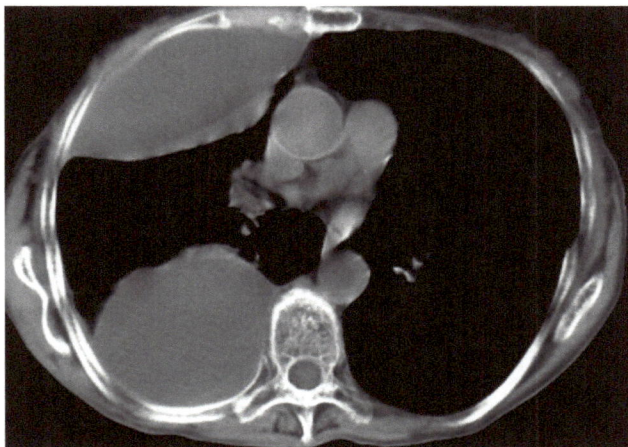

Fig. 2. Complex pleural effusion related to ovarian cancer.

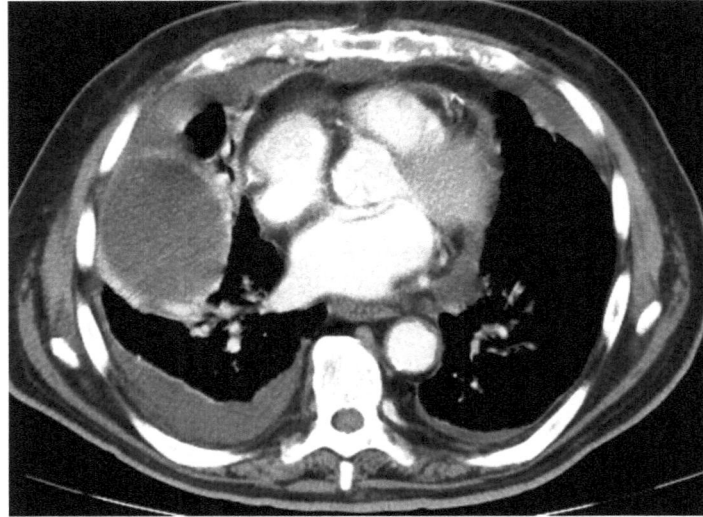

Fig. 3. Fibrinopurulent empyema thoracis treated by VATS under local anesthesia/sedation.

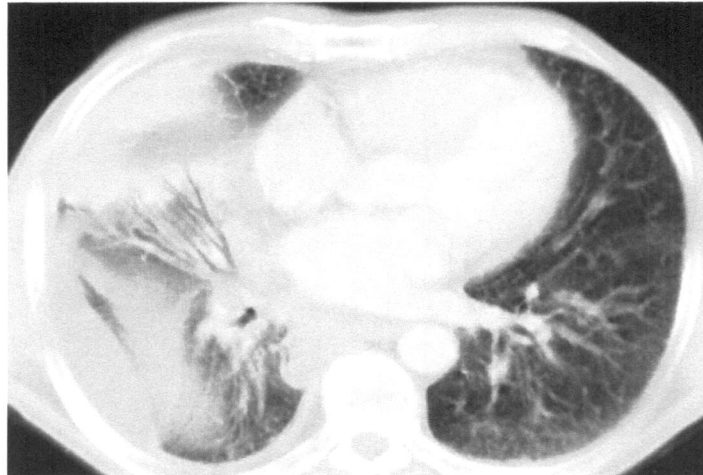

Fig. 4. Primary lung amyloidois.

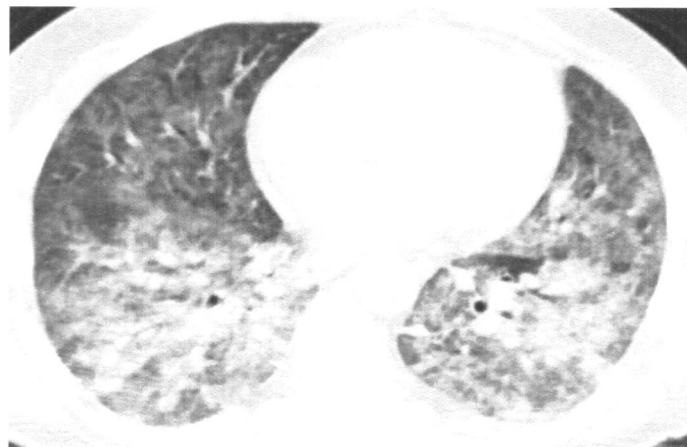

Fig. 5. Mixed cytomegalovirus and pneumocystis carinii infection in a patient with HIV.

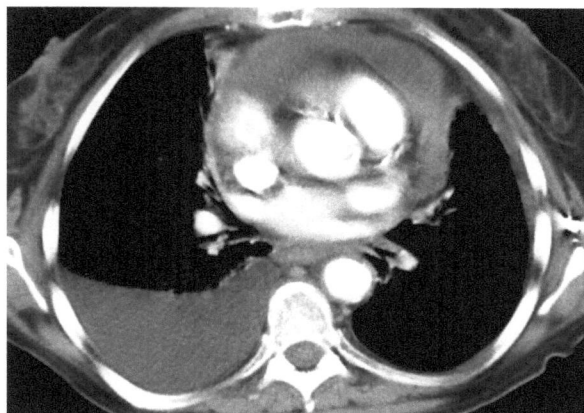

Fig. 6. Pleural-pericardial effusion successfully managed by VATS under local anesthesia.

Table 2. Cases treated by VATS under local anesthesia and sedation at the Geisinger Medical Center.

CONDITION	TOTAL CASES	(%)
Malignant pleural effusion	**142**	**37**
Lung cancer	66	46
Breast cancer	24	17
Mesothelioma	10	7
Endometrial/Ovarian cancer	9	6
Esophageal	6	4
Colon	4	3
Prostate	4	3
Lymphoma	4	3
Gastric	3	2
Other	12	8
Benign pleural effusion	**98**	**25.5**
Chronic pleuritis	67	68
Chronic pleuritis, radiotherapy	18	18
Renal failure	7	7
Ascites	6	6
Empyema	**74**	**19.2**
Lung Disease	**40**	**10.4**
Usual interstitial pneumonitis	7	17
Chronic aspiration pneumonia	4	10
Granuloma	4	10
Interstitial disease	4	10
Lung cancer	3	7.5
Pneumoconiosis	3	7.5
Metastatic cancer	3	7.5
Cytomegalovirus pneumonitis	2	5
Bronchiolitis obliterans organizing pneumonia	2	5
Bacterial pneumonitis	2	5

Table 2: cont....

Chemotherapy toxicity	2	5
Other, 1 each (aspergillus, primary amyloidosis, bronchiectasis, pneumocystis)	4	10
Chronic hemothorax	**13**	**3.5**
Pericardial effusion	**7**	**1.8**
Metastatic non-small cell lung cancer	4	57
Metastatic small cell lung cancer	3	43
Mesothelioma	**4**	**1**
Chylothorax	**2**	**<1**
Lung abscess	**2**	**<1**
Mediastinal mass (metastatic breast cancer)	**1**	**<1**
Pneumothorax	**1**	**<1**

No patient required conversion to thoracotomy. Diagnosis was achieved, without need for additional procedure, in all cases of biopsy; 2 patients (3% of 74) required a subsequent procedure for empyema. No patient had awareness or memory of the operation. There were 10 complications (3%): cerebrovascular accident 2, atrial fibrillation 2, persistent air leak 2, and 1 each empyema, transient renal failure (attributed to ketorolac), transient respiratory failure, and urinary tract infection. There were no deaths due to operation. Within 30 days of operation 1 patient died from overanticoagulation and 9 from underlying disease: advanced lung cancer (3), congestive heart failure (2), multiple organ failure (2), cytomegalovirus and pneumocystis in an HIV positive patient (1), primary amyloidosis (1).

COMMENT

For a subset of our patient population we are returning VATS to its beginnings, as a simple, straightforward procedure to manage pleural problems. The addition of suitable sedating drugs and sophisticated instruments, *e.g.*, endoscopic staplers, allows us to broaden our range to include lung biopsy, treatment of loculated empyema, and pericardial window procedures. General anesthesia and endotracheal intubation are a luxury rather than a necessity for many video-assisted thoracic operations, and this luxury is not entirely free. Admittedly, the collapsed quiet lung is easier to palpate (*e.g.*, to find a solitary pulmonary nodule); this also facilitates access to the mediastinum and better overall visualization. Lengthy procedures are possible. However, deep anesthesia ---with its hemodynamic consequences and slower recovery--- is often necessary for the patient to tolerate an endotracheal tube, particularly a double-lumen tube. Muscle paralysis is usually needed. There is more potential for drying of the airway.

Despite published reports every year few surgeons consider that tracheal trauma, and even esophageal trauma, can occur with endotracheal intubation. In 2005 Gomez-Car [17] reviewed 90 cases of iatrogenic tracheobronchial injury from seven series. Conti [18] in 2006 discussed 30 consecutive cases over a 12-year period. Schneider [19] in 2007 reported 29 cases from a single institution over a 10 year period. A recent review by Minambres [20] found 182 reported cases of postintubation tracheal rupture over 40 years, with a mortality of 22% and significant morbidity. The admittedly small risk of this trauma is eliminated by allowing the patient to breathe spontaneously without a tube. In addition, many of these procedures are performed for palliation in patients with advanced malignancy, making risk higher Patients as old as 100 years and as large as 140 kg tolerate this technique and its obligatory unilateral pneumothorax. For some patients the lung has already been partially collapsed due to effusion or empyema. In addition, the ipsilateral lung receives both less ventilation and less perfusion with the patient in lateral position, resulting in less physiologic shunt than anticipated. Chhajed [21] reported that hypoventilation does occur with an awake technique: mean pCO_2 increased a mean 13 mmHg to 52.3 mmHg (range 37 to 77 mmHg) and oxygen saturation decreased a mean of 4.6% (range 1 to 14%). Others [5] have reported little change in oxygen saturation. Our patients, even those with severe generalized interstitial lung disease, tolerated these procedures.

CONCLUSION

Sedating drugs are important supplements to disciplined local anesthesia and careful manipulation of instruments. An occasional patient will cough but none move or experience discomfort. These operations require no special skills and are routinely performed by residents under our guidance. Our anesthesiology staff have come to prefer this approach and express disappointment when we request general anesthesia for a more complicated case.

Pompeo and Mineo have pioneered the use of a related technique, epidural analgesia with light sedation and spontaneous ventilation. They have documented decreased anesthesia and operating room time [10, 13], decreased hospital length of stay [10, 12, 13], decreased cost [6, 12], and increased patient satisfaction [6, 10]. Others have also reported decreased operating room time [5] and decreased length of stay [5, 7].

Other surgeons who perform awake VATS have reported excellent results with the epidural analgesia technique noted above and with nebulized lidocaine to suppress cough [22]; we have not found these to be necessary. We do not routinely employ Bilevel Positive Airway Pressure (BIPAP) *via* facemask or nasal mask [23] but have continued this for several patients who came to the operating room with it.

Our recommendation to centers wishing to start this practice is to begin with treating large unilateral pleural effusions and early empyemas, then progress to multiloculated empyema, lung biopsy, and pericardial window procedures.

In conclusion, VATS utilizing local anesthesia and sedation is well-tolerated, safe, and valuable for a number of indications.

ACKNOWLEDGMENT

Part of the information included in this chapter has been previously published by the author in the European Journal of Cardiothoracic Surgery, Volume 30, Issue 3, September 2006, Pages 529-532.

REFERENCES

[1]   Jacobaeus HC. The practical importance of thoracoscopy in surgery of the chest. Surg Gynecol Obstet 1922;34:289-96.

[2]   Bethune N. Pleural poudrage. A new technique for the deliberate production of pleural adhesions as a preliminary to lobectomy. J Thorac Surg 1935;4:251-61.

[3]   Rusch VW, Mountain C. Thoracoscopy under regional anesthesia for the diagnosis and management of pleural disease. Am J Surg 1987;154:274-8.

[4]   Danby CA, Adebonojo SA, Moritz DM. Video-assisted talc pleurodesis for malignant pleural effusions utilizing local anesthesia and I.V. sedation. Chest 1998;113:739-42.

[5]   Nezu K, Kushibe K, Tojo T, Takahama M, Kitamura S. Thoracoscopic wedge resection of blebs under local anesthesia with sedation for treatment of a spontaneous pneumothorax. Chest 1997;111:230-5.

[6]   Elia S, Guggino G, Mineo D, *et al.* Awake one stage bilateral thoracoscopic sympathectomy for palmar hyperhidrosis: a safe outpatient procedure. Eur J Cardiothorac Surg 2005;28:312-7.

[7]   Al-Abdullatief M, Wahood A, Al-Shirawi N, *et al.* Awake anaesthesia for major thoracic surgical procedures: an observational study. Eur J Cardiothorac Surg. Aug 2007;32:346-50.

[8]   Macchiarini P, Rovira I, Ferrarello S. Awake upper airway surgery. Ann Thorac Surg 2010;89:387-90.

[9]   Migliore M, Giuliano R, Aziz T, *et al.* Four-step local anesthesia and sedation for thoracoscopic diagnosis and management of pleural diseases. Chest 2002;121:2032-5.

[10]   Pompeo E, Mineo D, Rogliani P, *et al.* Feasibility and results of awake thoracoscopic resection of solitary pulmonary nodules. Ann Thorac Surg 2004;78:1761-8.

[11]   Mineo TC. Epidural anesthesia in awake thoracic surgery. Eur J Cardiothorac Surg 2007;32:13-9.

[12]   Pompeo E, Tacconi F, Mineo D, Mineo TC. The role of awake video-assisted thoracoscopic surgery in spontaneous pneumothorax. J Thorac Cardiovasc Surg 2007;133:786-90.

[13]   Pompeo E, Mineo TC. Awake pulmonary metastasectomy. J Thorac Cardiovasc Surg 2007;133:960-6.

[14]   Tacconi F, Pompeo E, Mineo TC. Duration of air leak is reduced after awake nonresectional lung volume reduction surgery. Eur J Cardiothorac Surg 2009;35:822-8.

[15]   Tacconi F, Pompeo E, Fabbi E, Mineo TC. Awake video-assisted pleural decortication for empyema thoracis. Eur J Cardiothorac Surg 2010;37:594-601.

[16]   Katlic MR. Video-assisted thoracic surgery utilizing local anesthesia and sedation. Eur J Cardiothorac Surg 2006;30:529-32.

[17]   Gomez-Caro Andres A, Moradiellos Diez FJ, Ausin Herrero P, *et al.* Successful conservative management in iatrogenic tracheobronchial injury. Ann Thorac Surg 2005;79:1872-8.

[18]   Conti M, Pougeoise M, Wurtz A, *et al.* Management of postintubation tracheobronchial ruptures. Chest 2006;130:412-8.

[19]   Schneider T, Storz K, Dienemann H, Hoffmann H. Management of iatrogenic tracheobronchial injuries: a retrospective analysis of 29 cases. Ann Thorac Surg 2007;83:1960-4.

[20]   Minambres E, Buron J, Ballesteros MA, *et al.* Tracheal rupture after endotracheal intubation: a literature systematic review. Eur J Cardiothorac Surg 2009;35:1056-62.

[21]   Chhajed PN, Kaegi B, Rajasekaran R, Tamm M. Detection of hypoventilation during thoracoscopy: combined cutaneous carbon dioxide tension and oximetry monitoring with a new digital sensor. Chest 2005;127:585-8.

[22]   Guarracino F, Gemignani R, Pratesi G, *et al.* Awake palliative thoracic surgery in a high-risk patient: one-lung, non-invasive ventilation combined with epidural blockade. Anaesthesia 2008;63:761-3.

[23]   Iwama H. Application of nasal bi-level positive airway pressure to respiratory support during combined epidural-propofol anesthesia. J Clin Anesth 2002;14:24-33.

Awake Thoracic Surgery, 2012, 199-201

CHAPTER 16

Awake Thoracic Surgery: Future Perspectives

Eugenio Pompeo[*]

Department of Thoracic Surgery, Policlinico Tor Vergata University, Rome, Italy

Abstract: Awake thoracic surgery procedures have now been successfully performed in early series with satisfactory results.

Potential advantages include short hospitalization and immediate resumption of daily life activities, even in functionally compromised patients, as well as a minor impact on postoperative immune function and hormone stress response.

So far, awake anesthesia has been mainly employed to perform simple surgical procedures. In this setting, we have preferred thoracic epidural anesthesia but local anesthesia and paravertebral blocks are also promising alternatives, which have been successfully used.

Future perspectives might include ambulatory awake thoracic surgery programs as well as standardization of more complex awake surgical procedures such as thymectomy and anatomical lung resections.

The rapidly growing clinical experience and the accomplishment of properly controlled studies will provide more answers regarding the advantages and limits of this intriguing novel surgical approach when dealing with the various proposed indications.

Keywords: Awake thoracic surgery, VATS, epidural anesthesia, local anesthesia, complication.

Awake thoracic surgery has now been reliably employed for management of pleural effusion [1], bullectomy for spontaneous pneumothorax [2-5] and giant bullous disease [6], resection of pulmonary nodules [7], lung metastases [8] and lung cancer [9, 10]; pleural decortication [11], thymectomy [12, 13] and lung volume reduction surgery [14]. Early data indicate that awake thoracic surgery can assure a new patient-friendly and globally less invasive approach, which makes it possible to minimize both surgical and anesthesiological trauma resulting in immediate resumption of daily life activities and short hospitalization even in the most functionally compromised patients [14, 15].

Further potential advantages could also derive from findings of a reduced postoperative stress hormone response and a lesser impairment in lymphocytes activity that have already been anecdotally suggested in preliminary clinical studies [16, 17].

In this respect, if future investigations demonstrate that early immunologic surveillance is better preserved following awake thoracic surgery procedures, novel oncologic perspectives including a reduced risk of cancer spread as well as an easier and more prompt delivery of targeted systemic therapies might eventually translate into better outcome and survival [18].

So far, Thoracic Epidural Anesthesia (TEA) has been preferred by our awake thoracic surgery research group even though increasing interest towards awake thoracic anesthesia is leading to a better understanding of pros and cons of other non-general anesthesia techniques that include local anesthesia and paravertebral

*Address correspondence to Eugenio Pompeo: Department of Thoracic Surgery, Policlinico Tor Vergata University, Rome, Italy; Email: pompeo@med.uniroma2.it

blocks [1]. The latter in particular might make it possible to achieve widened thoracic analgesia as with TEA with less collateral effects.

Awake anesthesia has now been employed also to perform ambulatory thoracic surgery operations, which represents another potential future application of this rapidly evolving surgical field [19].

Other anesthesia options entailing deep sedation with maintenance of spontaneous ventilation and avoidance of endotracheal intubation have also been promisingly employed in a parallel manner with the ongoing experience on fully awake thoracic surgery [20].

Thus far, the most provocative indication for an awake surgical approach is its use in oncologic surgery. In fact, though limited resections have been successfully performed to remove isolated pulmonary metastases and peripheral lung cancer in patients considered at high-risk for general anesthesia [9], one further advance will clearly be represented by new standardized approaches allowing anatomical resection [10] to be safely accomplished.

The main concern raised against awake VATS procedures has been the fear that a surgical pneumothorax is poorly tolerable by spontaneously ventilating, awake patients. However, data that are progressively accumulating seem to contradict this empiric thought. Adequate ventilation is assured in most operated patients and satisfactory oxygenation has been easily maintained throughout the procedures even in severely emphysematous subjects [14].

A note of caution must be raised since as has already happened with other innovative surgical approaches, there may be the risk of an initial over-use with hazardous or unjustified indications. Complex major operation such as pneumonectomy [10] and even tracheal resection [21] have been successfully accomplished through sole TEA in awake subjects. The advantages of these extended indications probably need to be balanced against the patient's unpleasant feeling of witnessing her/his own major surgical demolition. Nonetheless, it is worth noting that Vischnevski [22] already reported on awake pneumonectomy and even esophagectomies performed under sole local anesthesia back in the 1950's.

Many physiopathological aspects related to a thoracic operation performed in an awake, spontaneously ventilating subject still need to be better elucidated and the real advantages, disadvantages and cost-effectiveness of each indication require further detailed investigation.

CONCLUSION

What is clearly evident to all of us is that surgery is changing and innovative non-surgical options are being actively investigated to treat several thoracic diseases, avoiding surgical trauma and even the need for hospitalization. This must not be considered an unfavorable phenomenon but rather a stimulus for thoracic surgeons to accept the challenge becoming more and more flexible, joining anesthesiologists and other investigators in a properly oriented, multidisciplinary effort to develop less invasive surgical methods [23, 24] carried out using less invasive types of anesthesia. This towards an ideal attempt of making thoracic surgery an easily accepted, maximally effective and optimally tolerated, *nearly-physiologic* event.

REFERENCES

[1]   Piccioni F, Langer M, Fumagalli L, *et al.* Thoracic paravertebral anesthesia for awake video-assisted thoracoscopic surgery. Anaesthesia 2010 [Epub ahead of print].

[2]   Nezu K, Kushibe K, Tojo T, *et al.* Thoracoscopic wedge resection of blebs under local anesthesia with sedation for treatment of spontaneous pneumothorax. Chest 1997;111:230-5.

[3]   Yokoyoma T, Tomoda M, Kanbara T, *et al.* Epidural anesthesia for a patient with catamenial pneumothorax. Masui 2001;50:290-2.

[4]   Sugimoto S, Date H, Sugimoto R, *et al.* Thoracoscopic operation with local and epidural anesthesia in the treatment of pneumothorax after lung transplantation. J Thorac Cardiovasc Surg 2005;130:1219-20.

[5]   Pompeo E, Tacconi F, Mineo D, Mineo TC. The role of awake video-assisted thoracoscopic surgery in spontaneous pneumothorax. J Thorac Cardiovasc Surg 2007;133:786-90.

[6]   Pompeo E, Tacconi F, Frasca L, Mineo TC. Awake thoracoscopic bullaplasty. Eur J Cardiothorac Surg 2010 [epub ahead of print].

[7]   Pompeo E, Mineo D, Rogliani P, Sabato AF, Mineo TC. Feasibility and results of awake thoracoscopic resection of solitary pulmonary nodules. Ann Thorac Surg 2004;78:1761-8.

[8]   Pompeo E, Mineo TC. Awake pulmonary metastasectomy. J Thorac Cardiovasc Surg 2007;133:960-6.

[9]   Pompeo E, Mineo TC. Awake operative videothoracoscopic pulmonary resections. Thorac Surg Clin 2008;18:311-20.

[10]   Al-Abdullatief M, Wahood A, Al-Shirawi N, *et al.* Awake anesthesia for major thoracic surgical procedures: an observational study. Eur J Cardiothorac Surg 2007;32:346-350.

[11]   Tacconi F, Pompeo E, Fabbi E, Mineo TC. Awake videoassisted pleural decortication for empyema thoracis. Eur J Cardiothorac Surg 2010;37:594-601.

[12]   Tsunezuka Y, Oda M, Matsumoto I, Tamura M, Watanabe G. Extended thymectomy in patients with myasthenia gravis with hygh thoracic epidural anesthesia alone. World J Surg 2004;28:962-965.

[13]   Matsumoto I, Oda M, Watanabe G. Awake endoscopic thymectomy via an infrasternal approach using sternal lifting. Thorac Cardiovasc Surg. 2008;56:311-3.

[14]   Pompeo E, Mineo TC. Two-year improvement in multidimensional body mass index, airflow obstruction, dyspnea and exercise capacity index after nonresectional lung volume reduction surgery in awake patients. Ann Thorac Surg 2007;84:1862-9.

[15]   Watanabe G, Yamaguchi S, Tomiya S, Ohtake H. Awake subxyphoid minimally invasive direct coronary artery bypass grafting yielded minimum invasive cardiac surgery for high risk patients. Interact Cardiovasc Thorac Surg. 2008; 7: 910-2.

[16]   Vanni G, Tacconi F, Sellitri F, *et al.* Impact of awake videothoracoscopic surgery on postoperative lymphocyte responses. Ann Thorac Surg 2010;90:973-978.

[17]   Tacconi F, Pompeo E, Sellitri F, Mineo TC. Surgical stress hormones response is reduced after awake videothoracoscopy. Interact Cardiovasc Thorac Surg 2010;10:666-71.

[18]   Petersen RP, Pham D, Burfeind WR, *et al.* Thoracoscopic lobectomy facilitates the delivery of chemotherapy after resection for lung cancer. Ann Thorac Surg. 2007 ;83:1245-9.

[19]   Rocco G, Romano V, Accardo R, *et al.* Awake single-access (uniportal) video-assisted thoracoscopic surgery for peripheral pulmonary nodules in a complete ambulatory setting. Ann Thorac Surg 2010;89:1625-7.

[20]   Katlic MR, Facktor MA. Video-assisted thoracic surgery utilizing local anesthesia and sedation: 384 consecutive cases. Ann Thorac Surg 2010;90:240-5.

[21]   Macchiarini P, Rovira I, Ferrarello S. Awake upper air way surgery. Ann Thorac Surg 2010;89:387-91.

[22]   Petrovsky BV. Role of local anesthesia according to Vischnevsky in thoracic surgery. Anesth Analg 1952;9:75-9.

[23]   Tagaya N, Kasama K, Suzuki N, Taketsuka S, Horie K, Kubota K. Video-assisted bullectomy using needlescopic instruments for spontaneous pneumothorax. Surg Endosc 2003;17:1486-7.

[24]   Kim HK, Jo WM, Jung JH, *et al.* Needlescopic lung biopsy for interstitial lung disease and indeterminate pulmonary nodules: a report on 65 cases. Ann Thorac Surg 2008;86:1098-103.

Subject Index

A

ACTH	20,23,27
Acute lung injury (ALI)	34,36-38
Acynetobacter	143
Adult respiratory distress syndrome (ARDS)	36,38
Air-leak	96,134,136,148
Anterior mediastinum	158,165,167,171,172
Anxiety	4,77,111,112,123,169,170,182
Arrhythmia	45,51,92,96,123

B

Blebs	6,89,131,135,137
Buckingham, W.W.	3,4,83,150
Bulky (mediastinal masses)	165-169,172,173
Bullae	89,90,98,131,133,135,137
Bullous emphysema	96,98,132

C

Carlens (tube)	4
Claude-Bernard-Horner (syndrome)	145
Cortisol	20,23,24,27-29,39,48,166
Cruise, F.	5,122,145

D

Decortication (pleural)	6,123,141-154 (overview),192

E

Emphysema-like changes (ELC)	131,134,135,137
Emphysema	6,9,11,12,14,15,21,46,80,83,84,88-104
Empyema (pleural)	3,5,6,141-154 (overview),192,193
Epidural abscess	49,150

G

General anesthesia	3,5,6,9,25,26,28,29,34-42,192
Graham, E.	3,145

H

Hypercarbia, hypercapnia (permissive)	15,92,97,101,112,150
Hyperhydrosis	See "Sympathectomy"
Hypoxia	3,14,34-36,38,126,133,150

I

Intercostal block	112,123,134,147,182,191
Interleukin 6 (IL-6)	21,25,26,28,29
Interleukin (overview)	20,21,38,166
Interstitial lung disease	12,15,105-118,132,196

J

Jacobaeus, H.	5,122,146,191

L

Lidocaine	51,53,55,123,134,157,159,170,182,197
Lung cancer	5,21,74,75,77,82,83,120,200
Lung volume reduction surgery	88-104 (overview)
Lymphocytes	20,22,23,28,29

M

Metastasectomy	77,79,81,82,84
Myasthenia gravis	59,155-164 (overview)
Mycobacterium	143,150

N

Natural killer cells	23,24,27-29,146
Nodules (lung).	6,74-87 (overview),192
Novocaine	3,4

O

One-lung ventilation (OLV)	25,27-29,34-36,38,97
Opioids	23,46,50,52-54,57,59
Ossipov, B.	4

P

Paravertebral block	44,59,60-62
Pleural effusion	5,10,64,119-129,141,142,145,147,166,191
Pneumothorax (spontaneous, secondary)	5,6,30-140
Pneumothorax (surgical, intraoperative)	4,9-18,78,94,97,113,123-126,134,145,148,162,181

R

Ropivacaine	26,50-54,58,62

S

Staphilococcus Aureus	143
Sternotomy (in awake patients)	156-158
Sympathectomy	6,177-191 (overview)
Systemic Inflammation Response Syndrome (SIRS)	19,24,25,27

T

Talc pleurodesis	119,123,126,127,136,137
Thoracic epidural anesthesia (TEA)	28,39,44-73,156,200
Thoracotomy (in awake patients)	149,150
Thymectomy	156-164
Tracheal rupture	100,196
Tuohy, needle	54,55,60,157

V

Ventilator-related lung injury	24,125,146
Vischnevski, A.	4,200